Early Modern Medicine

This collection offers readers a guide to analyzing historical texts and objects using a diverse selection of sources in early modern medicine. It provides an array of interpretive strategies while also highlighting new trends in the field.

Each chapter serves as a study of a different type of source, including the benefits and limitations of that source and what it can reveal about the history of medicine. Contributors provide practical strategies for locating and interpreting sources, putting texts and objects into conversation, and explaining potential contradictions. A wide variety of sources, including account books, legal records, and personal letters, provide new opportunities for understanding early modern medicine and developing skills in historical analysis. Together, the chapters highlight emerging methodologies and debates, while covering a range of themes in the field, from reproductive health to hospital care to household medicine.

With wide geographical breadth, this book is a valuable resource for students and researchers looking to understand how to better engage with primary sources, as well as readers interested in early modern history and the history of medicine.

Olivia Weisser is Associate Professor of History at the University of Massachusetts Boston where she teaches and writes about the history of health and healing in the 1500s–1700s. Her first book, *Ill Composed* (2015), examined how gender shaped patients' perceptions of sickness. She is finishing a new book on the history of venereal disease.

The Routledge Guides to Using Historical Sources

How does the historian approach primary sources? How do interpretations differ? How can such sources be used to write history?

The *Routledge Guides to Using Historical Sources* series introduces students to different sources and illustrates how historians use them. Titles in the series offer a broad spectrum of primary sources and, using specific examples, examine the historical context of these sources and the different approaches that can be used to interpret them.

Sources for the History of Emotions
A Guide
Edited by Katie Barclay, Sharon Crozier-De Rosa and Peter N. Stearns

Games of History
Games and Gaming as Historical Sources
Apostolos Spanos

Doing Spatial History
Edited by Riccardo Bavaj, Konrad Lawson and Bernhard Struck

Sources in the History of Psychiatry, from 1800 to the Present
Edited by Chris Millard and Jennifer Wallis

Sources for Studying the Holocaust
A Guide
Edited by Paul R. Bartrop

Early Modern Medicine
An Introduction to Source Analysis
Edited by Olivia Weisser

For more information about this series, please visit: https://www.routledge.com/Routledge-Guides-to-Using-Historical-Sources/book-series/RGHS

Early Modern Medicine

An Introduction to Source Analysis

Edited by
Olivia Weisser

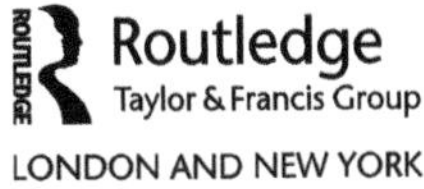

LONDON AND NEW YORK

Designed cover image: Woman applying a medicinal leech to her forearm, woodcut from a 1639 treatise by Joannis Mommarti. Everett Collection Historical/Alamy Stock Photo

First published 2024
by Routledge
4 Park Square, Milton Park, Abingdon, Oxon OX14 4RN

and by Routledge
605 Third Avenue, New York, NY 10158

Routledge is an imprint of the Taylor & Francis Group, an informa business

© 2024 selection and editorial matter, Olivia Weisser; individual chapters, the contributors

The right of Olivia Weisser to be identified as the author of the editorial material, and of the authors for their individual chapters, has been asserted in accordance with sections 77 and 78 of the Copyright, Designs and Patents Act 1988.

All rights reserved. No part of this book may be reprinted or reproduced or utilised in any form or by any electronic, mechanical, or other means, now known or hereafter invented, including photocopying and recording, or in any information storage or retrieval system, without permission in writing from the publishers.

Trademark notice: Product or corporate names may be trademarks or registered trademarks, and are used only for identification and explanation without intent to infringe.

British Library Cataloguing-in-Publication Data
A catalogue record for this book is available from the British Library

Library of Congress Cataloging-in-Publication Data
Names: Weisser, Olivia, editor.
Title: Early modern medicine : an introduction to source analysis / edited by Olivia Weisser.
Description: Abingdon, Oxon ; New York, NY : Routledge, 2024. | Series: Routledge guides to using historical sources | Includes bibliographical references and index.
Identifiers: LCCN 2023042794 (print) | LCCN 2023042795 (ebook) | ISBN 9780367557232 (hbk) | ISBN 9780367557225 (pbk) | ISBN 9781003094876 (ebk)
Subjects: LCSH: Medicine—History—Sources. | Medicine—History—16th century. | Medicine—History—17th century. | Medicine—History—18th century. | Medicine—History—19th century.
Classification: LCC R145 .E27 2024 (print) | LCC R145 (ebook) | DDC 610.9/031—dc23/eng/20231201
LC record available at https://lccn.loc.gov/2023042794
LC ebook record available at https://lccn.loc.gov/2023042795

ISBN: 978-0-367-55723-2 (hbk)
ISBN: 978-0-367-55722-5 (pbk)
ISBN: 978-1-003-09487-6 (ebk)

DOI: 10.4324/9781003094876

Typeset in Times New Roman
by codeMantra

Contents

Contributors

Laurinda Abreu is Professor of History at the University of Évora where her research specialty is the history of poor relief and health care in the early modern period. She is the author most recently of "Health care and the spread of medical knowledge in the Portuguese empire" in *Medical History*.

Sandra Cavallo is Emerita Professor of Early Modern History at Royal Holloway University of London. She works on the social and cultural history of early modern Italy and, in particular, on medicine and the body, gender, homelife, and material culture.

Zachary Dorner is a historian of medicine and commerce. He is the author of *Merchants of Medicines: The Commerce and Coercion of Health in Britain's Long Eighteenth Century* (2020) and is Assistant Professor of History at the University of Maryland, College Park.

Mary E. Fissell is Professor in the Department of the History of Medicine at the Johns Hopkins University, with appointments in the history of science and the history departments. Her scholarly work focuses on how ordinary people in early modern England understood health, healing, and the natural world.

Stefanie Hunt-Kennedy is Associate Professor at the University of New Brunswick. She is an award-winning historian and author of *Between Fitness and Death: Disability and Slavery in the Caribbean* (2020). Her research explores disability and madness, and the intersecting histories of race, gender, and class in the British Caribbean.

Lauren Kassell is Professor of History of Science at the European University Institute and Professor of History of Science and Medicine at the University of Cambridge. She is a historian of science and medicine, with expertise focused on everyday medicine and the occult sciences in early modern England.

Sebestian Kroupa is Assistant Professor in the Department of Social Studies of Medicine at McGill University. He is a historian of pre-modern medicine and the life sciences in cross-cultural contexts, with a particular focus on the Indian and the Pacific Oceans.

Elaine Leong's research centers upon medical and scientific knowledge transfer and production. Her first book, *Recipes and Everyday Knowledge: Medicine, Science, and the Household in Early Modern England* (2018), examines "household science," or quotidian investigations of the natural world. Her current book is titled *Reading Rivière in Early Modern England.*

Elizabeth W. Mellyn is Associate Professor of History at the University of New Hampshire. Her publications include *Mad Tuscans and Their Families: A History of Mental Disorder in Early Modern Italy*. She is currently at work on a history of Florence's first hospital devoted to caring for the mentally ill.

Elise A. Mitchell is a historian of the early modern Black Atlantic and Assistant Professor in the Department of History at Swarthmore College. Broadly, her work examines the social and cultural histories of slavery, the body, medicine and healing, disease, race, and gender in the early modern Atlantic World.

Alisha Rankin is Professor of History at Tufts University. Her research interests include early modern European history, the history of science and medicine, the history of pharmacy, and women's history. Her latest book is *The Poison Trials: Wonder Drugs, Experiment, and the Battle for Authority in Renaissance Science* (2021).

Carolin Schmitz is a historian of early modern Spain, specializing in the social and cultural history of medicine and the history of the patient. Her current research interest lies in how medicine in its pluralistic form was shaped by, and affected, diverse members of early modern communities.

Miri Shefer-Mossensohn is Professor of Middle Eastern history at Tel Aviv University. She specializes in Ottoman & Turkish Studies, with a focus on the history of medicine, health, and wellbeing.

Sharon T. Strocchia is Professor of History at Emory University. She has published widely on women, family, religion, health, and society in fifteenth- and sixteenth-century Italy. Strocchia is the author or editor of five books, including the award-winning *Forgotten Healers: Women and the Pursuit of Health in Late Renaissance Italy* (2019).

Olivia Weisser is Associate Professor of History at the University of Massachusetts Boston where she teaches and writes about the history of health and healing in the 1500s–1700s. Her first book, *Ill Composed* (2015), examined how gender shaped patients' perceptions of sickness. She is finishing up a new book on the history of venereal disease.

Rebecca Whiteley is a British Academy Postdoctoral Fellow at the University of Birmingham. She works on the intersections of visual and material culture, history of medicine, and social history. She has published widely on early modern midwifery illustration and more recently works on nineteenth-century cultures of sex and medicine.

Anna Winterbottom works on the early modern Indian Ocean region and the European colonial presence there, with a focus on the history of medicine, science, and environment. She is the author of *Hybrid Knowledge in the Early East India Company World* (2016).

Yi-Li Wu is Associate Professor of Women's and Gender Studies and History at the University of Michigan, where she studies society, culture, and the body in late imperial China. She is the author of *Reproducing Women: Medicine, Metaphor, and Childbirth in Late Imperial China* and is completing a monograph on the history of medicine for injuries and wounds.

Introduction

Olivia Weisser

"More analysis!" Perhaps, as a student, you have received this comment on a paper. Perhaps, as an instructor, you have written it. This can be a challenging directive, however well intended. What does analysis *really* mean? Historians know it when they see it, and students are expected to know how to do it. Yet, despite being so central to historical scholarship, analysis is not a skill that historians tend to teach or even talk about explicitly. Instead, we use language that masks the work of analysis, either by framing it by what it is not ("less summary") or by falling back on euphemisms ("read against the grain"). Most of us know how to describe and narrate, but not everyone knows how to "read against the grain." Analysis takes different forms depending on the research question and the source. This book introduces a broad range of primary sources for studying the history of medicine spanning 1500–1800 and guides readers through the rewarding intellectual work of how to analyze them.

Most students first learn analysis in introductory writing courses. Valuable books on academic research and writing teach the skill in broad terms: how to "read for a problem," find meaning in a source, locate claims, and so on.[1] This book offers a discipline-specific version of those approaches. It is a guide that caters to historical inquiry and to sources in the history of medicine, in particular. Centered on the early modern period, the 18 essays in this volume both model analysis and provide instruction on how to actually do it, including how to find, read, and interpret a wide range of sources; put texts and objects into conversation; and explain potential contradictions. Chapters serve as guides to sources, outlining their benefits, limits, and what they can and cannot tell us about the history of medicine, as well as practical strategies for how to use them. Some chapters offer the nuts and bolts of how to locate sources by way of bibliographies, databases, and tips for navigating archives. Readers can dip into the book for support and inspiration; each chapter is a toolkit that can be applied to a wide variety of sources and topics. The result is not a primary source reader nor an overview of the field – though readers may find both such uses – so much as a manual on the messy, wide-ranging, rewarding art of historical analysis.

Chapters introduce a variety of analytical methods, some covering the same moves in different ways. Several chapters, for instance, model literary techniques that consider the relationship between a source's form and content. Mary Fissell's

DOI: 10.4324/9781003094876-1

chapter centers on a single ballad, or song, about sex, pregnancy, and childbirth. The chapter explains how to analyze the ballad both by interpreting its content (the lyrics), as well as its form as a material object (its physical size, font, imagery, reproduction techniques, and so on). Even the tune, Fissell shows, could convey meanings that complicated the ballad's content. Olivia Weisser's chapter focuses on stories of sickness recorded in life writing, such as diaries, autobiographies, and memoirs. One way to approach these sources, the chapter shows, is to consider how the conventions and intentions of different genres of life writing informed authors' self-constructions on the page. Elaine Leong's chapter, likewise, looks at the content of a popular medical book alongside its many "book parts" – title page, dedication, index, table of contents – to discern the author's goals and likely readership.

These and other chapters cover many more analytical strategies, too, including how to read for silences, locate and explain patterns, and triangulate sources to build context and meaning, to name just a few. Elise Mitchell models this last method using newspaper advertisements, and in doing so shows how ephemeral documents can reveal information that was not necessarily intended by their authors. We learn from one advertisement, for example, about an enslaved woman named Anna who worked as a nurse at a plantation hospital where she specialized in bloodletting. Elizabeth Mellyn showcases this same move in a very different way. A brief and seemingly opaque admission record to a mental health hospital in Florence contains a knotty set of competing interests. And Alisha Rankin brings readers on a detective hunt through the archives to make sense of an otherwise flummoxing account of a poison experiment performed on dogs inserted into a manuscript recipe book.

In demonstrating how to conduct analysis, the book also introduces readers to diverse sources for studying the history of medicine. Those newer to the field may assume that historical sources must be explicitly medical, derived from healthcare practices or provision. Of course, medical sources are incredibly valuable, and this volume devotes an entire section to them. Miri Shefer-Mossensohn looks at the complexities of learned writing by Ottoman physicians, and Lauren Kassell explains how to approach a massive and newly accessible collection of early modern medical casebooks. Both of these chapters demonstrate how to approach writing by practitioners to piece together past constructions of medical knowledge and the extent to which we can recover actual clinical practices. Other chapters address less obvious sources for studying the history of medicine, including those that are not about health and healing per se but can be just as relevant all the same: legal cases, family letters, account books, and ship logs. Sharon Strocchia shows how various kinds of religious writing by Italian nuns – long overlooked by historians of medicine – contain abundant information about health-related issues, from the demographics of disease to the cultural meanings of pain. Strocchia's chapter, and this book as a whole, invites readers to think broadly and creatively about what might or might not "count" as a source for studying medicine in the past.

In addition to providing a guide to analysis and an introduction to potential primary sources, the book showcases new trends in the field. Each chapter centers on a single type of source, but in doing so offers a sense of the historical debates and methods that led historians to approach texts or objects in particular ways or even to consider them as sources at all. Although the essays that follow are not meant to provide a historiographical overview, together they map more recent methodologies, sources, and debates in the field, all the while pointing toward exciting directions for the future.

If this book had been published 30 years ago, for example, it likely would have been centered entirely on primary sources written by male physicians and natural philosophers. Over the past few decades, historians of medicine have moved well beyond such a focus, not only by accounting for other types of healers but also by embracing a broader view of healing itself. Historians have found that early modern women provided care in a wide variety of contexts (domestic, culinary, cosmetic, religious) that were not always delineated as strictly medical. Sandra Cavallo, whose chapter here looks at family letters, has shown the significance of viewing early modern health and healing as a realm that encompassed both prevention and cure. Such shifts in the field have led to new ways of thinking about embodied experiences and have invited historians to consider non-medical spaces as important sites of healthcare and medical inquiry. Convents, kitchens, courts, and workshops, historians have shown, were places associated with healthcare and knowledge production on par with hospitals, laboratories, and consultation rooms.[2]

An older but nonetheless important shift in the field involved accounting for the lives and experiences of the dispossessed. This turn initially took the form of "history from below" and a focus away from the words and lives of learned physicians and toward the thoughts and experiences of ordinary patients. Since the 1980s, scholars have examined how various cultural forces, such as gender norms, family dynamics, and religious differences, came to shape everyday experiences of healthcare.[3] Several of the chapters here model such modes of interpretation and demonstrate how to analyze sources to capture the beliefs and experiences of ordinary men and women. There also has been significant attention paid to the working poor who did not, or could not, write for posterity. Capturing the health histories of non-elite men and women is a key benefit of legal records, despite their being heavily mediated and formulaic. To overcome such challenges, Carolin Schmitz's chapter outlines concrete strategies for reading court cases for their "cultural truths" as opposed to their "historical truths." Schmitz shows how different kinds of cases and courts can provide varied information about medicine, and how historians can read for patterns to ascertain the likelihood that the events related in cases actually happened. Laurinda Abreu introduces readers to the rewards and challenges of another mediated source, the documents left behind by charitable societies for the poor run by local authorities in Portugal. These administrative records must be read carefully, Abreu shows, to recover the lives of the poor while also accounting for the clerks and scribes who compiled them.

Reflecting a somewhat more recent "material turn," chapters explain how to "read" objects and images as historical sources. Those interested in the forms, uses, and meanings of medical illustrations should turn to Rebecca Whiteley's discussion of a midwifery text. Whiteley outlines how an image can illuminate an author's aims, sometimes by way of landscape, intentional details, and choice of production technique. Yi-Li Wu's chapter on a Chinese surgical manual also includes tips for analyzing images, including how to interpret potential discrepancies between illustrations and texts. Lack of detail in an image, for example, might be a deliberate move to emphasize the primacy of a text. Medical images served functions other than descriptive ones, and historians of medicine should treat them, these chapters show, as more than window dressing. They are complex sources that require sophisticated interpretative strategies.

Readers wishing to learn more about objects and how to interpret them as sources can consult Anna Winterbottom's essay on Sri Lankan healing containers, which range from amulets to coconut cups. Elaine Leong's chapter, too, is instructive by showing us what the physicality of a book can reveal about its production and use. Stefanie Hunt-Kennedy's chapter likewise models newer developments in the field by outlining how to read familiar sources anew through the lens of disability. Historians have long viewed the history of disability and the history of medicine as distinct subfields.[4] Yet, as Hunt-Kennedy shows, each has much to gain from the other – in this case, careful analysis of travelogues, slave ship surgeons' records, and runaway advertisements shows how congenital illness, labor accidents, and malnutrition underwrote the oppression of enslaved Africans in the Caribbean.

The geographical breadth of this book, too, points to more recent approaches in the history of medicine and the field of history writ large, as scholars have looked beyond national borders to trace the movements of people, diseases, drugs, and ideas.[5] The geographical focus of the book broadens typical associations between "early modern" and Western Europe. Medical commerce and knowledge traveled and borrowed elements from multiple traditions, and recovering those complexities can require moving away from arbitrary borders and a Eurocentric focus. Miri Shefer-Mossensohn's essay on the Turkish- and Arabic-speaking Middle East shows how a mixture of traditions and languages comprised medical writing and practices in the early modern Ottoman Empire. Sebestian Kroupa's chapter offers a local version of a global story using missionary pharmacopoeias in the Philippines, which reveal how new medical specimens altered long-enduring healing traditions. Zachary Dorner tracks economic sources, such as ship logs and account books, across an ocean. The paper trails that merchants left behind, Dorner shows, were key components of the complex tangle of empire, science, and commercial venture at the heart of the era's drug trade.

Chapters here likewise cover a wide range of topics, including hospitals, poor relief, clinical work, pain, malpractice, experiments, disability, household medicine, sexuality, surgery, patients' experiences, childbirth, medical retailing, and more. One book cannot do everything, of course. There is no chapter on plague nor alchemy and some analytical methods, such as newer approaches that draw on paleo-genetics and bioarcheology, are absent. But this book does not purport to do everything. Rather than provide a comprehensive overview, it is meant to be used in a modular way, as a menu of topics, sources, and analytical strategies that readers can mix and match to suit their particular needs. Those interested in

Chinese medicine or the history of surgery would do well to start with Yi-Li Wu's chapter on a bone-setting manual, for example. Yet Wu's chapter is also instructive for readers with completely different interests, as it offers insights into how to conduct a close reading of a text that are widely applicable to other types of sources. Likewise, readers may not be working on the same hospital as Elizabeth Mellyn nor the same cases as Lauren Kassell, and yet the approaches modeled in those two chapters – how to find and explain patterns in a large dataset and how to imagine multiple perspectives and/or events outside the written record – can be applied to many types of sources. Readers need not be working on the exact topic, source, or geographical focus of each chapter to find value in it.

This book is not an introduction to early modern medicine so much as a guide. And the key skill at its core is analysis, a skill that historians seldom teach or talk about in a disciplined way, but one that they arguably value above all others. Analysis can turn a piece of historical writing that is descriptive and thin into one that is persuasive and trenchant. It allows historians to say something interpretive about sources, rather than merely report or summarize them. The chapters in this volume, in a multitude of ways, unlock the mysteries of how to do that analytical work. They disclose the questions that historians ask themselves as they begin working with a source, the silent assumptions that historians make, and the numerous ways of explaining and contextualizing sources to imbue them with meaning. If you have a topic but are not sure how to approach it, or you have a source but do not know what to do with it – perhaps it is too terse or too obvious or maybe too confusing – then this book is for you.

Notes

1 Classics include Anthony Brundage, *Going to the Sources: A Guide to Historical Research and Writing*, 5th Edition (Hoboken, NJ: Wiley-Blackwell, 2013); Wayne Booth, Gregory G. Colomb, Joseph M. Williams, Joseph Bizup, and William T. Fitzgerald, *The Craft of Research*, 4th Edition (Chicago, IL: University of Chicago Press, 2016). Citations here are intentionally brief. Readers are encouraged to consult substantive chapters for fuller lists of secondary literature on various types of sources and themes.

2 Sandra Cavallo and Tessa Storey, *Healthy Living in Late Renaissance Italy* (Oxford: Oxford University Press, 2013). See Sara Margaret Ritchey and Sharon T. Strocchia eds., *Gender, Health, and Healing, 1250–1550* (Amsterdam: Amsterdam University Press, 2020); Sharon T. Strocchia, *Forgotten Healers: Women and the Pursuit of Health in Late Renaissance Italy* (Cambridge, MA: Harvard University Press, 2019); Elaine Leong, *Recipes and Everyday Knowledge: Medicine, Science, and the Household in Early Modern England* (Chicago, IL: University of Chicago Press, 2018); Mary E. Fissell, "Introduction: Women, Health, and Healing in Early Modern Europe," *Bulletin of the History of Medicine* 82 (2008): 1–17.

3 See Roy Porter's work, especially, "The Patient's View: Doing Medical History from Below," *Theory and Society* 14 (1985): 175–98. For a few examples since the 1980s, see: Sharon Howard, "Imagining the Pain and Peril of Seventeenth-Century Childbirth: Travail and Deliverance in the Making of an Early Modern World," *Social History of Medicine* 16 (2003): 367–82; Lisa W. Smith, "Reassessing the Role of the Family: Women's Medical Care in Eighteenth-Century England," *Social History of Medicine* 16 (2003): 327–42; Olivia Weisser, *Ill Composed: Sickness, Gender, and Belief in Early Modern England* (New Haven, CT: Yale University Press, 2015); Mary E. Fissell,

Patients, Power, and the Poor in Eighteenth-Century Bristol (Cambridge: Cambridge University Press, 1991).

4 For a useful overview of disability studies and its relationship to the history of medicine, see Beth Linker, "On the Borderland of Medical and Disability History: A Survey of the Fields," *Bulletin of the History of Medicine* 87 (2013): 499–535.

5 For a few recent examples, see Pratik Chakrabarti, *Materials and Medicine: Trade, Conquest and Therapeutics in the Eighteenth Century* (Manchester: Manchester University Press, 2015); Benjamin Breen, *The Age of Intoxication: Origins of the Global Drug Trade* (Philadelphia: University of Pennsylvania Press, 2019).

Part I

Institutions

1 The Transatlantic Business of Medicine

Zachary Dorner

The relationship between medicine and commerce can feel obvious in our twenty-first-century present, but the two have a long, intertwined history that can be just as apparent if you know where to look. Take, for example, the pharmaceutical multinational GlaxoSmithKline (GSK). Beneath its sleek exterior, GSK's West London headquarters holds an older reminder of the close relationship between medicine and commerce in the form of letters, invoices, and account books from Plough Court pharmacy, one of eighteenth-century London's foremost manufacturers of medicines. Thanks to a convoluted series of mergers and acquisitions beginning in the mid-nineteenth century, Plough Court became a part of what would eventually become GSK (GSK, itself, being the result of a 2000 merger of Glaxo Wellcome and SmithKline Beecham). GSK's is hardly unique among the origin stories of big pharma. As people have pursued health and purchased medicines to do so, whether from Plough Court or GSK, they have participated in the development of medicine as global business and, important for our inquiry here, left records as they did so. The archive of the medicine trade demonstrates the ways accounting practices helped to make disparate items appear comparable on paper and thereby able to be exchanged in the real world. It also illuminates medicines in motion across a busy Atlantic world from laboratories to ships and eventually to ailing people. Though such business records can require a specialized vocabulary to unlock, learning that vocabulary and learning how to use it effectively reveals evidence of the profit, power, and possibilities that have shaped and continue to reshape the parameters of healthcare.

Each chapter in this volume offers a primer on the contexts, vocabularies, or tools required to understand certain sources in the history of medicine. What follows here will do the same for early modern business records from the European and transatlantic medicine trades. Since the term *business record* can be such a capacious one, this chapter provides an overview of the types of sources categorized under that heading and some examples of the approaches suited to their analysis. Many kinds of records passed through an early modern business office or "counting house," all stored in particular ways (many of which make work difficult for a researcher): some were cut or folded, others copied or transcribed, and still others reused or destroyed (see Figure 1.1).[1] Over the intervening years, they have been subject to water damage, funguses, hungry mice, and overlooked as prosaic

DOI: 10.4324/9781003094876-3

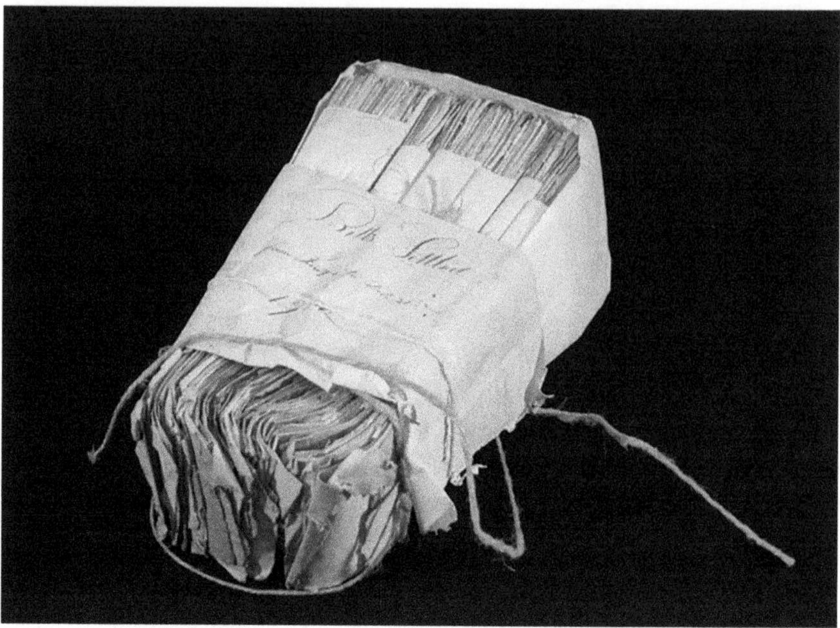

Figure 1.1 Day-to-day business records – such as bills, invoices, correspondence, and receipts – could be stored in a number of ways during the eighteenth century that make them appear reluctant to divulge their stories. Some were pressed onto a spike and others, seen here, were folded, bound, and labeled after relevant information had been copied into other records. "Bills Settled from Jany 1 to Dec. 31 1780," Arnold Family Business Records, the John Carter Brown Library. Image courtesy of the John Carter Brown Library.

(read: boring) sources of historical inquiry. Moreover, business information was not consistently written down, and even when it was, was not always deemed worth preserving in an archive. Consider all the receipts, checks, tickets, shopping lists, notes, and other scraps that pass through your lives in a day, a week, or a year. They can pile up and soon seem insignificant. In one notable case, accounts of the English East India Company's drug trade from 1730 to 1784 were destroyed with other seemingly "useless records" in 1860 to clear space for newer paperwork in the company's storage room.[2] Yet, no matter how small, torn, stained, poorly written, or mundane they may seem, these pieces of paper were crucial to moving things around and getting stuff done in the past because of the information they conveyed.

Paper greased the wheels of transoceanic commerce in an age of empires. After all, business records were useful things – termed "paper technologies" by historians who study capitalism – produced to help complete transactions, ensure debts were paid, or move things from one place to another.[3] Business, whether shipping a barrel of rum, a crate of hats, or a chest of cinchona tinctures, was bound by the time it took letters to cross distances and the kinds of promises that could be conveyed in ink. Some scholars have deemed Europe's eighteenth century a "papered century" of rampant print culture and an unprecedented traffic in commercial instruments, including banknotes, bills of exchange, price currents, and stocks.[4] Trading, especially across long distances, also required familiarity with many types of money and credit since locations around the Atlantic world used different currencies and standards of measure. A shortage of hard money – metal coins or specie – meant that bartering goods or services became the principal means of resolving transactions. This could be accomplished by letter, confirmed with a receipt, and then logged in a ledger. Often the only things exchanged in practice were the numbers written on the page of an account book, rather than any piece of gold or silver.[5] Debits and credits, what one owed or was owed, therefore organized interpersonal relations, and the letters, account books, invoices, and other papers that kept track of them became powerful tools of world building.

As druggists, chemists, and apothecaries in Europe began to participate more and more in this commercial landscape during the seventeenth and eighteenth centuries, they started to do business like merchants did in a shift that generated a lot more paperwork for them (and historians of medicine) to parse. This marked something of a departure for many apothecaries from centuries of smaller scale artisanal practice to bulk trade across longer distances. New techniques were not always easy to remember. The apprentice William Jepson kept a list of "Rules to be remembered in Trade" in his diary, including that he should "keep but one Ledger & Journal" to record his transactions.[6] The eighteenth century saw the coalescence of something resembling a coherent, though complicated, system of trade. Readers may be familiar with some parts of this system – the transatlantic slave trade, for instance – but the medicine trade constituted it as well. European medicine manufacturers looked more akin to merchants than provincial craftspeople in terms of their overseas distribution of goods, reliance on financial tools, deployment of labor, ties to the state, and recordkeeping practices. London's medicine exports, for example, grew at a rate of more than five percent annually, outpacing the growth rate of many other colonial export trades. Exports of medicines to some transoceanic destinations rose almost 300 percent from the 1720s, peaking in the early 1770s at more than a million pounds weight per year.[7] Medicines thus linked an increasingly connected Atlantic world. Everything that left a London laboratory or counting house embodied imported ingredients, human labor, and capital investment and had to be packaged, insured, and documented before it could go out to overseas patient populations of free and unfree people in locations where fear, death, and a desire for health acknowledged neither skin color nor rank.

At first glance, a page from an account book, such as the merchant Samuel Nightingale's (see Figure 1.2), can appear like abstract art. Due to their unpredictable shapes and sizes, variable conditions, specialized terminologies, and unfamiliar layouts, business records can seem quite daunting (and I say this from experience!).[8] Sometimes, the sheer volume of paper can be overwhelming, and other times incomplete or missing accounts infuriate. Despite these challenges, the scale of paperwork generated by long-distance commerce offers many rewards. Following the money, real or imaginary, recorded on the pages of early modern account books, invoices, inventories, bills, and other materials – the paper technologies of

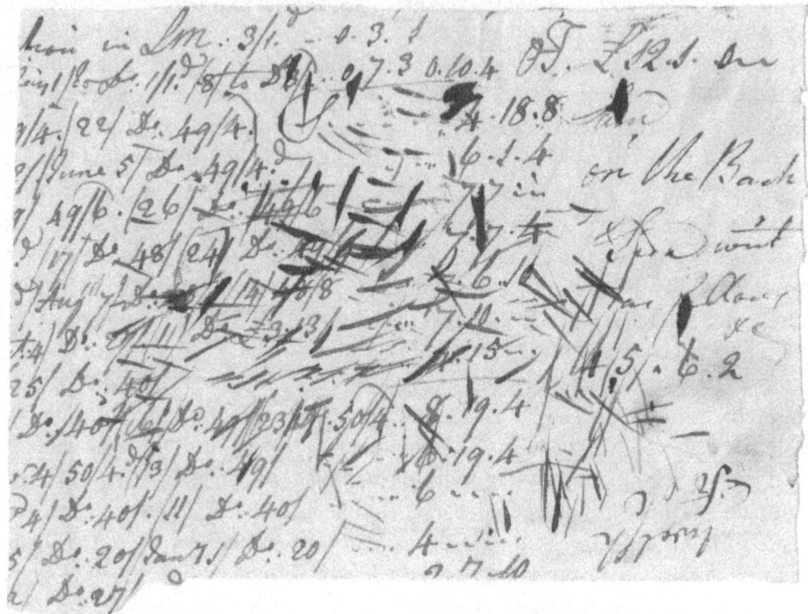

Figure 1.2 This loose page from Samuel Nightingale's (1715–1786) day book illustrates the merchant's marginal calculations and ink blotting while entering transactions into his book – think of scratch paper. Monetary symbols for pounds sterling (£), shillings (s), and pence (d) are visible on the page (the slash mark denotes s/d), as is the common shorthand for ditto ("D°"). Samuel Nightingale, [Scribble Scrap from Daybook], MSS 588 SG1 S3 B1 F3 (RHi X174350A), Rhode Island Historical Society. Image courtesy of the Rhode Island Historical Society.

the medicine trade – uncovers the outlines of a global medicine trade dependent on shipping routes, imperial institutions, and financial innovations that had real consequences for the ways people understood their health and that of others.

The Alchemy of Accounting

Account books can be difficult to describe because the category includes such a range of items. One could hold a record of shop transactions, household purchases, and debts; a list of human cargo and plantation provisions; or a family history, for example. Nevertheless, as Tara Bynum's classic article shows, account books constitute a literary genre that can reveal all kinds of everyday lived experiences and social connections.[9] As material things, account books could be large, sturdy leatherbound tomes or small, flimsy affairs. They could be written in one hand or many, cover a short or long time, and be legible or hopelessly messy. Spellings could also be inconsistent, with abbreviations and shorthand styles specific to the author. Such variation and idiosyncrasy defy the simple categorization of many account books. These sources took so many forms in the past because it was up to their users to determine the books' precise forms based on their needs, though some common characteristics can help us decipher their contents.

Account books were also more than simply tools to keep track of who owed whom and how much. They enabled one thing to be equated in value to another completely different thing through what can look like mundane lists but with the proper interpretation emerge as powerful means of transmutation. Take, for example, the following collection of people and goods traded for each other: 156 gallons of rum, a barrel of flour, 300 bunches of onions, six iron bars, and several Bambara women. Other lists like it can be found throughout the account books of the transatlantic slave trade wherein writing down people and goods in terms of each other made them exchangeable but also obscured the pain and violence such accounting caused across the Atlantic world. The paper technology of an account book, in other words, acted as "the philosopher's stone in what [Stephanie] Smallwood calls the 'alchemy' of converting countless individuals into something known as 'a parcel of negroes,'" notes the historian Seth Rockman.[10] Medicines, too, appear in such lists and changed hands for all sorts of commodities including the proceeds of plantation labor and the transatlantic slave trade. By recognizing the power of rendering real things (people, goods, the natural world) as lines on an account, business records can reveal much about the lives of those who used them and appear within them.

Many people across the Atlantic world kept one or more account books to organize the day-to-day business that comprised their lives. Techniques of mercantile bookkeeping pervaded literate culture in Europe from the sixteenth century onward. Shakespeare, for example, instructed his beloved to "commit whatever may be forgotten to a series of tables or books" in a sonnet. Bookkeeping manuals recommended that merchants keep two principal volumes: a rough account book that was a daily record of transactions, called a day book, journal, or waste book; and a more formal book into which the daily transactions would be copied, known as a ledger.[11] The first book served as a memory aid for the entry of information into the second. Several more specialized account books could also be used in service of trade, such as order, invoice, or wages books that condensed aspects of the business into a single, accessible volume. Personal account books also recorded quotidian activities such as purchasing groceries or health-related expenses. Thus, the producer, distributor, and consumer sides of the medicine trade can each be found in account books depending on where you choose to look.[12]

The first level of accounting, the day book, collected details from the loose papers of trade – the invoices, receipts, and bills – into a chronological record of transactions that would later be totaled and "posted" into the ledger. For instance, each page of the Harvard-trained physician Joseph Osgood's day book begins with the location and the date above a running list of transactions with a section for each customer (designated by the abbreviation "Dr," meaning debitor or debt register; in other words, those in debt to Osgood). This list offers details about Osgood's customers as well as the goods and services he provided to them – pulverized rhubarb or an elixir of camphor, for instance, as well as visits and attendance (for which he charged extra if on a Sunday). The costs of those items, identified by the word "to," are tallied in the right margin divided by three vertical lines to denote pounds, shillings, and pence from left to right. Historians might use the book, then, to analyze a colonial doctor's livelihood or, perhaps, trends in medicine costs across a particular geography (among many other possibilities) depending on the specificity of data contained in the source. Osgood's account book, for example, records a lot of contextual data pertaining to his customers, whereas others abbreviate and generalize to a greater extent in lieu of details about people, goods, or locations. The data to be gleaned from account books varies quite widely despite the similar techniques used to record them.

When an account book does contain sufficient detail, networks of exchange and of obligation begin to emerge. When one person owes another, that debt represents a connection between those people, affecting their interactions until it is fulfilled. As can be seen in the bottom left margin of the July 14, 1770, page of Osgood's day book (see Figure 1.3), Richard Perl of Boxford, Massachusetts, owed Osgood for ten medical visits, several emetic pills made of ipecac, and various elixirs valued at more than 17 shillings. In return, Perl provided Osgood not with coins but rather 12¾ pounds (lb) of veal and 5¼ pounds of lamb, presumably from his own livestock. The word "by" is used in these cases to signify the form by which someone has repaid their debt to the account book holder, Osgood in this example. It is also the transformative word by which veal and lamb were rendered commensurable with medicines and medical services to be exchanged for each other as represented by a notation in an account book.

All this daily transaction information would then be collected in a ledger that offers an overarching view of a business or, in other cases, a household or institution. The ledger served to align all of one's accounts to determine if one had been paid what one was owed and vice versa. This was accomplished through the practice of double-entry bookkeeping where every transaction is entered into the ledger twice, once as a debit (Dr) and once as a credit (Cr) since to be balanced properly every entry needs its opposite. Because they are essentially aggregations, however, ledgers usually contain less granular detail than the separate account books. In contrast to chronological day books, ledgers are arranged by account, such as individuals or a common expense like rent, on pages that list brief summaries of the transactions extrapolated from other business records. If a customer purchased a quantity of merchandise, the goods would be registered as a debit on the left side of the page ("to" something) for the customer's account ("Dr" for debitor) and the payment given for the goods ("by" something) would appear as a credit on the right side ("Cr" for creditor). In the ledger account of Martin Brimmer, an apothecary in Boston, with the London merchants Hughes & Whitelock, "stock" noted on the right side of the page under the Cr column represents the goods Brimmer received from the merchants whom he repaid with the "cash" entered on the left side under Hughes & Whitelock's Dr column (see Figure 1.4). Note that from this ledger alone one cannot determine which medicines Brimmer received in these transactions. Even though Brimmer was the one receiving goods from Hughes & Whitelock, because it was his ledger the account reads as though the merchants owed him for

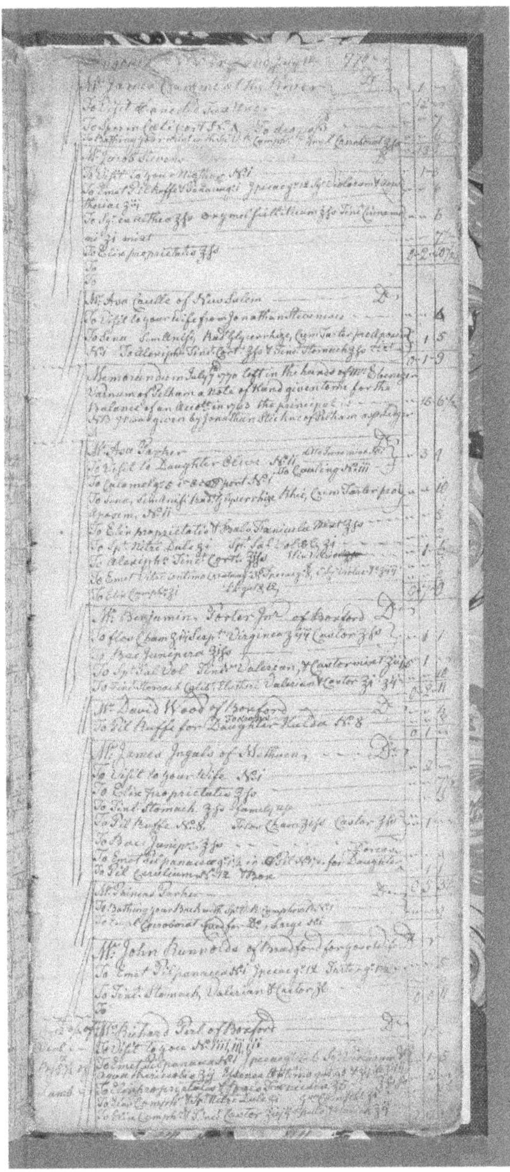

Figure 1.3 Osgood's transaction with Perl at the bottom of the page shows how debts were often recorded in account books in terms of money that usually never existed beyond the page and that were satisfied by the exchange of goods or services to balance the book debt. In this case, lamb and veal repaid medicines and care. The z's, i's, and other notations after the names of medicines represent measures of liquid volume as part of the apothecaries' system of weights and measures. Day Books of Joseph Osgood and son George, 1770–1796, vol. 1, f 1.K.77, Boston Medical Library, Francis A. Countway Library of Medicine (Boston, MA). Image courtesy of Countway Medicine Rare Books.

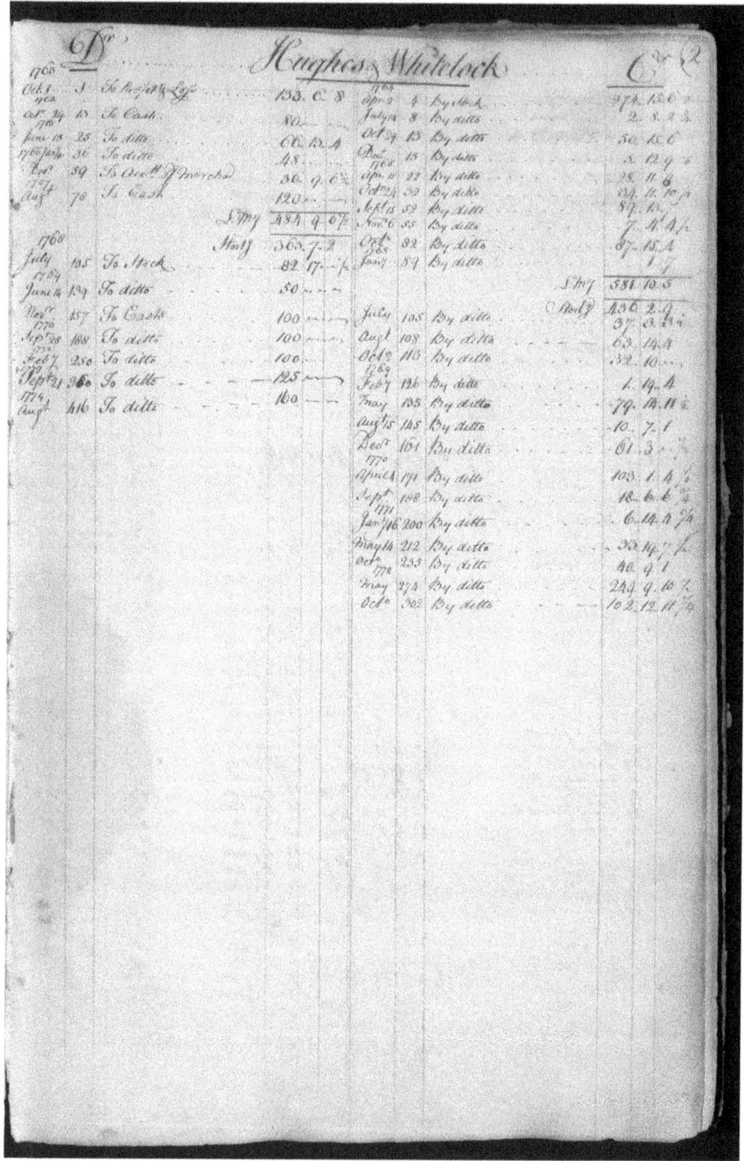

Figure 1.4 Values are calculated on the right side of the Cr and Dr columns in both local Massachusetts money and British pounds sterling (both denoted by the same symbol, £, which can be confusing), illustrating the profusion of currencies across the Atlantic world at the time as well as the inconvenient reality for traders that even currency was not always worth the same in one place as another. If one needed to find a particular account in a ledger, he could check the index which most featured to ease usage. Martin Brimmer Account Ledger, Special Collections Research Center, W&M Libraries, William and Mary. Image courtesy of William and Mary.

cash and repaid him by merchandise. Thus, who wrote the ledger determines whose side of the story you see in an archive.

Ideally, the debits and credits recorded in each of the ledger's accounts would be equal when the book was periodically balanced. Balanced accounts would have equal totals in their debit and credit columns, thereby signaling that all relevant information had been entered. A balanced account, and thus no apparent surplus or deficit, does not suggest a lack of profit or loss by whomever kept the ledger. Rather, surpluses or deficits from a particular account would be denoted by a credit or debit to that account and then a corresponding debit or credit to the ledger's "profit & loss" account.[13] Balancing one's books was also an important consideration since the ledger was open to inspection by trading partners, in contrast to the day book and other business papers that could be destroyed or reused once their contents were copied. Proper bookkeeping thus served to enforce collective commercial norms and display the trustworthiness of individuals who wished to buy, sell, lend, or receive a loan.[14] Ledgers could be transformative of objects and people on many levels.

Medicines in Motion

The business archive of Plough Court pharmacy at GSK offers an opportunity to find medicines in motion across the early modern Atlantic world by weaving together these kinds of business records. The pharmacy's bundles of invoices and receipts would have been compiled into order books that record domestic and overseas shipments of bulk medicines to institutional customers including London hospitals, Royal Navy ships, and Jamaican plantations, just to name a few. By contrast, the pharmacy's day-to-day accounts (sometimes collected in what was called a "practical journal") chronicle over-the-counter sales of pills, tinctures, plasters, and various other remedies to a local network of patients. These usually small transactions would be entered as line items into the cash or shop account in the pharmacy's ledger, while the large shipments detailed in the order book would be posted to their purchaser's separate account in the ledger. For example, an order of 30 pounds weight of elixir of vitriol, a mixture of sulfuric acid and alcohol used as a treatment for scurvy, in 60 half pound bottles for the Royal Navy on June 26, 1777 was entered as "goods" and "sundries" to the Dr side of the Commissioners of Sick and Wounded Seamen's account in the ledger for which they would repay Plough Court by cash or something else on the Cr side of the page. Summary accounts in the ledger, such as bills payable, bills receivable, cash, profit and loss, or charges on trade were used to make sense of all the information contained in individual accounts.[15]

Merchants of medicines kept track of their stock in trade through written inventories of goods on hand and invoices of goods sent out. While some of this information would be captured in account books, inventories and invoices offer a more detailed look at the items traded as well as the production and distribution processes enabling that trade. From inventories, we can picture the bright aloe and gnarled guaiacum roots displayed in Thomas Corbyn's shop window and the glass case in the middle of the floor containing acrid salts and aromatic oils. In contrast to this tidy shop floor, Corbyn's home, storerooms, and laboratories were a mess. Plants, chemicals, and packaging choked the hallways of his London home, while his counting house was piled high with vials, corks, glassware, baskets, casks, bags, brown paper, and other shipping supplies. At another property, bottles of vitriol, benzoin, and other chemical spirits lay in the stables near the laboratory. These items would become the products noted on the pages of his day books, order books, and ledgers.[16] In my own work, I have used inventories and invoices to illustrate the medicine trade's global reach yet local realities as embodied by the fragrant, colorful clutter of London's pharmacies from this period. Wills, probate records, insurance policies, and bankruptcy records are other types of inventories that can be useful in studying early modern business since they list a person's property at a particular moment in time as one way to evaluate success, for example. To pay for all this material, participants in the medicine trade, like other traders, relied on borrowing money, such as via loans and mortgages, which generated their own stacks of paperwork to be uncovered in an archive.[17]

Whereas inventories can reveal the goods sitting in a shop, warehouse, or laboratory, invoices show items moving around. Invoices are best understood as one of a broader assortment of paper technologies to minimize risk of loss in maritime trade. Merchants tracked their cargoes with invoices and shipping receipts called "bills of lading," while captains and crews noted shipboard events in logbooks and journals (see Figure 1.5). Invoices kept by the partnership of Lacey Primatt and John Maud, for example, illustrate the many supply chains for raw materials stretching across Europe toward Asia. Their invoices also demonstrate the calculations required to determine insurance rates, shipping costs, commission charges, duties, and exchange rates at various stages of long-distance trade. In an invoice for jalap resin, a yellow-brown powder of tuberous roots, imported from Amsterdam, the partners added insurance, duties, and freight costs while also exchanging Dutch florins into British pounds sterling. The medicine trade required fluency, or at least familiarity, with a variety of systems of weights, measures, and monies as goods crossed geographical, cultural, and political boundaries.[18] Recipes also offer a way to assess the raw materials and human labor that went into the medicines made in laboratories and then sold elsewhere.[19]

The early modern medicine trade's global reach appears from a holistic view of the location data contained in business records such as bills of lading, invoices, and account books (see Figure 1.6). One can also quantitatively assess the trade's scale from a governmental perspective. Taxes on trade offered significant revenues to the British state in this period, so it should come as no great surprise that the Treasury sought to understand and then tax the import and export of medicinal commodities. London's Port Books offer a view of the city's seventeenth-century maritime commerce, and the Naval Office Shipping Lists and Customs Records provide a measure of colonial and metropolitan trade during the eighteenth century. This period also saw the emergence of a business press across the Atlantic world that published commercial statistics in a variety of formats.[20] Official trade statistics offer an important, though incomplete, measure of the medicine trade because they capture

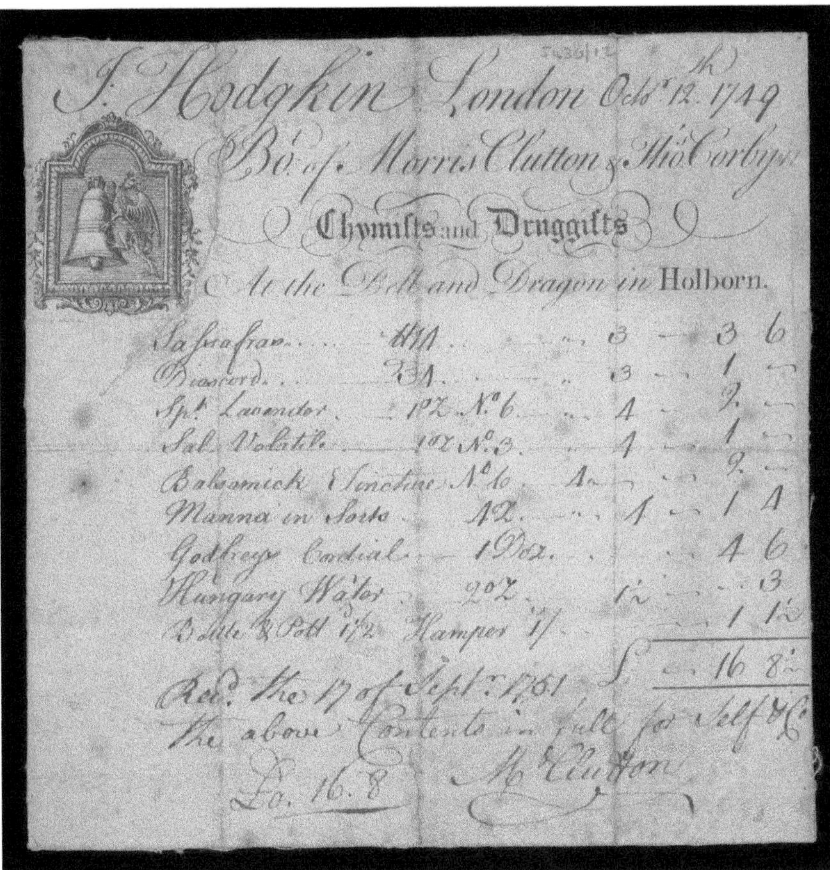

J. Hodgkin London Octr 12. 1749
Bo. of Morris Clutton & Thos Corbyn
Chymists and Druggists
At the Bell and Dragon in Holborn.

Sassafras	℔ij	3	3 6
Diascord.	℥j	3	1 –
Spt Lavender	1oz No 6	4	2 –
Sal Volatile	1oz No 3	4	1 –
Balsamick Tincture No 6		1½	9 –
Manna in Sorts	1℔	1	1 4
Godfreys Cordial	1 Doz.		4 6
Hungary Water	2oz	1½	3
Bottle & Pott 1½ Hamper 1/			1 1½
		£	– 16 8

Recd the 17 of Sept 1751
the above Contents in full for Self & Co.
M Clutton
£0. 16. 8

Figure 1.5 This receipt for goods purchased by J. Hodgkin at Thomas Corbyn's shop offers a representative example of an eighteenth-century receipt. The goods are listed on the left with their quantities, unit prices, and total prices in subsequent columns moving toward the right. These items would all have been found in one of the contemporaneous inventories of Corbyn's property. Abbreviations for various weights, measures, and monies can be seen throughout. [Corbyn & Co. receipt], 1749, MS 5436/12, Corbyn & Co. Papers, Wellcome Collection. Image courtesy of the Wellcome Collection.

only legal trade and miss smuggling – by definition, trade that avoided state taxes and scrutiny – which could account for a substantial portion of business depending on the context. Customs records also encourage us to consider the ways things in the past were classified and taxed because of those classifications.

Quantitative business records offer only one perspective of the medicine trade that should be paired with what historian Stephanie Smallwood calls the "more hidden, internal transcript" of the trade's human story by also reading letters and other qualitative sources.[21] Plough Court pharmacy, for instance, would have been awash in a sea of paper, including bundles of letters coming in and going out, needing to

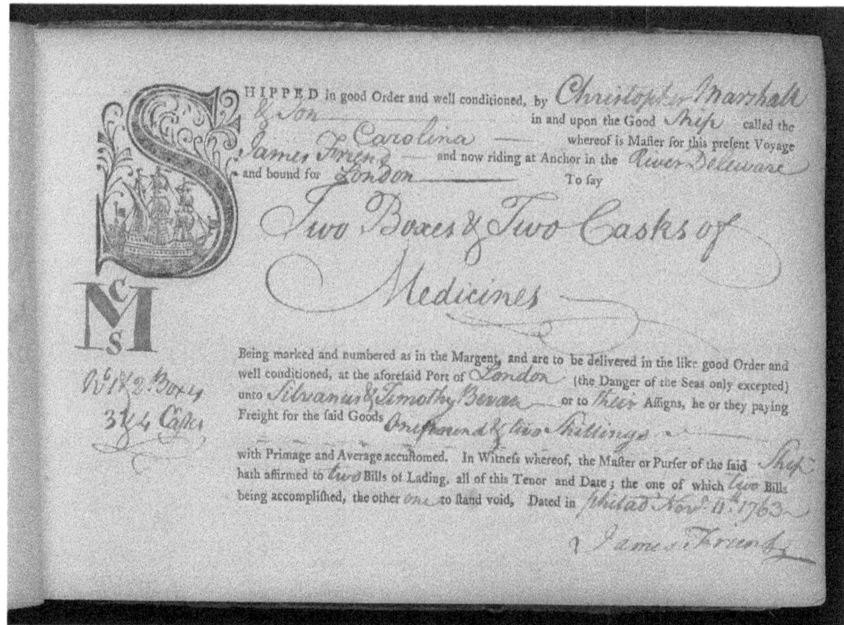

SHIPPED in good Order and well conditioned, by Christopher Marshall & Son in and upon the Good Ship called the Carolina whereof is Master for this present Voyage James Friend and now riding at Anchor in the River Delaware and bound for London To say

Two Boxes & Two Casks of Medicines

McM S

No 1 & 2 Boxes
3 & 4 Casks

Being marked and numbered as in the Margent, and are to be delivered in the like good Order and well conditioned, at the aforesaid Port of London (the Danger of the Seas only excepted) unto Silvanus & Timothy Bevan or to their Assigns, he or they paying Freight for the said Goods One pound & two Shillings

with Primage and Average accustomed. In Witness whereof, the Master or Purser of the said Ship hath affirmed to two Bills of Lading, all of this Tenor and Date; the one of which two Bills being accomplished, the other one to stand void, Dated in Philad Nov 11th 1763

James Friend

Figure 1.6 Preprinted forms were often used for commercial documents, like this bill of lading, and sold in convenient books. In this example from 1763, the Philadelphia merchant of medicine Christopher Marshall records a shipment of medicines (two boxes and two casks) he has sent via the ship Carolina to London for Silvanus and Timothy Bevan, the brothers in charge of the Plough Court pharmacy at the time. Per bookkeeping standards this shipment would have been entered in Marshall's ledger as a debit (Dr) to the Bevan brothers' account. Christopher Marshall's Bills of Lading, p. 11, [Am.916], Historical Society of Pennsylvania. Reproduced with permission from the Historical Society of Pennsylvania.

be copied into letter books that were sold in standard sizes and shapes for mass consumption in eighteenth-century London.[22] Merchants of medicines shared strategies for making products alongside tips for selling: what would be accepted as payment, at what interest rate, and where, for example. They also took their business correspondence as an opportunity to discuss their pains and worries. Sometimes a personal note or a request was added hastily in a letter's margin, or a price list scrawled just before the letter was sealed. Such details could be significant for the merchant trying to buy low or sell high and can be significant for historians searching for details often excluded from messages by the conventions of formal letter writing. Historians have read emergent cultures and world views of merchants in the concerns, goals, and opinions expressed in early modern correspondence. If you find an interesting source, whether it is a letter or an invoice, for instance, try to cross-reference the individuals mentioned in it to see where the story takes you. In my case, following up on a familiar name helped me to reattribute a Barbadian account book mislabeled in an archive, and thereby put its contents into new perspective.

Embodied Histories

For all they can tell us, business records represent only a particular slice of the medicine trade that captures people literate and numerate enough to keep such records and lucky or powerful enough that those records have been preserved. In other words, who typically appears in the business archive does not represent the full range of people who made, applied, and engaged with medicines in the early modern world, nor does the business archive fully capture the diversity of people's relationships with medicine – topics all covered elsewhere in this volume and elsewhere in scholarship.[23] Structural power differentials based on categories of race and gender, coupled with a legal system designed to codify those perceived distinctions, also make it challenging, though far from impossible, to uncover those who did not possess the power or freedom to leave their own business records. For example, coverture laws imposed on married women, whereby their legal identities and much of their property were subordinated to those of their husbands, often prevented female consumers from appearing in account books under their own names. Many women had to use their husband's account when making local purchases. Medical practitioners operating outside of sanctioned, pre-professional boundaries, whether a Black ritual practitioner in the Caribbean or an herbwoman in England, are less likely to be found in business records except in oblique ways given their limited access to credit and other official mechanisms of transacting business.[24]

Nevertheless, this wider world can still often be found in the business archive. In the ledgers of Plough Court pharmacy, for example, appear accounts with herbalists, chemists, bottle merchants, grinders, turners, oilmen, box makers, coopers, scale makers, sassafras cutters, vinegar merchants, gardeners, and distillers – the people upon whom merchants of medicines relied for the packaging, raw materials, expertise, and services required for a robust trade. Though we lack their voices, we can begin to see a medicine trade vibrant with tradespeople, so-called cunning women, and indigenous informants who lived and worked across the Atlantic world.[25] Similarly, the experiences of unfree men, women, and children can also be glimpsed in the pages of such records. The account books of plantation doctors record the names, locations, and treatments given to (or forced upon) bound laborers in the Caribbean. In another case, a 1767 invoice from James Carter to the College of William and Mary reveals the medicines and attendance purchased for those enslaved by the college, including applying plasters to what could have been whipping injuries. An instance of smearing ointment or extracting a tooth seen in an account book or invoice takes on more critical significance when read within the embodied context of the many connections between medicine, enslavement, power, and profit in the eighteenth-century Atlantic world.[26]

The physical experience of making, packing, and shipping goods can get lost amid the transactions or even be deliberately hidden from view in the business archive. Wage books and recipes from some of London's laboratories, however, tell us that scores of men worked over hot coals, sweating, breathing in fumes, and drinking beer for hydration to manufacture medicines in the eighteenth century. Some received steady wages for years while others worked for a month or two only to fade back into the ranks of London's economically precarious working poor.[27] Others still, such as the unnamed man who "was terribly burnt" when a distillation gone awry set fire to the apothecary shop where he worked, paid dearly for their labor.[28] Across the Atlantic Ocean in Massachusetts, colonial merchants of medicines relied on apprenticed, indentured, and enslaved labor for their businesses. In one case, William Jepson trusted the expertise of a boy he enslaved "to make most of [his] Plasters and unguents [Tinctures] and Elixirs."[29] We can only surmise if Mark and Quarts, enslaved by the apothecary William Hunter in Newport, Rhode Island, or those men and women enslaved by the apothecary Joseph Gamble Jackman in Speightstown, Barbados, similarly toiled over stills, carried heavy loads, or rolled pills in the medicine trade.[30]

Such examples underscore the importance of recognizing the tendency of business records to obscure certain experiences and even to transform people into abstract quantities of labor or rum, depending on the account book. How then should we balance that dehumanizing risk against everything business records have to offer the history of medicine? One answer lies in the empathic reading of qualitative and quantitative sources together to recognize who and what is left out of those accounts and to better identify traces of them when they do appear. Historian Marisa Fuentes, for example, reconstructs vivid scenes of eighteenth-century Barbados from the perspectives of women who appear only briefly, if at all, in the archive of their enslavers, though whose archival absences can tell us so much about the contexts in which they lived, worked, suffered, loved, and attended to their health.[31] A second answer lies in understanding the business archive as not just a passive record of trade but rather an active tool of trade, and the transformations that accompanied it can help us relocate people's decisions, opportunities, and constraints within a sea of paper.

Conclusion

To conclude this chapter, I pose a rhetorical question: how should considering the business archive change your perspective of the history of medicine? The examples offered here reflect an approach to the history of medicine that asks how things worked in addition to what they meant and probes the ways health and healing became commodities to be bought and sold on a global scale. Business records also illuminate the transoceanic infrastructures behind the intimate act of ingesting a bitter tincture of cinchona, for example. Entire networks of debt and obligation existed that encouraged promises to pay and failures to do so; opportunities and dead ends; hopes for health for some and brutal labor for others. The medicine trade did not just happen on its own. There were always people behind the movement of things whose experiences paperwork can reveal if we know how to read for them. Thinking in terms of commerce, though, does not mean retreating into a world of numbers; it can also suggest valuable approaches that acknowledge both individual experience and quantitative data. In the business archive of the transatlantic medicine trade, we find the influence of material concerns about shipping and payment, for instance, on abstract things like how we understand our bodies, those of our families or neighbors, and the world around us. Medicine and commerce are inseparable then as now.

Notes

1 John Carter Brown Library, "Mind Your Business: Records of Early American Commerce at the John Carter Brown Library" (Sept.–Dec. 2012), www.brown.edu/Facilities/John_Carter_Brown_Library/exhibitions/business/index.html.
2 Papers Relating to the Destruction of Useless Records (1858–1881), IOR/H/722, pp. 253, 257-259, India Office Records and Private Papers, Archives and Manuscripts, British Library.
3 "Forum: The Paper Technologies of Capitalism," *Technology and Culture* 58, no. 2 (2017): 487–569.
4 Miles Ogborn, *Indian Ink: Script and Print in the Making of the English East India Company* (Chicago, IL: University of Chicago Press, 2007); Lindsay O'Neill, *The Opened Letter: Networking in the Early Modern British World* (Philadelphia: University of Pennsylvania Press, 2015), 87; Richard D. Brown, *Knowledge Is Power: The Diffusion of Information in Early America, 1700–1865* (Oxford: Oxford University Press, 1989), 112. "Papered century" or "paper century," depending on the translation, quoted in Marc Shell, *Art & Money* (Chicago, IL: University of Chicago Press, 1995), 66; John J. McCusker, "Colonial Paper Money," in *Studies on Money in Early America*, ed. Eric P. Newman and Richard G. Doty (New York: American Numismatic Society, 1976), 94.
5 On the scarcity of money, see Craig Muldrew, "'Hard Food for Midas': Cash and Its Social Value in Early Modern England," *Past & Present* 170 (2001): 78–120.
6 William Jepson Diary, 1753, Massachusetts Historical Society.
7 Zachary Dorner, *Merchants of Medicines: The Commerce and Coercion of Health in Britain's Long Eighteenth Century* (Chicago, IL: University of Chicago Press, 2020), 44–46.
8 The history of finance is coming back into style, see Stephen Mihm, "Follow the Money: The Return of Finance in the Early Republic," *Journal of the Early Republic* 36, no. 4 (2016): 783–804, 784, 790.
9 Tara Bynum, "Caesar Lyndon's Lists, Letters, and a Pig Roast: A Sundry Account Book," *Early American Literature* 53, no. 3 (2018): 839–49.
10 Seth Rockman, "Forum: The Paper Technologies of Capitalism, Introduction," *Technology and Culture* 58, no. 2 (2017), 495 ("philosopher's stone"); Stephanie Smallwood, *Saltwater Slavery: A Middle Passage from Africa to American Diaspora* (Cambridge, MA: Harvard University Press, 2007), 10 ("alchemy"), 97–100; Marcus Rediker, *The Slave Ship: A Human History* (New York: Viking, 2007), 12.
11 Jacob Soll, "From Note-Taking to Data Banks: Personal and Institutional Information Management in Early Modern Europe," *Intellectual History Review* 20, no. 3 (2010): 361; Angus Vine, "Commercial Commonplacing: Francis Bacon, the Waste-Book, and the Ledger," *English Manuscript Studies, 1100–1700* 16 (2011): 197–98 ("commit whatever").
12 For examples of patient or consumer perspectives, see Patrick Wallis and Teerapa Pirohakul, "Medical Revolutions? The Growth of Medicine in England, 1660–1800," *Journal of Social History* 49, no. 3 (2016): 510–31; Elaine Leong, "Making Medicines in the Early Modern Household," *Bulletin of the History of Medicine* 82, no. 1 (2008): 145–68; Ben Mutschler, *The Province of Affliction: Illness and the Making of Early New England* (Chicago, IL: University of Chicago Press, 2020).
13 How-to manuals written for apprentices and young traders tend to be helpful tools for reading pre-modern accounting, for example: Benjamin F. Foster, *A Concise Treatise on Commercial Bookkeeping, Elucidating the Principles and Practice of Double Entry and the Modern Methods of Arranging Merchants' Accounts*, 2nd ed. (Boston, MA: Perkins &

Marvin, 1837). For other tips see Robert J. Wilson III, "Early American Account Books: Interpretation, Cataloguing, and Use," Technical Leaflet 140, *History News* 36, no. 9 (Sept. 1981): 21–28; Christopher Densmore, "Understanding and Using Early Nineteenth Century Account Books," *Midwestern Archivist* 5, no. 1 (1980): 5–19; Historical Society of Pennsylvania, "Subject Guide: Financial Records Guide and Glossary," updated May 28, 2015, portal.hsp.org/subject-guides/subject-guide-13.

14 Mary Poovey, *A History of the Modern Fact: Problems of Knowledge in the Sciences of Wealth and Society* (Chicago, IL: University of Chicago Press, 1998), 29–91.

15 [Bundles of letters, vouchers, orders, agreements], c. 1790, AH197, Allen & Hanburys Manuscripts, GlaxoSmithKline (hereafter GSK); Order Book (1776–1777), AH140, Allen & Hanburys Manuscripts, GSK; Ledgers, AH207, AH226, AH228, Allen & Hanburys Manuscripts, GSK; Practical Journal (1782–1790), AH201, Allen & Hanburys Manuscripts, GSK.

16 Inventories and Valuations of Stock, 1761–1770, MS 5452/1-9, esp. MS 5452/5, Corbyn & Co. Papers, Wellcome Collection.

17 For example: [Bond to Thomas Talwin], 1755, MS 5439/1/1, Corbyn & Co. Papers, Wellcome Collection. On mortgages, see S. D. Smith, *Slavery, Family, and Gentry Capitalism in the British Atlantic: The World of the Lascelles, 1648–1834* (Cambridge: Cambridge University Press, 2006), ch. 6–7.

18 Primatt's and Maud's invoice book also contains recipes, which is another reminder that business records are frequently difficult to catalog because they could serve multiple functions at the same time. Primatt & Maud Invoice Book (1753–1806), MS 5858, Wellcome Collection. Perhaps the greatest resource for historians of exchange in the early modern Atlantic world is John J. McCusker, *Money and Exchange in Europe and America, 1600–1775: A Handbook* (Chapel Hill: University of North Carolina Press, 1978).

19 Manufacturing Recipe Book (c. 1782), MS 5447, Corbyn & Co. Papers, Wellcome Collection.

20 For advice on working with customs data, see John J. McCusker, "The Current Value of English Exports, 1697 to 1800," *William and Mary Quarterly* 28, no. 4 (1971): 607–28; Patrick Wallis, "Exotic Drugs and English Medicine: England's Drug Trade, C. 1550–C. 1800," *Social History of Medicine* 25, no. 1 (2012): 20–46. Sources of customs data include the Ledgers of Imports and Exports, America (CUST 16/1) and the Ledgers of Imports and Exports, England and Wales (CUST 3/1-82), both held at the National Archives of the UK. Data from the colonial side can be found in sources such as the Naval Office Shipping Lists for Massachusetts (MS N-1635) at the Massachusetts Historical Society.

21 Smallwood used this phrase in the context of the transatlantic slave trade, see Smallwood, *Saltwater Slavery*, 4–5.

22 Mark Boonshoft, "Letterbooks, Indexes, and Learning about Early American Business," *New York Public Library Blog* (20 July 2015), www.nypl.org/blog/2015/07/20/letterbooks-in-early-american-business.

23 For example: Mary E. Fissell, *Patients, Power, and the Poor in Eighteenth-Century Bristol* (Cambridge: Cambridge University Press, 1991); James Sweet, *Domingo Álvares, African Healing, and the Intellectual History of the Atlantic World* (Chapel Hill: University of North Carolina Press, 2011).

24 Pablo F. Gómez, "Incommensurable Epistemologies?: The Atlantic Geography of Healing in the Early Modern Caribbean," *Small Axe* 18, no. 2 (2014): 95–107; Ellen Hartigan-O'Connor, *The Ties That Buy: Women and Commerce in Revolutionary America* (Philadelphia: University of Pennsylvania Press, 2009), ch. 3–4.

25 Ledgers (1789–1796, 1797–1808), AH228, AH226, Allen & Hanburys Manuscripts, GSK.

26 [Invoice to William & Mary College from James Carter], 1767, box 5, folder 2, Office of the Bursar Records, Special Collections Research Center, W&M Libraries, William and Mary; for additional context, see Sharla M. Fett, *Working Cures: Healing, Health, and*

Power on Southern Slave Plantations (Chapel Hill: University of North Carolina Press, 2002).
27 Wages Books (1762–1770, 1770–1825), MSS 5444 & 5445, Corbyn & Co. Papers, Wellcome Collection; Flor. Benzoin Costing, May 1760, MS 5448/2, Corbyn & Co. Papers, Wellcome Collection.
28 *Weekly Miscellany* (London, UK), 13 Oct. 1733, [3].
29 Silvester Gardiner to William Jepson, 26 May 1758, case 7, box 29, folder 5, Simon Gratz Autograph Collection, Historical Society of Pennsylvania.
30 Inventory of the personal estate of the late William Hunter, 7 Feb. 1777, vault A, box 90, folder 9, William Hunter Papers, Newport Historical Society; "Joseph Gamble Jackman Inventory," 6 Oct. 1786, Barbados Department of Archives, Black Rock.
31 Marisa J. Fuentes, *Dispossessed Lives: Enslaved Women, Violence, and the Archive* (Philadelphia: University of Pennsylvania Press, 2016).

Bibliography

Primary Sources

Allen & Hanburys Manuscripts. GlaxoSmithKline, London, UK.
"Bills Settled from Jany 1 to Dec. 31 1780." Arnold Family Business Records. John Carter Brown Library, Providence, RI.
Christopher Marshall's Bills of Lading. Am.916. Historical Society of Pennsylvania, Philadelphia, PA.
Corbyn & Co. Papers. Wellcome Collection, London, UK.
Day Books of Joseph Osgood and son George (1770–1796). f 1.K.77. Boston Medical Library. Francis A. Countway Library of Medicine, Boston, MA.
Foster, Benjamin F. *A Concise Treatise on Commercial Bookkeeping, Elucidating the Principles and Practice of Double Entry and the Modern Methods of Arranging Merchants' Accounts*. 2nd ed. Perkins & Marvin, Boston, MA, 1837.
Inventory of the personal estate of the late William Hunter (7 Feb. 1777). Vault A, box 90, folder 9. William Hunter Papers. Newport Historical Society, Newport, RI.
[Invoice to William & Mary College from James Carter]. Box 5, folder 2. Office of the Bursar Records. Special Collections Research Center. W&M Libraries. William and Mary, Williamsburg, VA.
"Joseph Gamble Jackman Inventory" (6 Oct. 1786). Barbados Department of Archives, Black Rock, Barbados.
Ledgers of Imports and Exports, America. CUST 16/1. National Archives, Kew.
Ledgers of Imports and Exports, England and Wales. CUST 3/1-82. National Archives, Kew.
Martin Brimmer Account Ledger. Special Collections Research Center. W&M Libraries. William and Mary, Williamsburg, VA.
Naval Office Shipping Lists for Massachusetts. MS N-1635. Massachusetts Historical Society, Boston, MA.
Papers Relating to the Destruction of Useless Records (1858–1881). IOR/H/722. India Office Records and Private Papers. Archives and Manuscripts. British Library, London, UK.
Primatt & Maud Invoice Book (1753–1806). MS 5858. Wellcome Collection, London.
[Scribble Scrap from Daybook]. MSS 588 SG1 S3 B1 F3 (RHi X174350A). Rhode Island Historical Society, Providence, RI.
Silvester Gardiner to William Jepson (26 May 1758). Case 7, box 29, folder 5. Simon Gratz Autograph Collection. Historical Society of Pennsylvania, PA.
Weekly Miscellany (London, UK). 13 Oct. 1733.
William Jepson Diary (1753). Massachusetts Historical Society, Boston, MA.

Secondary Sources

Boonshoft, Mark. "Letterbooks, Indexes, and Learning about Early American Business." *New York Public Library Blog* (20 July 2015). www.nypl.org/blog/2015/07/20/letterbooks-in-early-american-business.

Brown, Richard D. *Knowledge Is Power: The Diffusion of Information in Early America, 1700–1865*. Oxford: Oxford University Press, 1989.

Bynum, Tara. "Caesar Lyndon's Lists, Letters, and a Pig Roast: A Sundry Account Book." *Early American Literature* 53, no. 3 (2018): 839–49.

Densmore, Christopher. "Understanding and Using Early Nineteenth Century Account Books." *Midwestern Archivist* 5, no. 1 (1980): 5–19.

Dorner, Zachary. *Merchants of Medicines: The Commerce and Coercion of Health in Britain's Long Eighteenth Century*. Chicago, IL: University of Chicago Press, 2020.

Fett, Sharla M. *Working Cures: Healing, Health, and Power on Southern Slave Plantations*. Chapel Hill: University of North Carolina Press, 2002.

Fissell, Mary. *Patients, Power, and the Poor in Eighteenth-Century Bristol*. Cambridge: Cambridge University Press, 1991.

"Forum: The Paper Technologies of Capitalism." *Technology and Culture* 58, no. 2 (2017): 487–569.

Fuentes, Marisa J. *Dispossessed Lives: Enslaved Women, Violence, and the Archive*. Philadelphia: University of Pennsylvania Press, 2016.

Gómez, Pablo F. "Incommensurable Epistemologies?: The Atlantic Geography of Healing in the Early Modern Caribbean." *Small Axe* 18, no. 2 (2014): 95–107.

Hartigan-O'Connor, Ellen. *The Ties That Buy: Women and Commerce in Revolutionary America*. Philadelphia: University of Pennsylvania Press, 2009.

Historical Society of Pennsylvania. "Subject Guide: Financial Records Guide and Glossary." Updated May 28, 2015. portal.hsp.org/subject-guides/subject-guide-13.

John Carter Brown Library. "Mind Your Business: Records of Early American Commerce at the John Carter Brown Library" (Sept.–Dec. 2012). www.brown.edu/Facilities/John_Carter_Brown_Library/exhibitions/business/index.html.

Leong, Elaine. "Making Medicines in the Early Modern Household." *Bulletin of the History of Medicine* 82, no. 1 (2008): 145–68.

McCusker, John J. "Colonial Paper Money." In *Studies on Money in Early America*, edited by Eric P. Newman and Richard G. Doty, 94–104. New York: American Numismatic Society, 1976.

McCusker, John J. "The Current Value of English Exports, 1697 to 1800." *William and Mary Quarterly* 28, no. 4 (1971): 607–28.

McCusker, John J. *Money and Exchange in Europe and America, 1600–1775: A Handbook*. Chapel Hill: University of North Carolina Press, 1978.

Mihm, Stephen. "Follow the Money: The Return of Finance in the Early Republic." *Journal of the Early Republic* 36, no. 4 (2016): 783–804.

Muldrew, Craig. "'Hard Food for Midas': Cash and Its Social Value in Early Modern England," *Past & Present* 170 (2001): 78–120.

Mutschler, Ben. *The Province of Affliction: Illness and the Making of Early New England*. Chicago, IL: University of Chicago Press, 2020.

Ogborn, Miles. *Indian Ink: Script and Print in the Making of the English East India Company*. Chicago, IL: University of Chicago Press, 2007.

O'Neill, Lindsay. *The Opened Letter: Networking in the Early Modern British World*. Philadelphia: University of Pennsylvania Press, 2015.

Poovey, Mary. *A History of the Modern Fact: Problems of Knowledge in the Sciences of Wealth and Society*. Chicago, IL: University of Chicago Press, 1998.
Rediker, Marcus. *The Slave Ship: A Human History*. New York: Viking, 2007.
Rockman, Seth. "Forum: The Paper Technologies of Capitalism, Introduction." *Technology and Culture* 58, no. 2 (2017): 487–505.
Shell, Marc. *Art & Money*. Chicago, IL: University of Chicago Press, 1995.
Smallwood, Stephanie. *Saltwater Slavery: A Middle Passage from Africa to American Diaspora*. Cambridge, MA: Harvard University Press, 2007.
Smith, S. D. *Slavery, Family, and Gentry Capitalism in the British Atlantic: The World of the Lascelles, 1648–1834*. Cambridge: Cambridge University Press, 2006.
Soll, Jacob. "From Note-Taking to Data Banks: Personal and Institutional Information Management in Early Modern Europe." *Intellectual History Review* 20, no. 3 (2010): 355–75.
Sweet, James. *Domingo Álvares, African Healing, and the Intellectual History of the Atlantic World*. Chapel Hill: University of North Carolina Press, 2011.
Vine, Angus. "Commercial Commonplacing: Francis Bacon, the Waste-Book, and the Ledger." *English Manuscript Studies, 1100–1700* 16 (2011): 197–218.
Wallis, Patrick. "Exotic Drugs and English Medicine: England's Drug Trade, C. 1550–C. 1800." *Social History of Medicine* 25, no. 1 (2012): 20–46.
Wallis, Patrick and Teerapa Pirohakul. "Medical Revolutions? The Growth of Medicine in England, 1660–1800." *Journal of Social History* 49, no. 3 (2016): 510–31.
Wilson III, Robert J. "Early American Account Books: Interpretation, Cataloguing, and Use." Technical Leaflet 140, *History News* 36, no. 9 (1981): 21–28.

2 Medicine in the Convent

Sharon T. Strocchia

Between 1500 and 1650, tens of thousands of women across the Italian peninsula lived in religious communities, more than any other region in Europe. In mid-sixteenth century Florence, roughly one in every eight adult women lived in a convent, while close to 54 percent of Venetian aristocratic women became nuns in the seventeenth century. Similar patterns pertained in other major Italian cities in the same years.[1] The vast majority of these well-born women could read and write in the vernacular; some were also versed in the Latin classics that became increasingly available in vernacular print. Thanks to this high level of literacy and immersion in written culture, which probably was unmatched anywhere in Europe, Italian nuns produced a multitude of texts spanning a wide range of genres, often penned in their own hands. These women dispatched countless letters to friends and family, kept chits and account books, wrote frequent administrative reports, and authored spiritual poems and plays, foreign language dictionaries, histories of the world, and imaginative devotional literature.[2]

Among nuns' voluminous writings are two types of narrative sources – convent chronicles and necrologies – that lend themselves to a wide range of health-related inquiries. These topics run the gamut from the demographics of disease and social constructions of disability to illness management, pharmaceutical practices, mental health, and the cultural meanings of pain and suffering. It should be noted that neither chronicles nor necrologies explicitly intended to convey clinical information or medical thinking about these and other issues. Nevertheless, these narratives communicated important insights into the practice of early modern medicine and the subjective experiences of illness in the course of reporting other information.

Each type of source reveals a different dimension of health and healing in line with its intrinsic objectives. Convent chronicles aimed to identify a community's distinctive features as well as key turning points in its history. Organized chronologically, these narratives recounted an institutional history from the community's foundation to the present day or to some other pivotal point in its past, such as a major change in administrative oversight.[3] Because they focused on relations with the outside world, convent chronicles portray nuns primarily in their guise as "agents of health": that is, as active, informed healthcare practitioners who lacked a formal title, much like other practitioners who relied on practical skills and knowledge within a pluralistic medical market.[4] They highlight religious women

DOI: 10.4324/9781003094876-4

in action as they diagnosed illness, developed treatment plans, experimented with medical recipes, ran commercial apothecary shops, dispensed medical advice via letters and visits, and nursed sick members of their communities. Dozens of nuns' chronicles written in the fifteenth and sixteenth centuries are still extant in archives across the Italian peninsula. Other texts have been lost to the ravages of time; only a few surviving manuscripts have been published and fewer still have been translated into English.[5]

By contrast, necrologies convey information centered on the personal health of the women who populated religious houses. This inward-looking focus stemmed from the purposes of necrologies as a source type. At base, these documents were collections of obituaries celebrating the lives of individual nuns shortly after their death; they originated as simple calendars of the dead that helped religious communities keep track of anniversary masses performed for the soul of the deceased.[6] Over time, these remembrances acquired new purposes. Read aloud at mealtime or at commemorative celebrations, poignant stories of singular lives provided inspirational role models while also reinforcing a sense of community. In Renaissance Italy, these accounts frequently acquired great emotional depth. The nuns who authored them commonly added intimate personal details or biographical notes about the sisters in religion with whom they had worked, prayed, laughed, suffered, and shared meals for many years. Since Renaissance nuns took responsibility for their own care in order to preserve religious reclusion, they were the ones who nursed their colleagues through repeated bouts of illness. These firsthand bedside experiences gave nuns profound insight into each other's bodies, which sharpened their diagnostic skills, while at the same time familiarizing them with an individual's strengths and fears. The life stories told in obituaries thus combine the force of eyewitness testimonies with the subjective insights of patient narratives. Even though obituaries were not written by patients themselves but were mediated by their caregivers and other nuns, they nevertheless provided windows into "the inner worlds and imaginations" of sufferers and the companions who cared for them. Consequently, necrologies offer an important source base for scholars writing medical history "from below," in which the task of recovering patients' perceptions and subjective attitudes toward illness takes center stage.[7]

Despite their differing objectives, these memory books – one communal, the other individual – worked as complements to each other. Sometimes they were sewn together into a single manuscript to form a living archive of memory binding nuns to their predecessors.[8] Composite tomes ranged from slender compilations to magnificent manuscripts, depending on the size and status of the community. Both source types enjoyed enormous geographical reach beyond Italy.[9] Numerous female religious communities in other parts of Europe maintained house chronicles and necrologies, and these transplanted genres were especially influential in shaping institutional record keeping as Catholicism expanded globally into the Americas after 1500.[10]

In approaching these narratives as sources for early modern medical history, we should keep three key points in mind. First, because of their shared interest in storytelling, convent chronicles and necrologies must be read as literary compositions as well as historical records. The constructed nature of these sources means that they should not be taken at face value; instead, readers should approach them like other complex narratives, keeping particular tropes and narrative conventions in mind while paying close attention to gaps, silences, and contradictions. For instance, the Florentine chronicle of Le Murate, penned by Sister Giustina Niccolini in 1598, presented a well-researched account of historical events spanning almost 200 years, drawing on the now-lost convent archive. A self-assured stylist, Niccolini selected which details to include, what themes to emphasize, and the order in which to present them. Writing this chronicle thus afforded Sister Giustina considerable agency and creativity in its construction. Because of her deep personal devotion, she remarked with unusual frequency on the soaring spirituality of other convent residents, which, in turn, garnered many favors from well-born patrons and churchmen alike. This emphasis did not prevent Niccolini from recounting internal conflicts or the gritty realities of convent life, but it did give her interpretation of events a decidedly spiritual inflection.[11] Other nun-authors working with the same evidence probably would have painted a slightly different picture.

Second, convent chronicles and necrologies were celebratory texts that aimed to showcase positive traits and achievements – fortitude, resilience, good judgment, spiritual heroics – while glossing over errant or unwelcome behaviors. Take the example of Sister Bartolomea da Firenzuola, a nun in the Florentine convent of San Jacopo di Ripoli who died in 1578 at the young age of 24. According to her obituary, Sister Bartolomea was afflicted by severe episodes of what we would now call epilepsy (*mal caduco*). The increasing frequency of these episodes "rendered her almost monstrous because of the unexpected, dangerous falls" she experienced, some of which injured her face. Despite this "great affliction" that reduced her to a "most dreadful state," Sister Bartolomea was determined to fulfill her convent duties, earning high praise from her colleagues. Part of the point in recording the severity of her condition was to emphasize the sheer grit with which she managed it.[12] Given the celebratory nature of these texts, scholars need to crosscheck their content against other types of evidence such as account books, tax petitions, and judicial proceedings in order to gauge their accuracy and contextualize possible exaggerations. This is not to say that these sources fabricated evidence outright, but simply acknowledges the particular perspectives that condition historical narratives of all kinds.

Finally, it is essential to understand exactly why convent chronicles and necrologies have been overlooked as sources for medical history. For the most part, scholars have categorized them as "religious" materials whose main value lies in writing the histories of monastic communities or female spirituality. As a result, the medical work performed in these institutions has been discounted as non-professional; moreover, nuns' medical skills have either been devalued or naturalized as "women's work." If we set aside our preconceptions about the religious content of these sources and focus instead on what nuns actually did to heal their colleagues, we find that convent chronicles and necrologies paint a valuable portrait of everyday healthcare practices and women's medical skills in Renaissance Italy. Other types of religious sources, such as saints' lives, miracle stories, canonization proceedings, visitation records, and spiritual autobiographies, can yield similar dividends when viewed through a medical lens.

Once we recognize that coding sources in a certain way can hamper historical inquiry, it becomes apparent that convent chronicles and necrologies actually offer several advantages over more conventional types of medical evidence. First, these multi-layered narratives are especially valuable for documenting women's health histories as both patients and practitioners. They place women at the speaking center, in contrast to the silencing effect induced by other early modern sources such as guild rolls and civic records. Both types of narrative recount stories nuns told about themselves, their lives, and their communities, in which their healing activities and personal experiences of illness loom large.[13] Using the forgotten voices captured in chronicles and necrologies enables us to write more robust and accurate histories of health and healing in the early modern world.

A second advantage is that these sources typically cover long, continuous time spans – often several centuries – which is rare for the early modern period. For example, the chronicle of Santa Caterina da Siena in the central Italian town of Pistoia treated the years from its establishment in 1494 to its suppression in 1784. Stretching even further in time was the history related in the Florentine chronicle of San Jacopo di Ripoli, which ran from the convent's foundation in 1282 to its transformation into an educational conservatory for girls in 1785.[14] This long trajectory not only allows historians to pinpoint crucial turning points like epidemics; it also has important methodological implications for how we write medical history. Tracing complex problems and themes over a long duration invites the use of multiple scales of analysis, from micro to macro. We can use convent narratives to probe micro-level issues like individual and familial responses to illness and medical decision-making, as well as larger questions regarding public health challenges, information networks, and medical provisioning in cities and countryside. Similarly, scholars can call on these sources when grappling with macro-level inquiries into broad systems of knowledge making, overarching disease regimes, and their cultural meanings. From a methodological standpoint, the availability of comparable information over many centuries – what historians have called the *longue durée* – encourages the use of both quantitative and qualitative methods, as discussed below.

We can better appreciate both the historical value and inevitable limitations of each source type by comparing the information they provide about a common topic, such as the practice of pharmacy in the convent. Pharmacy was a particularly inviting activity for early modern women, since making medicines was considered an essential part of their household duties. Preparing medicinal herbs, learning distillation techniques, and trying out new remedies paved the way for more extensive experimental practices among female householders and informal medical practitioners.[15] Making medicines also had important commercial dimensions for women across the social spectrum that are just beginning to be recognized.[16] Italian convent chronicles reveal that pharmaceutical work – growing and distilling medicinal herbs, compounding prescription medicines, preparing ready-made products – provided one of the chief sources of revenue for early modern religious communities. Such hands-on engagement should not be surprising, since Renaissance religious women were heirs to a long tradition in herbal medicine, having prepared and administered remedies to members of their own communities throughout the Middle Ages.

This therapeutic tradition took a new turn, however, when it became commercialized around 1500.[17] In response to swelling convent populations and shrinking revenues, scores of female religious houses across Italy established commercial pharmacies that generated much-needed income. By producing and selling remedies to the public, Renaissance nuns both augmented the medical resources available in Italian urban society and acquired roles of public significance beyond the spiritual realm. After 1600, convent pharmacies across the peninsula grew in both number and reputation. Many became renowned for making standard remedies as well as proprietary "secrets" and wellness products like soaps, tonics, and perfumes. In short, these apothecary shops retailed a product line comparable to guild pharmacists.[18] Until recently, these female-run businesses have been overlooked and undervalued by medical historians, in part because nuns' pharmaceutical work has been seen as a charitable activity, rather than as a skilled professional endeavor. The evidence of convent chronicles forces us to reconsider this narrow definition of what constitutes medical work in the early modern period.

The chronicle kept by the Florentine nuns of Le Murate – the city's largest convent, housing 200 women – offers a deeper look at these apothecary shops and the medical resources they provided to Italian urban society. In 1598, Sister Giustina Niccolini completed her history of the house from its origins as a female hermitage to her own day, using original archival records that have since been lost.[19] Niccolini maintained that the nuns had already begun to explore the commercial possibilities of pharmacy by the 1460s, when they built "the lower rooms of the pharmacy, [which were] fitted out for distillation and other necessary things, with the equipment and furnishings used in those endeavors." Over the next half-century, the Murate nuns extended their business by building on relationships with established suppliers and clients. In the 1520s, the enterprising abbess Bonifazia Risaliti wanted "to improve her convent in ways that would be useful and profitable," and so decided to make "some improvements in our pharmacy," especially in "the earthenware vessels used to confect [remedies] and other pertinent things used in that craft."[20] These alterations fueled the rapid growth of the business, including the development of new products – ointments, distillates, syrups, pills, and purgatives – that fully immersed the convent in contemporary market culture.

Using pharmacy as a lens through which to read the Murate chronicle sheds new light on the organization of workspaces, production processes, and technologies. Renaissance pharmacies typically featured two or three separate rooms: the dispensary for displaying and selling products, which were stored in beautiful maiolica jars like the ones shown in Figure 2.1; the actual production site or "kitchen" where medicinal herbs and flowers were distilled and medicines compounded; and sometimes an adjacent area for storing medicinals and ready-made products. The Murate pharmacy had to be rebuilt several times in the late sixteenth century due to flood damage resulting from its location in a low-lying area of the city. The chronicle

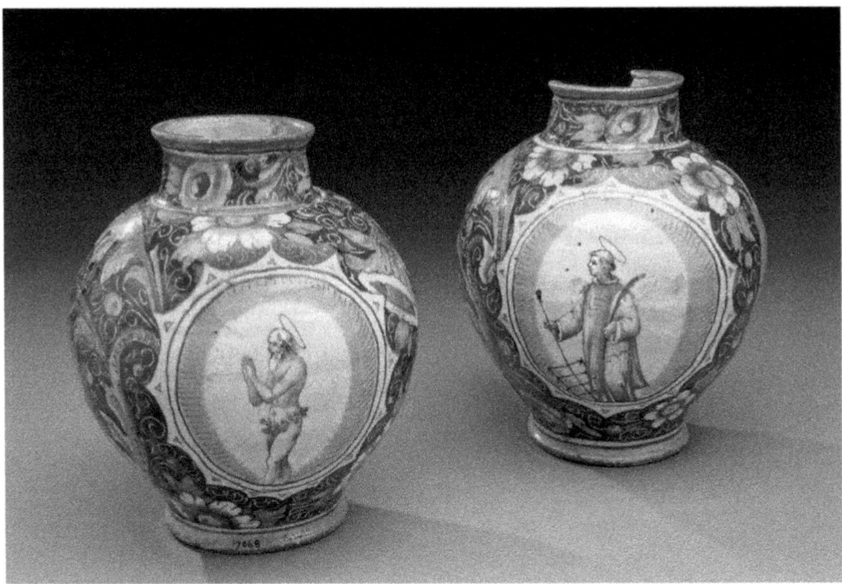

Figure 2.1 Pharmacy jars depicting the saints John the Baptist and Lawrence, Venice, 1501. Courtesy of the Science Museum, London.

tells us that the epic flood of the Arno River in 1557 destroyed the dispensary, infirmary, all of the medicinals, other storerooms, portions of the church, and much of the convent archive. To recover their business quickly, the nuns prioritized the construction of a spacious new storage room on an upper floor "to keep the medicinal items safe."[21]

In subsequent chapters, Niccolini noted that the Murate nuns capitalized on this disaster by investing heavily in specialized distillation equipment to satisfy consumer demand. Within the next decade, they installed a massive brick apparatus called a pyramid in the ground-floor stillroom. This innovative device probably resembled one of the furnaces popularized by the physician-botanist Pietro Andrea Mattioli in his printed works on distillation (Figure 2.2). Operational by 1581, this furnace allowed dozens of glass alembics or lead distilling bells to be placed over a single fire, thereby dramatically increasing the volume that could be obtained from a single process. The adoption of this commercial-grade apparatus in a female institutional setting underscores both the diffusion of innovative technologies and women's firsthand exposure to early scientific culture in Renaissance Italy. Niccolini goes on to recount other episodes in the pharmacy's evolution, especially after it was damaged yet again in 1589.[22]

This evidence detailing nuns' robust engagement in pharmacy work clearly disrupts conventional views about women's limited participation in both early modern market culture and the culture of experimentation. Despite providing this precious information, the Murate chronicle does not indicate how nuns actually produced and transferred the skills and knowledge necessary to run a commercial enterprise,

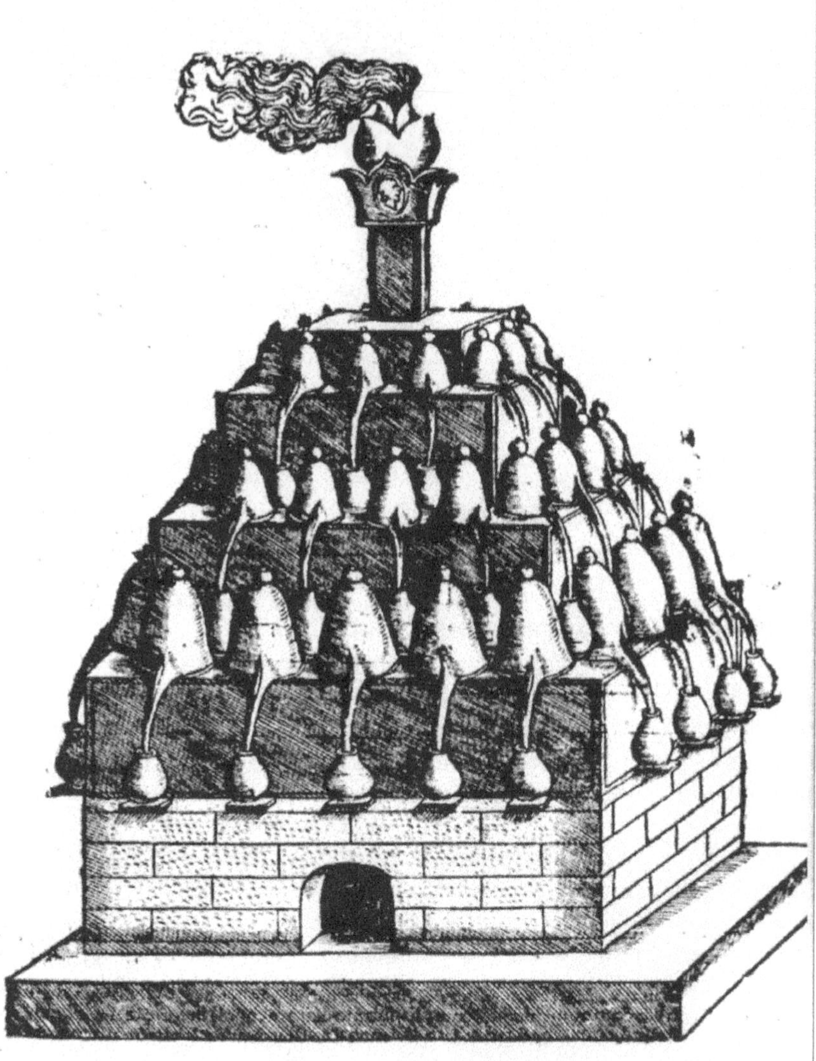

Figure 2.2 Pyramid furnace for distillation. Pietro Andrea Mattioli, *Del modo di distillare le acque da tutte le piante*. Venice, 1604. Courtesy of the Department of Special Collections, Memorial Library, University of Wisconsin-Madison.

since Niccolini's goal was to show how the workshop fit into the overall arc of convent history. To understand these knowledge transfers, we must turn to the more granular life stories presented in convent necrologies. Using chronicles and necrologies in tandem to fill in gaps and silences allows scholars to construct a more complete picture of women's medical work while analyzing forms of early modern knowledge production.

Here, a close reading of one necrology entry that pays careful attention to content, tone, and rhetorical strategies speaks volumes about the circulation of pharmaceutical knowledge in religious communities. The remembrance penned for Sister Giovanna Ginori (d. 1579), the head apothecary at the Florentine house of Santa Caterina da Siena, reveals that apprenticing with a more advanced practitioner played a key role in sustaining the healing arts in Italian convents. This traditional mode of craft training helped learners develop embodied knowledge about materials and processes. According to her obituary, Ginori apprenticed in the pharmacy for six years; after this probation period, she reportedly "became so expert at the job that the other nuns decided amongst themselves not to confer any other convent office upon her." Highlighting Ginori's exclusive focus on this role, her obituary articulates Renaissance notions of expertise, in which deep hands-on experience enhanced a practitioner's legitimacy. The next sentence stating that Ginori ran the pharmacy for 37 years added even greater luster to her reputation, since it verified her continued competence as a top-tier pharmacist. The obituary also stressed that, over this long period, she became "extremely knowledgeable about medicinals and botanicals," despite the fact that she had acquired skills and knowledge empirically. Emphasizing her widespread reputation as an expert practitioner, the remembrance claimed that "anyone wishing to take advantage of good medicinal products" sought her advice. The accompanying detail noting that she freely dispensed medical advice at the pharmacy counter highlighted her compassion as well as her expertise. The narrative closed by remarking that Ginori had trained two "excellent apprentices" who mastered her "way of working with great understanding," thereby creating an ongoing legacy for her and the community.[23] By subjecting this short narrative to a close reading, we gain fresh insights not only into early modern healthcare practices but also into the ways that unlicensed female healers achieved social recognition.

While many of the health-related topics addressed in convent narratives lend themselves to this kind of close reading, they also are amenable to other methodological approaches, including quantitative analysis. Using the data points embedded in narratives makes it possible to move from micro-level evidence to macro-level findings and conclusions. For instance, scholars have pooled the demographic information included in nuns' obituaries, such as age and time in the convent, to establish comparative life expectancies, patterns of morbidity, and cause of death for a significant subset of the Italian female population. The breadth of convent information is especially valuable given the relative paucity and fragmented nature of other Italian civic records such as birth and death notices. Demographic analyses based on convent narratives reveal that Italian nuns lived astonishingly long lives that far exceeded the lifespan of wives and mothers of all classes, even when adjusting for death in childbirth.[24]

Taking an aggregate approach to the same sources also sheds new light on the history of infectious diseases. Bubonic plague presented the greatest disease threat to Europeans from its initial catastrophic appearance in 1347 to the early 1700s, when this scourge finally subsided. The first waves of plague in the fourteenth and fifteenth centuries hit convent populations hard, but most communities across the peninsula recovered and even exceeded previous population levels by the 1480s.[25] Physical reclusion provided a protective buffer for nuns by limiting their contact with outsiders, although communities like Le Murate also adopted preventive measures to limit exposure, such as dipping coins in vinegar to disinfect them.[26]

By culling data about cause of death from these sources, we learn that tuberculosis rather than plague figured as the most prominent disease threat in female religious houses after 1500. Skyrocketing convent populations led to serious overcrowding, providing ideal conditions for the spread of respiratory ailments like pulmonary tuberculosis. Dramatic symptoms made this ancient disease easy to spot. Obituaries from the Venetian convent of Corpus Domini, for example, noted that suffering nuns "became consumptive and often threw up globs of blood;" other nuns endured a "wasting fever and consumption" that left them "extremely thin."[27] Tuberculosis featured as the leading cause of death at San Vincenzo in Prato, according to the house chronicle, while 62 out of over 200 nuns living at Santa Caterina da Siena contracted the disease during their lifetimes.[28] The Florentine necrology of San Jacopo di Ripoli indicates that tuberculosis, influenza, and other respiratory ailments accounted for at least 40 percent of the 152 deaths whose symptoms are recorded.[29] Read through a quantitative lens, these narratives demonstrate that, while enclosure may have protected religious women from the ravages of plague, it did not spare them from deadly respiratory infections. To reduce the burden of illness, convent officers tried to create healthier living environments when possible by enlarging the windows of nuns' rooms and attending to other aspects of ambient air.[30]

In addition, maladies of a chronic or recurrent nature appear with some frequency in both chronicles and necrologies, although it is more difficult to quantify them precisely. Since these afflictions left a smaller footprint in the historical record than infectious diseases, information about these conditions, especially if it includes detailed empirical observations, is critical for reconstructing the range of early modern illness experiences. Accounts of malarial fevers, sciatica, skin ailments, cataracts, kidney stones, and blinding headaches abound in convent sources. Because many nuns lived to an advanced age, they suffered from chronic ailments like cancer or had debilitating strokes that left them paralyzed or unable to speak. A considerable number experienced dementia that prevented them from confessing and taking the sacraments.[31] Set in the therapeutic space of the convent infirmary, these accounts present illness as an opportunity for sustained reflection about religious values and the brevity of life.

Interwoven with this spiritualization of illness, however, are vital clues about illness management. Convent narratives communicate crucial evidence about the course of specific diseases and the hierarchy of resort on which nuns relied; they also lay out the basic timeline for diagnosis and treatment as well as therapeutic protocols that frequently blended naturalistic and spiritual healing. For example, Sister Caterina da Fiesole, a serving nun living in the same convent as the pharmacist Giovanna Ginori discussed earlier, suffered from many illnesses but was particularly aggrieved by an inflammation of the kidneys that forced her to sleep upright in bed. After the inflammation manifested outwardly as swellings on the skin, the nuns called in two physicians who recommended surgery, which was performed on 13 May 1582. Although the surgery went well, her condition worsened; "day by day the [surgical] wound took on a terrible ugly color" accompanied by "the sharpest pain." Sustained by constant prayer and her colleagues' ministrations, Sister Caterina died ten days after surgery at the age of 39.[32] Hundreds of other examples, all presented in a similar format, greatly expand our evidentiary base by supplementing the limited, sometimes idiosyncratic observations noted in physicians' casebooks.

In evaluating this information, historians of health and medicine must take into account key differences between early modern disease categories and modern biomedical ones. Diseases are not merely biological entities but are also social and cultural constructions whose meanings must be firmly situated in their historical context. Indeed, scholars have recognized the pressing need to problematize retrospective diagnosis in order to write authentic, contextualized medical histories.[33] Attempts to grapple with this issue include adopting contemporary names for past diseases, such as "the pox" or the "French Disease" rather than the modern designation of syphilis.[34] Although discussions of this issue have centered largely on perceptible disease and disability, these considerations apply equally or even especially well to the unseen mental disorders recorded in convent chronicles and necrologies. In fact, nowhere is the issue of retrospective diagnosis more vexed than in the case of mental illness. Behaviors that were commonplace in female religious communities of the day – visions, ecstasies, fasts, hearing voices – would have been interpreted in dramatically different ways in other times and places. These spiritual gifts were signs of sanctity in Renaissance Christianity, not madness. We risk distorting the historical record and failing to appreciate past lives if we evaluate culturally specific behaviors by modern-day criteria rather than by historical ones. Complicating the picture is the fact that early modern monasteries and convents provided one of the few options for the care of mentally disordered persons beyond the family, especially before the foundation of specialized hospitals in the late seventeenth century.[35]

Convent narratives recorded numerous instances of madness and melancholy – the two basic categories into which early modern people divided mental disorders.[36] Of the two, melancholic states appear with much greater frequency, particularly in necrologies. Although Renaissance Europeans believed that cases of melancholy were on the rise, it is not entirely clear what they meant when they described others as melancholic, owing to the conceptual plasticity of the term and the varied social uses to which it could be put. By the sixteenth century, melancholy simultaneously denoted a humoral temperament, a physical illness, and a dangerous spiritual condition arising from a diseased or disordered imagination. According to the eminent physician Girolamo Mercuriale (1530–1606), melancholy was more prevalent among men but more acute among women. It struck religious women with particular force because they spent "the greater part of their life in quiet and meditation," which produced noxious vapors that rose to the brain and corrupted it.[37] Although learned medical opinion held that melancholy primarily affected the elderly, convent sources indicate that these disorders struck nuns at all stages of life, regardless of social class or monastic lifestyle. Melancholy imposed heavy burdens of illness on religious communities by interfering with the harmonious functioning of communal life and by distracting nuns from prayer and normal work duties. More severe forms of mental illness demanded constant oversight to prevent afflicted nuns from harming themselves or others.[38]

Convent narratives offer some of the most intimate portraits of melancholic states available for the early modern period. Some of the extended sketches recorded in necrologies are reminiscent of modern microhistories in their attempt to capture the essentials of plot, character, and context in a few brief strokes; these vignettes require a keen eye along with a particular approach to reading in order to discern their medical details. To take one example: the Florentine nuns of San Jacopo di Ripoli attributed the frequent melancholy of Sister Raffaella del Maestro (d. 1572) to the fact that she suffered from epilepsy and severe dropsy for 50 of her 70 years.[39] Sketching her life story after her death, her co-religionists explained her despondence as an understandable reaction to chronic pain and physical limitations. These fragments allow us to access forgotten voices from the past as people confronted the realities of an unseen illness; they also provide a point of entry into thinking about the everyday remedial options for mental disorders available to early modern people.

Here, the evocative postmortem portrait of Sister Maria Benigna del Corso (d. 1583) painted by her peers at Santa Caterina da Siena in Florence reveals some of the strategies Renaissance people used to manage mental illness. The nuns noted that, after the young woman contracted a fever that left her bedridden, "she began to suffer from melancholic humors to such a degree that the other nuns decided not to burden her with any convent office for her own peace of mind." Despite its good intentions, this strategy backfired. Instead of relieving her condition, "this deprivation greatly worsened her illness because it distressed her terribly not to be involved in convent business and [to do] chores, since she would have worked willingly." Convent officers subsequently tasked her with assisting the doorkeeper with her duties, but her melancholy only deepened in this role. Soon Sister Maria Benigna experienced a full-blown psychological crisis "because she was extremely timid and was concerned about appearing to discharge her office well." Adopting a psychosocial explanation, her peers believed that the crux of the problem was excessive concern for reputation: "by thinking too much about herself and every one of her actions, she nourished her illness in this way." The community found a workable solution by directing her to stay in the choir as long as she wished and to sweep the convent whenever she felt her dark moods gather. This plan hinged on the notion that Sister Maria Benigna could regulate her own moods; most likely, other nuns monitored her behavior.[40] This episode provides keen insight into the ways in which early modern people constructed an explanatory framework for mental disorders and tried to address them in behavioral terms based on trial and error.

In conclusion, convent chronicles and necrologies offer unexpectedly rich sources for writing the history of health and healing in the early modern period. These multi-layered narratives encompass a wealth of health-related topics that run the gamut from gendered pharmacy practices to the experience and treatment of infectious diseases and everyday ailments. This diversity lends itself to a variety of historical approaches ranging from close reading to quantification that can be used singly or in combination. In fact, the sheer number and type of topics that can be addressed using chronicles and necrologies encourage what one scholar has called a "methodological fuzziness" that productively borrows from many different historical approaches.[41] As indicated above, these methods run the gamut from analyzing the nuances of language and using gender as a primary lens to constructing economic or demographic trend lines.

Convent chronicles and necrologies not only expand the evidentiary source base for writing the history of early modern medicine, but they also challenge longstanding preconceptions about the knowledge and training of medical practitioners who acquired their practical skills outside university lecture halls or guild workshops. By placing women at the speaking center, these sources disrupt conventional definitions and interpretations of women's medical work while giving voice to their subjective experiences as sufferers. Covering long time spans, convent chronicles and necrologies invite the creative use of multiple scales of analysis that span the spectrum from individual life stories to dominant disease regimes. Whether using the valuable evidence of convent narratives to evaluate infectious diseases or mental disorders, scholars must take the problematic nature of retrospective diagnosis into account in order to capture culturally contingent meanings of health and healing. In sum, these sources open a valuable window onto the lived experience of people in the past while presenting an impressive sweep of research possibilities for students and scholars alike.

Notes

1 Jutta Gisela Sperling, *Convents and the Body Politic in Late Renaissance Venice* (Chicago, IL: University of Chicago Press, 1999), 18; Sharon T. Strocchia, *Nuns and Nunneries in Renaissance Florence* (Baltimore, MD: Johns Hopkins University Press, 2009), 2.

2 Elissa B. Weaver, *Convent Theatre in Early Modern Italy: Spiritual Fun and Learning for Women* (Cambridge: Cambridge University Press, 2002), 9–48.

3 K.J.P. Lowe, *Nuns' Chronicles and Convent Culture in Renaissance and Counter-Reformation Italy* (Cambridge: Cambridge University Press, 2003), 5–60, provides an excellent introduction to this source type. Anne Winston-Allen provides a comparative geographical perspective in *Convent Chronicles: Women Writing about Women and Reform in the Late Middle Ages* (University Park: Pennsylvania State University Press, 2004).

4 Monica H. Green coined this term in "Bodies, Gender, Health, Disease: Recent Work on Medieval Women's Medicine," *Studies in Medieval and Renaissance History*, ser. 3, 5 (2005): 1–46.

5 Lowe, *Nuns' Chronicles*, 6. One highly informative example of this genre has been published as *Memoriale di Monteluce: Cronaca del monastero delle Clarisse di Perugia dal 1448 al 1838*, ed. and intro. Ugolino Niccolini (Perugia: Edizioni Porziuncola, 1983).

6 See, for instance, Biblioteca Riccardiana, Florence. Mss. Moreni. 317, a calendar begun in 1336 by the Florentine convent of San Niccolò Maggiore and continued sporadically in a similar vein until 1591.

7 Olivia Weisser, "Histories of the Pox," *History Compass* 2021, doi: 10.1111/hic3.12681 (accessed July 7, 2021). On history from below, see Roy Porter, "The Patient's View: Doing Medical History from Below," *Theory and Society* 14 (1985): 175–98.

8 See, for example, Sister Bartolomea Riccoboni, *Life and Death in a Venetian Convent: The Chronicle and Necrology of Corpus Domini, 1395–1436*, trans. Daniel E. Bornstein (Chicago, IL: University of Chicago Press, 2000). The Florentine convent of San Jacopo di Ripoli also kept a combined memory book, which included lists of convent officers. The latter is conserved at the Archivio di Stato, Florence (hereafter abbreviated as ASF). San Jacopo di Ripoli. Vol. 23.

9 Gertrude Jaron Lewis has studied nine fourteenth-century German "sister-books," whose contents are comparable to Italian convent necrologies, in *By Women, for Women, about Women: The Sister-Books of Fourteenth-Century Germany* (Toronto: Pontifical Institute of Mediaeval Studies, 1996). Some Italian male religious houses also kept necrologies in Latin rather than the vernacular; Stefano Orlandi, *Necrologio di S. Maria Novella, 1235–1504*, 2 vols. (Florence: L.S. Olschki, 1955).

10 Asunción Lavrin, *Brides of Christ: Conventual Life in Colonial Mexico* (Stanford, CA: Stanford University Press, 2008); James M. Córdova, "Images beyond the Veil: Funeral Portraits and Sacred Materialities in New Spain's Nunneries," *Res: Anthropology and Aesthetics* 67–68 (2016/2017): 256–72. See also *Journey of Five Capuchin Nuns*, ed. and trans. Sarah E. Owens (Toronto: University of Toronto Press, 2009), which recounts the early eighteenth-century foundation of a Capuchin convent in Lima by Spanish nuns.

11 Sister Giustina Niccolini, *The Chronicle of Le Murate*, ed. and trans. Saundra Weddle (Toronto: Centre for Reformation and Renaissance Studies, 2011).

12 Biblioteca Nazionale Centrale, Firenze (hereafter cited as BNCF). Ms. Landau Finaly. 72, fols. 218v–220v.

13 Sara Ritchey, *Acts of Care: Recovering Women in Late Medieval Health* (Ithaca, NY: Cornell University Press, 2021), argues for the importance of narratives in reconstructing the therapeutic body knowledge and caregiving expertise of religious women in the late medieval Low Countries.

14 Elettra Giaconi, *Il monastero domenicano di S. Caterina da Siena a Pistoia dalla fondazione alla soppressione (1477–1783). Cronaca e documenti* (Florence: Nerbini, 2005–2006); Judith C. Brown, "Everyday Life, Longevity, and Nuns in Early Modern Florence," in *Renaissance Culture and the Everyday*, ed. Patricia Fumerton and Simon Hunt (Philadelphia: University of Pennsylvania Press, 1999), 115–38.

15 Alisha Rankin, *Panaceia's Daughters: Noblewomen as Healers in Early Modern Germany* (Chicago, IL: University of Chicago Press, 2013); Elaine Leong, "Making Medicines in the Early Modern Household," *Bulletin of the History of Medicine* 82 (2008): 145–68.

16 Tessa Storey, "Face Waters, Oils, Love Magic and Poison: Making and Selling Secrets in Early Modern Rome," in *Secrets and Knowledge in Medicine and Science, 1500–1800*, ed. Elaine Leong and Alisha Rankin (Burlington, VT: Ashgate, 2011), 143–63.

17 Sharon T. Strocchia, *Forgotten Healers: Women and the Pursuit of Health in Late Renaissance Italy* (Cambridge, MA: Harvard University Press, 2019), 89–102.

18 Gianna Pomata, "Medicina delle monache. Pratiche terapeutiche nei monasteri femminili di Bologna in età moderna," in *I monasteri femminili come centri di cultura fra Rinascimento e Barocco*, ed. Gianna Pomata and Gabriella Zarri (Rome: Edizioni di storia e letteratura, 2005), 331–63; Strocchia, *Forgotten Healers*, 102–09. "Secrets" were proprietary remedies that had been developed empirically, often through trial and error. For products retailed by guild pharmacists, see James Shaw and Evelyn Welch, *Making and Marketing Medicines in Renaissance Florence* (Amsterdam: Rodopi, 2011).

19 Niccolini, *Chronicle of Le Murate*, 1–29. The original manuscript is conserved as BNCF. II. II. 509.

20 BNCF. II. II. 509, fols. 88r, 98v–99v; *Chronicle of Le Murate*, 88–89, 179, 195; Strocchia, *Forgotten Healers*, 95–96.

21 BNCF. II. II. 509, fols. 139v–140r; *Chronicle of Le Murate*, 197–99, 264–65; Strocchia, *Forgotten Healers*, 153–54.
22 BNCF. II. II. 509, fols. 141r–142r; *Chronicle of Le Murate*, 267–68; Strocchia, *Forgotten Healers*, 155–57.
23 BNCF. Ms. Landau Finaly. 72, fol. 91r/v. See also Strocchia, *Forgotten Healers*, 132–49.
24 Brown, "Everyday Life, Longevity, and Nuns," 116.
25 Strocchia, *Nuns and Nunneries*, 6–10.
26 Strocchia, *Forgotten Healers*, 79.
27 *Life and Death in a Venetian Convent*, 71, 96–97, 99–100. Pawel Dobrowolski, "Piety and Death in Venice: A Reading of the Fifteenth-Century Chronicle and the Necrology of Corpus Domini," *Bulletino dell'Istituto storico italiano per il Medioevo* 92 (1985–1986): 295–324. Fredrika Jacobs discusses remedial options for tuberculosis sufferers in "Infirmity in Votive Culture: A Case Study from the Sanctuary of the Madonna dell'Arco, Naples," in *Representing Infirmity: Diseased Bodies in Renaissance Italy*, ed. John Henderson, Fredrika Jacobs, and Jonathan K. Nelson (London and New York: Routledge, 2021), 191–212.
28 Caterina de' Ricci, *S. Caterina de' Ricci: Cronache, diplomatica, lettere varie*, ed. Guglielmo Di Agresti (Florence: L.S. Olschki, 1969), lxxxvi–lxxxvii; Giaconi, *Il monastero domenicano di S. Caterina da Siena*, 89.
29 Brown, "Everyday Life, Longevity and Nuns," 127.
30 Strocchia, *Forgotten Healers*, 102.
31 Sharon T. Strocchia, "Savonarolan Witnesses: The Nuns of San Jacopo and the Piagnone Movement in Sixteenth-Century Florence," *Sixteenth Century Journal* 38.2 (2007): 393–418; Judith C. Brown, "Monache a Firenze all'inizio dell'età moderna. Un'analisi demografica," *Quaderni storici* 85 (1994): 117–52.
32 BNCF. Ms. Landau Finaly. 72, fols. 237r–238v.
33 Jon Arrizabalaga, "Problematizing Retrospective Diagnosis in the History of Disease," *Asclepio* 54 (2002): 51–70. See also the considered remarks by Jonathan K. Nelson, "Cancer in Michelangelo's *Night.* An Analytical Framework for Retrospective Diagnoses," in *Representing Infirmity*, 3–27.
34 Jon Arrizabalaga, John Henderson, and Roger French, *The Great Pox: The French Disease in Renaissance Europe* (New Haven, CT: Yale University Press, 1997), 1–19.
35 Elizabeth W. Mellyn, *Mad Tuscans and Their Families: A History of Mental Disorder in Early Modern Italy* (Philadelphia: University of Pennsylvania Press, 2014).
36 Two foundational works are Angus Gowland, "The Problem of Early Modern Melancholy," *Past & Present*, 191 (2006): 77–120, and H.C. Erik Midelfort, *A History of Madness in Sixteenth-Century Germany* (Stanford, CA: Stanford University Press, 1999).
37 Girolamo Mercuriale, *Il medico e la follia: cinquanta casi di malattia mentale nella letteratura medica italiana del Seicento*, ed. Alessandro Dini (Florence: Le Lettere, 1997), 46.
38 Sharon T. Strocchia, "The Melancholic Nun in Late Renaissance Italy," in *Diseases of the Imagination and Imaginary Disease in the Early Modern Period*, ed. Yasmin Haskell (Turnhout: Brepols, 2011), 139–58.
39 ASF. San Jacopo di Ripoli, Vol. 23, fol. 129v.
40 BNCF. Ms. Landau Finlay, Vol. 72, fols. 240v–241r.
41 Sarah Maza, *Thinking about History* (Chicago, IL: University of Chicago Press, 2017).

Bibliography

Arrizabalaga, Jon. "Problematizing Retrospective Diagnosis in the History of Disease." *Asclepio* 54 (2002): 51–70.

Arrizabalaga, Jon, John Henderson, and Roger French. *The Great Pox: The French Disease in Renaissance Europe.* New Haven, CT and London: Yale University Press, 1997.

Brown, Judith C. "Everyday Life, Longevity, and Nuns in Early Modern Florence." In *Renaissance Culture and the Everyday*, edited by Patricia Fumerton and Simon Hunt, 115–38. Philadelphia: University of Pennsylvania Press, 1999.

Brown, Judith C. "Monache a Firenze all'inizio dell'età moderna. Un'analisi demografica." *Quaderni storici* 85 (1994): 117–52.

Córdova, James M. "Images beyond the Veil: Funeral Portraits and Sacred Materialities in New Spain's Nunneries." *Res: Anthropology and Aesthetics* 67–68 (2016/2017): 256–72.

Dobrowolski, Pawel. "Piety and Death in Venice: A Reading of the Fifteenth-Century Chronicle and the Necrology of Corpus Domini." *Bulletino dell'Istituto storico italiano per il Medioevo* 92 (1985–1986): 295–324.

Giaconi, Elettra. *Il monastero domenicano di S. Caterina da Siena a Pistoia dalla fondazione alla soppressione (1477–1783). Cronaca e documenti.* Florence: Nerbini, 2005–2006.

Gowland, Angus. "The Problem of Early Modern Melancholy." *Past & Present* 191 (2006): 77–120.

Green, Monica H. "Bodies, Gender, Health, Disease: Recent Work on Medieval Women's Medicine." *Studies in Medieval and Renaissance History*, ser. 3, 5 (2005): 1–46.

Jacobs, Fredrika. "Infirmity in Votive Culture: A Case Study from the Sanctuary of the Madonna dell'Arco, Naples." In *Representing Infirmity: Diseased Bodies in Renaissance Italy*, edited by John Henderson, Fredrika Jacobs, and Jonathan K. Nelson, 191–212. London and New York: Routledge, 2021.

Journey of Five Capuchin Nuns, edited and translated by Sarah E. Owens. Toronto: University of Toronto Press, 2009.

Lavrin, Asunción. *Brides of Christ: Conventual Life in Colonial Mexico.* Stanford, CA: Stanford University Press, 2008.

Leong, Elaine. "Making Medicines in the Early Modern Household." *Bulletin of the History of Medicine* 82 (2008): 145–68.

Lewis, Gertrude Jaron. *By Women, for Women, about Women: The Sister-Books of Fourteenth-Century Germany.* Toronto: Pontifical Institute of Mediaeval Studies, 1996.

Lowe, K.J.P. *Nuns' Chronicles and Convent Culture in Renaissance and Counter-Reformation Italy.* Cambridge: Cambridge University Press, 2003.

Maza, Sarah. *Thinking about History.* Chicago, IL: University of Chicago Press, 2017.

Mellyn, Elizabeth W. *Mad Tuscans and Their Families: A History of Mental Disorder in Early Modern Italy.* Philadelphia: University of Pennsylvania Press, 2014.

Memoriale di Monteluce: Cronaca del monastero delle Clarisse di Perugia dal 1448 al 1838, edited and introduction by Ugolino Niccolini. Perugia: Edizioni Porziuncola, 1983.

Mercuriale, Girolamo. *Il medico e la follia: cinquanta casi di malattia mentale nella letteratura medica italiana del Seicento*, edited by Alessandro Dini. Florence: Le Lettere, 1997.

Midelfort, H.C. Erik. *A History of Madness in Sixteenth-Century Germany.* Stanford, CA: Stanford University Press, 1999.

Nelson, Jonathan K. "Cancer in Michelangelo's *Night.* An Analytical Framework for Retrospective Diagnoses." In *Representing Infirmity: Diseased Bodies in Renaissance Italy*, edited by John Henderson, Fredrika Jacobs, and Jonathan K. Nelson, 3–27. London: Routledge, 2021.

Niccolini, Sister Giustina. *The Chronicle of Le Murate*, edited and translated by Saundra Weddle. Toronto: Centre for Reformation and Renaissance Studies, 2011.

Orlandi, Stefano. *Necrologio di S. Maria Novella, 1235–1504*, 2 vols. Florence: L.S. Olschki, 1955.

Pomata, Gianna. "Medicina delle monache. Pratiche terapeutiche nei monasteri femminili di Bologna in età moderna." In *I monasteri femminili come centri di cultura fra Rinascimento e Barocco*, edited by Gianna Pomata and Gabriella Zarri, 331–63. Rome: Edizioni di storia e letteratura, 2005.

Porter, Roy. "The Patient's View: Doing Medical History from Below." *Theory and Society* 14 (1985): 175–98.

Rankin, Alisha. *Panaceia's Daughters: Noblewomen as Healers in Early Modern Germany.* Chicago, IL: University of Chicago Press, 2013.

Ricci, Caterina de'. *S. Caterina de' Ricci: Cronache, diplomatica, lettere varie*, edited by Guglielmo Di Agresti. Florence: L.S. Olschki, 1969.

Riccoboni, Sister Bartolomea. *Life and Death in a Venetian Convent: The Chronicle and Necrology of Corpus Domini, 1395–1436*, translated by Daniel E. Bornstein. Chicago, IL: University of Chicago Press, 2000.

Ritchey, Sara. *Acts of Care: Recovering Women in Late Medieval Health.* Ithaca, NY and London: Cornell University Press, 2021.

Secrets and Knowledge in Medicine and Science, 1500–1800, edited by Elaine Leong and Alisha Rankin. Burlington, VT: Ashgate, 2011.

Shaw, James and Evelyn Welch. *Making and Marketing Medicines in Renaissance Florence.* Amsterdam: Rodopi, 2011.

Sperling, Jutta Gisela. *Convents and the Body Politic in Late Renaissance Venice.* Chicago, IL: University of Chicago Press, 1999.

Storey, Tessa. "Face Waters, Oils, Love Magic and Poison: Making and Selling Secrets in Early Modern Rome." In *Secrets and Knowledge in Medicine and Science, 1500–1800*, edited by Elaine Leong and Alisha Rankin, 143–63. Burlington, VT: Ashgate, 2011.

Strocchia, Sharon T. *Forgotten Healers: Women and the Pursuit of Health in Late Renaissance Italy.* Cambridge, MA: Harvard University Press, 2019.

Strocchia, Sharon T. "The Melancholic Nun in Late Renaissance Italy." In *Diseases of the Imagination and Imaginary Disease in the Early Modern Period*, edited by Yasmin Haskell, 139–58. Turnhout: Brepols, 2011.

Strocchia, Sharon T. *Nuns and Nunneries in Renaissance Florence.* Baltimore, MD: Johns Hopkins University Press, 2009.

Strocchia, Sharon T. "Savonarolan Witnesses: The Nuns of San Jacopo and the Piagnone Movement in Sixteenth-Century Florence." *Sixteenth Century Journal* 38.2 (2007): 393–418.

Weaver, Elissa B. *Convent Theatre in Early Modern Italy: Spiritual Fun and Learning for Women.* Cambridge: Cambridge University Press, 2002.

Weisser, Olivia. "Histories of the Pox." *History Compass* 2021, doi: 10.1111/hic3.12681 (accessed July 7, 2021).

Winston-Allen, Anne. *Convent Chronicles: Women Writing about Women and Reform in the Late Middle Ages.* University Park: Pennsylvania State University Press, 2004.

3 The Curious Case of the Two Antonios

What Hospital Records Can and Cannot Tell Us

Elizabeth W. Mellyn

Florence. December, 1756. Tuscany's criminal justice minister, Domenico Colombi, sends a letter to Niccolò Martelli, the superintendent of Florence's mental hospital, Santa Dorotea. Colombi requests that two men be admitted. The first is a well-to-do Florentine named Antonio Corsini. According to his relative Giuseppe Nardi, Antonio "has succumbed to madness." Nardi asks that Colombi instruct Santa Dorotea to admit Antonio with the assurance that he would personally cover the cost of Antonio's care. Colombi complies. He orders Santa Dorotea to welcome the "raving mad" Antonio Corsini "to be cured of his disease and maintained" in hospital at Nardi's expense.[1] Antonio Corsini is sent to Santa Dorotea (Figure 3.1).

In the same letter, Colombi mentions "a Florentine named Caterina dell'Ara, wife of Antonio Bianconi." Her husband, she claims, is also insane. Like Nardi, she asks that *her* Antonio "have a place" in Santa Dorotea, too. Through Colombi, the government grants this request as well, ordering Martelli to admit the "demented" Antonio Bianconi. Because the couple is poor, *this* Antonio is admitted at public rather than private expense in accord with state law.[2]

Here begins a three-year saga centered on two allegedly insane men, separated by wealth and status, and brought together under the same roof by alleged insanity in Tuscany's first hospital devoted solely to the care of the severely mentally ill. Both men were evaluated by the hospital's physicians upon entry, during their stays, and upon discharge. Both men were released only to be admitted a second time. Two years after his initial admission, Antonio Corsini's estate administrator wrote to Santa Dorotea claiming that his charge "had fallen again into his usual fixations."[3] The hospital would accept Corsini, but with the provision that he could be released into his administrator's custody to "take the air."[4] "Through this experiment," Colombi reported, they would learn "if the recovery of this *maniac* could be made stable."[5] A letter written a year later suggests the experiment worked. One of Santa Dorotea's physicians claimed that Corsini's transfer "to enjoy country air… freed him from false ideas and from the melancholic fixations that oppressed him."[6] From that point, Antonio Corsini disappears from Santa Dorotea's records.

Likewise, two years after Caterina dell'Ara requested to have her husband committed, she claimed that Antonio Bianconi had "fallen again into his earlier frenzies." Like Corsini, Bianconi entered Santa Dorotea a second time, but into the hands of a different fate.

DOI: 10.4324/9781003094876-5

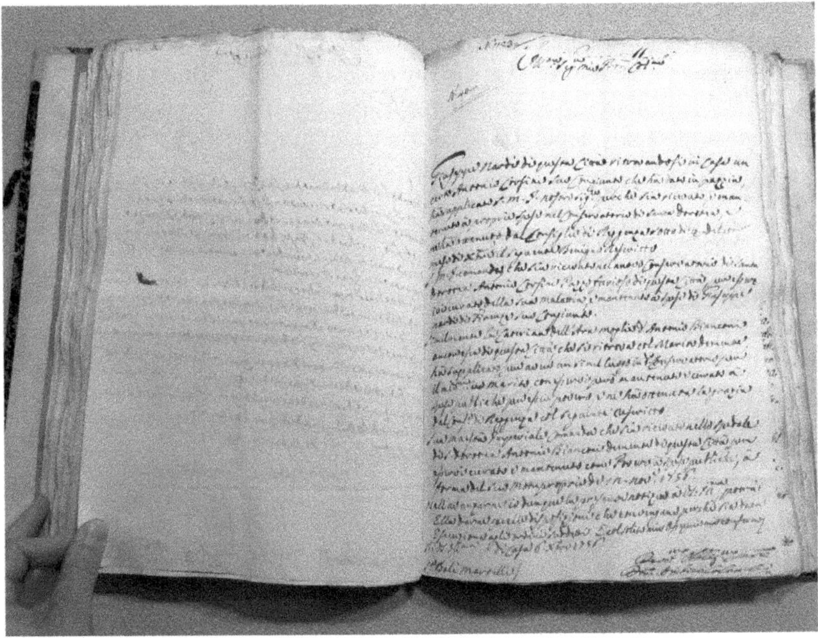

Figure 3.1 Letter from Domenico Brichieri Colombi to Niccolò Martelli. ASF, Santa Dorotea, 2, Motupropri, Rescritti, ed altri Documenti appartenti allo Spedale di Santa Dorotea, no. 40.

Where the wealthy Corsini exited the hospital on his feet into the custody of his estate administrator and the pleasures of the Tuscan countryside, the poor Bianconi exited in a coffin, headed for burial in a common parish grave.

***

When I first read the entangled stories of the two Antonios – one rich, the other poor, both allegedly insane – I felt excitement. It seemed like I had some rare and tangible glimpse into the lives of these two troubled men even though details about them were scant.

I wondered: who were they? How and with whom did they measure out their days? What course of events induced their families to have them admitted to a mental hospital? How did the hospital's physicians decide that they warranted treatment there? And once in the hospital, what was their daily care and who delivered it? Could they move around? Were they somehow restrained? Who fed them? Who bathed them or changed their linens? Why did one of the Antonios die? And why was Colombi, the state's justice minister, directly involved in the administration of a mental hospital? By what right did he compel the hospital's superintendent to admit or discharge patients? And by what obligation did the superintendent comply?

From these relatively brief letters, a more complex and intriguing narrative about mental health and the beginnings of institutional mental healthcare in early modern Europe began to take shape in my mind as I read ten, then a hundred, and finally over 4000 admission and discharge letters. But I could not stop there. These letters represented only about a fifth of Santa Dorotea's total written record.[7] The hospital's 146-year lifespan lives on in 65 bulky registers, containing tens of thousands of pages.

When I realized just how many documents there were to wade through, I felt a mounting sense of despair. Surely it would take multiple lifetimes to analyze such a massive trove. If I really wanted to write a history of Tuscany's first mental hospital, I would have to find some way of using this material systematically and efficiently. In this essay, I use the sources that relate the tale of the two Antonios to illustrate three approaches I developed to make writing Santa Dorotea's history with that mammoth collection of documents possible.

The first approach is twofold. I separated the records by type – founding documents, hospital statutes, governing board minutes, patient intake and discharge books, admission and discharge letters, financial records, and hospital-related government decrees – and then read for patterns within each category. By this method, I observed that the case of the two Antonios shared important characteristics with other patient letters. Like other patients, the two Antonios had different constellations of family and friends around them, managing or failing to manage their care. Each of these letters brought together a diverse cast of characters around the alleged illness of a single person. In them, I caught fleeting glimpses of household struggles to provide care for insane relatives, the challenges administrators faced in running a hospital, encounters between doctors and patients, the construction of disease categories and treatment strategies, and the use of institutional health care by government authorities as an instrument of public order.

It quickly became clear that many families shared similar struggles – the inability to provide round-the-clock care for a relative who threatened violence against self or others; fear that a relative might squander patrimony or might bring shame on a household. Certain diagnoses appeared again and again – mania and melancholy, terms that generally captured aggressive and depressive states respectively, were by far the most common. But there were also cases of erotic madness that only women seemed to experience, or a particularly violent form of mania described as wolf-like that was particular to men. Moreover, windows, rivers, and wells were perilous places for men and women bent on self-slaughter. Despite religious prescriptions against suicide, families often sought a place in Santa Dorotea for suicidal relatives in hopes that they would be prevented from completing the act.

The second approach was to observe overlaps, linkages, and relationships between different types of records. The immense volume of an institutional archive can be daunting, but it adds depth and substance to the history a scholar will eventually write. Patient registers and ledgers that record patient fees, for example, helped me reconstruct the hospital's patient population and determine individual lengths of stay. From these sources, I learned that the Antonios shared the experience of admission to Santa Dorotea with some 2,220 other men and women from

1647 when it opened to its closure in 1788. Fee ledgers that outline what each patient was expected to pay based on an assessment of financial capacity also helped me to establish the socio-economic composition of the patient population. From these records, I observed that for the hospital's first century of operation it admitted mainly affluent fee-paying patients. In the 1740s, the Tuscan government restructured Santa Dorotea's finances so that the hospital could accept poorer patients.

Third, I thought in terms of individual voices and perspectives. Perhaps the easiest way to grasp this approach is to think of a choir. When you listen to choral music you see many people singing together, but hear a single, unified sound. That unity cloaks the different vocal parts. Sopranos, alto, tenors, and basses sing vastly different parts that together form a coherent whole. Similarly, hospital records contain many voices that can be identified and studied apart to animate the different perspectives and experiences that, taken together, make up the hospital's entire history. For a long time, it was the perspective of doctors that dominated hospital histories. The thick documentary record they left behind made them some of history's loudest voices. More recently, historians have shifted their focus to patients, families, and their social networks, considering the voices of medicine's consumers as equally important in understanding how ordinary people of the past experienced health and illness.

And so, I read Santa Dorotea's archival documents with the aim of capturing multiple points of view – patients and practitioners or caretakers, families and administrators, superintendents and government agents.

Armed with these three interpretive strategies, I was able to hear voices typically silent in history and make unexpected discoveries. On the first point, I was better able to hear the concerns of families seeking help for their troubled members. On the second point, I learned that the single most important players at the hospital were administrators whose concerns about overcrowding and financial sustainability shaped the hospital's admission policies. Second only to the interests of administrators were those of the state, which legally required the hospitalization of mentally ill persons who disturbed public peace. From that perspective, Santa Dorotea was an instrument of state order.

Administrators and judicial authorities far outranked the authority of physicians, who had to align their medical care both with the hospital's fiscal needs and the criminal justice apparatus of the Tuscan state. Men like Martelli and Colombi established the framework in which physicians practiced and patients were admitted, treated, and discharged.

This essay explores these three approaches to reading and interpreting hospital records whether you have thousands of pages like I did or maybe just a dozen. We will read the case of the two Antonios for patterns to recover the personalities and struggles buried within these documents and within the larger context of the archive. But the principal focus will be on capturing the four perspectives that the letters pertaining to the two Antonios unearth.

Making hospital records "speak" with many voices requires that the researcher imagine what it was like to be one of these historical actors even with the understanding that the information we excavate from our documents is partial, imperfect, and biased. By adopting the perspective of a hospital administrator or the head of the criminal justice system, or a physician, or a patient, or a patient's relative we begin to appreciate and understand the historical cultures from which they came and how those cultures shaped individual experience and the hospital's history. This chapter proceeds in three parts, using the historical actors we meet in the cases of the two Antonios to represent the interests at play. Niccolò Martelli is our lens onto hospital governance and administration, Domenico Colombi is the voice of the Tuscan state, Giovanni Targioni Tozzetti gives us insight into the role of physicians, and Antonio Corsini and his relatives shed light on patient and family experience.

Thinking Like an Administrator and a Magistrate

When Niccolò Martelli, Santa Dorotea's superintendent, received that letter from the grand duchy's criminal justice minister in December 1756 ordering him to admit the two Antonios, he immediately complied. The next day, the hospital's secretary recorded the entry of Signore Antonio Corsini of Florence on two facing pages of the institution's large patient registers – admissions on the left-hand page and discharges on the right. The record is brief. We learn that Corsini arrived at 6 pm. We learn also that the same Giuseppe Nardi who originally requested Antonio's admission agreed to pay 42 lire per month to cover Antonio's care. That cost broke down into 38 lire for food, a little over a lira for linens and regular shaves, and 3 lire for taxes. Nardi was also responsible for clothing, medicines, and any other incidental costs that accrued down the road. There was no cost for a bed since Antonio would bring his own.[8] The first admission record ends there without accompanying details about Corsini's medical diagnosis or his physical or mental condition (Figure 3.2).

The next entry belongs to Antonio Bianconi, husband of the poor Caterina dell'Ara, to whom the honorific "Signore" is not applied. An hour after the more affluent Corsini entered Santa Dorotea, Bianconi followed, crossing the same threshold into the hospital. In Bianconi's case, the secretary noted that his fees were to be paid by "the hospitals" by order of the grand duke.[9] And that's it. There are no further details, itemizations of costs, or information of who or what those "hospitals" were or how much they would pay to cover his cost of care. Like Corsini, the record was silent on Bianconi's health (Figure 3.3).

The first thing that struck me about these records was how much they had to say about fees relative to how little they had to say about medicine. This seemed like a problem for someone writing a history of medicine. My first instinct was to ignore the financial information and to search elsewhere for opinions physicians might have left behind about our two Antonios. I was quickly disappointed. For many early modern hospitals, the casebooks of physicians are rare sources. None exist for Santa Dorotea. The only significant discussion of patient health by physicians occasionally ends up in admission and discharge letters. And even in these rich narrative sources, physicians often only said briefly that admission or discharge was appropriate or inappropriate without deeper discussion. Antonio Corsini's record is already uncharacteristically detailed.

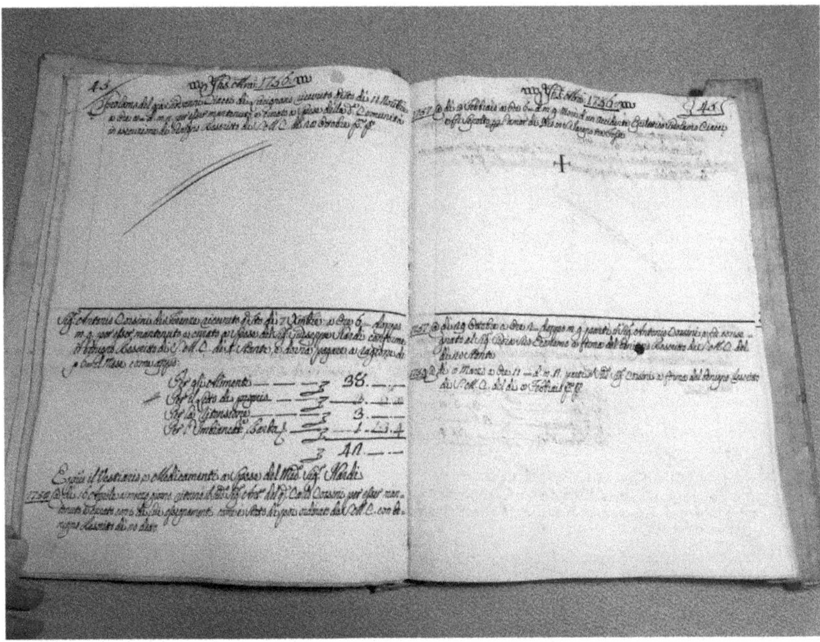

Figure 3.2 Record of Antonio Corsini's admission and discharge to and from Santa Dorotea. Corsini's record is on the bottom half of the two pages. ASF, Santa Dorotea, 35, Libro Registro di Malati A, fol. 45 verso facing recto.

When I could find no more medical information, I returned to the patient registers to try to think again about all that financial information. Corsini brought his own bed. That was interesting. As I read more, a pattern emerged. Wealthy people tended to bring their own beds. But what happened if you were too poor or just didn't have your own bed to bring? I wondered what kind of accommodations these patients received. That question stuck in my mind until, many months later, I happened upon invoices the hospital kept with mattress dealers. For those who could not bring their own beds, mattress dealers provided straw-stuffed mattresses of varying quality depending on the financial capacity of the patient. Without his own bed, Antonio Bianconi most likely slept on the lowest quality mattress the hospital dealer offered. Could a cheap perhaps dirty mattress have compromised his health? This question I could not answer.

The relative quality of patient mattresses may seem irrelevant, but it was one of those financial details that kept recurring in-patient admission and discharge registers much like they did in admission and discharge letters. I began to think that what hospital superintendents like Martelli really worried about daily was not diagnoses or treatment regimens, but money. Martelli's greatest preoccupation was how and by whom the hospital would get paid for its services. In fact, fees rather than treatment consistently dominate admission and discharge records.

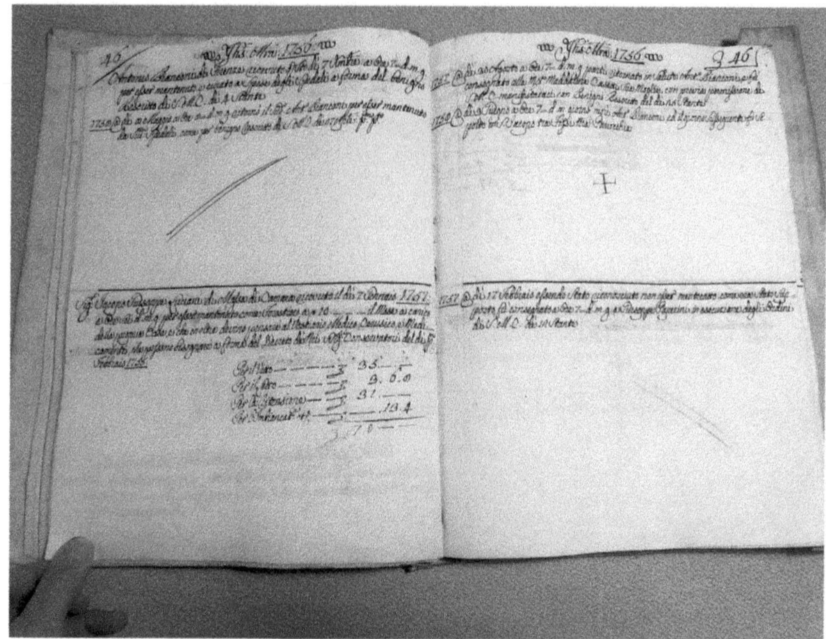

Figure 3.3 Record of Antonio Bianconi's admission and discharge to and from Santa Dorotea. Bianconi's record is on the top half of the two pages. The cross on the right-hand page indicates that he died in hospital. ASF, Santa Dorotea, 35, Libro Registro di Malati A, fol. 46 verso facing recto.

It was only when I tried to appreciate what it was like to be Martelli, a person responsible for executing Santa Dorotea's mission, that I began to understand that early modern hospitals were economic as well as healthcare institutions.[10] This point may sound obvious, but it was hidden by scholarship that tended to focus on physicians, patients, and medical practice rather than hospital administration and administrators. Archival documents were telling me that this focus was a barrier to understanding how early modern hospitals were really run. How to generate revenue to pay for patient care was the single most important factor shaping hospital policy, medical practice, and patient experience.

When we look through the eyes of Martelli, we see the hospital's managerial culture. This culture represented patients primarily as fee payers or resource consumers rather than as people suffering specific illnesses. Martelli's prime concern was how patients affected the hospital's bottom line. And so, he aimed to distinguish between patients who could pay for their care and patients who needed subsidy.

As a servant and representative of the Tuscan state, Colombi's focus was different. How the hospital funded its services was important, but his main concern was public order. His title in the grand ducal government was Auditore Fiscale, a kind of attorney general who oversaw the duchy's criminal courts and prisons.[11]

His mandate was to maintain peace. Some types of severely mentally ill men and women came to his attention because they threatened that peace. And so, through Colombi's eyes, we also begin to see that the hospital could be used as an instrument of state order. But, although Colombi could compel Martelli to admit a patient who was threatening public peace, I was also beginning to learn it was really the hospital's economically oriented outlook that shaped hospital operations as well as its discharge policies. To make this argument, I needed a better understanding of Santa Dorotea's financial structure. This took me back to its founding documents.

I was not surprised to find that Martelli's economically oriented outlook was already evident in the hospital's first statutes – or what we might call bylaws. By statute, Santa Dorotea was "to receive all those who are not of sound mind or commonly referred to as crazy (*pazzi*)."[12] The governing board was free to accept "men as well as women, clerical or lay, those from the city or dominion of Florence as well as those from any other place or dominion."[13] To support this large target population, hospital founders stipulated that higher fees charged to affluent patients would subsidize free care for the poor. Founders further required that legacies, gifts, testamentary bequests, or property given to the hospital be sold for cash and reinvested in local or regional financial markets.[14] In their opinion, this would both prevent fraud and allow the hospital to generate investment income.

This financial strategy seemed revolutionary to me, but was it revolutionary to early modern Tuscans? Secondary scholarship suggests that the answer was yes and no. The strategy was not revolutionary in the sense that social welfare and health-provisioning institutions had a long history in Europe that reached back into the Middle Ages. When we think of hospitals today, we call to mind medical institutions grounded in the practice, promotion, and research of biomedicine. We tend to think also of asylums or psychiatric institutions as being different from hospitals in the strict biomedical sense. Premodern European hospitals of all types, by contrast, had their origins not in medical care, but in poor relief.[15] They emerged within an intermeshing network of Christian charitable institutions devoted to the bodily and spiritual care of the poor.[16]

In Florence, where acute-care hospitals like Santa Maria Nuova played a vital role in treating the sick poor, other hospitals directed services specifically to orphans, widows, and vulnerable young girls or boys. These structures – some permanent, some temporary – emerged on the urban scene in the fifteenth and sixteenth centuries, respectively, forming a network of medical and charitable institutions designed to keep cities physically, spiritually, and morally clean.[17]

Santa Dorotea shared many of these characteristics, but it was unique in several ways. First, unlike most of Florence's hospitals, it was founded to aid people from the entire social spectrum, from the penniless to the prosperous. Second, where most of Tuscany's hospitals funded services by developing large patrimonies based on land, Santa Dorotea supported its expansive mission through a combination of maintenance fees charged to patients and financial investments.[18] This was a revolutionary solution to a perennial problem throughout Europe: building a hospital was easy. Making it financially sustainable in the long term was much harder.

Santa Dorotea was over 100 years old by the time Martelli admitted the two Antonios. Raising operating revenue had been a problem from the very beginning. In 1750, government officials launched a campaign to rebuild and reinvigorate Santa Dorotea. In a decree published in November of that year, servants of the Tuscan government acknowledged that the new improved Santa Dorotea would need funding sources to augment maintenance fees and investment returns. And so, it required Florence's other major hospitals to subsidize Santa Dorotea's budget. Santa Maria Nuova, San Matteo, San Paolo, and Bonifazio were to give Santa Dorotea a yearly stipend on the principle that putting the mentally ill in an institution designed for their treatment relieved other institutions from the burden of their care. This critical piece of information offers the key to identifying the "hospitals" in Antonio Bianconi's admission record.

This combined stipend supported Florentines, but the government did not think it adequate to support all of Tuscany's mad so, it demanded that the duchy's cities and towns bear the cost of supporting their own mentally ill through the Nove Conservatori del Dominio Fiorentino, the financial organ of the provincial domains.[19] "Remaining funds," a government decree stated, "were there to support the poor, but only in the case of necessary subsidy – and not otherwise – at the expense of the communities of which they were a part."[20] The justification was that these communities would save energy and resources by outsourcing care for the mad to a central institution like Santa Dorotea. The result would contribute to the rational economy of a public health network that was increasingly evolving into a centralized public health system.

But the new Santa Dorotea had another problem: overcrowding. The law of 1750 stated that the hospital had to accommodate at least 60 patients comfortably. This goal was attainable in theory since the new hospital boasted over 50 patient rooms of varying sizes. Yet, challenges quickly arose. Santa Dorotea was on the Arno, a river that tended to flood. On November 30, 1758, Niccolò Martelli wrote to the grand ducal government about the damages a catastrophic flood caused at the hospital.[21] "Among the many places in Florence damaged by the waters of the last overflowing of the Arno," Martelli reported, "one of those that has suffered the most was the hospital of Santa Dorotea." The waters had flooded the ground-floor patient rooms "at a height of almost four feet [2 braccia] for which reason they have remained uninhabitable for many months because of the humidity." These rooms, Martelli claimed, would have to be laid with new bricks "at great expense."[22] In these "unfortunate circumstances," Martelli continued, "it was necessary to move all the sick to higher floors and to put more people together in the same rooms." This was a grave situation indeed. Without those 18 ground-floor rooms, Martelli explained, "there were not rooms sufficient to care for 46 patients" – the population of the hospital at that time – while respecting the principles of separation by gender and class that statute required.[23]

They were not without a solution. Martelli observed that since there were only a very small number of *maniaci*, "who could live for a long time in the same room," the hospital would have to reduce patient numbers.[24] To do that, Martelli enlisted the help of the hospital's doctors and the hospital's chief caretaker. Together they would best determine which patients were in the greatest need of treatment in hospital and which could be safely discharged into the care of relatives or designated guardians without fear of creating "any disturbance to the public quiet or to their own health."[25] In this case, after examining patients who did not seem *furiosi*, the hospital's physician and the chief patient caretaker certified six patients for discharge. Martelli wrote that one "was completely cured from the diverse fixations that had molested her." Three others could "be securely consigned to their respective relatives since they had not for a long time given a sign of *frenesia*, but rather of a weak intellect and dim-wittedness [*melenso*]." Abbot Antonio Arfaroli of Pistoia had also "not manifested his insanity [*pazzia*]," but his case was not straight forward. At other times, he had succumbed to "false ideas" that he was being poisoned, which, in turn, caused him to descend into a "melancholic delirium." Still, he had financial resources enough that he could be released into the hands of a "secure person, who would watch him continually."[26] Martelli added that he could be readmitted at the first clear signs of insanity (*pazzia*). Except for one patient who was said to be completely cured, the others were *sufficiently* cured.

There was no guarantee that they would not fall ill again. Were that the case, their relatives could apply for readmission. Even after the 18 ground-floor rooms were renovated, Santa Dorotea experienced increasing requests for admission which translated into an increasingly large patient population. To match the flow of patients entering with those returning home, Martelli regularly asked Santa Dorotea's physicians for recommendations on which patients were cured "enough" to be released. In this respect, the hospital's needs for space and money were the most important aspects of the admission process. Once in the hospital, the practical needs of the hospital even influenced the construction of diagnoses. Mania could be interpreted as less severe if administrators needed to free up space. From Martelli's managerial perspective, discharge even at the risk of repeated readmission was preferable to overcrowding. This is where the sources bring to bear the role and perspective of hospital physicians – a group of earlier histories of medicine put front and center. Santa Dorotea's records suggest that their medical concerns were less central to the institution's daily operations than historians once thought.

Thinking Like a Physician

On January 27, 1759, Niccolò Martelli and Luca de' Medici, Santa Dorotea's superintendent and chief officer of daily operations respectively, wrote to the government. The topic was Antonio Corsini and what to do with him. "Because different types of diseases are included in the category of *demenza*," they began, "it is thus necessary that there be different cures and guidelines for each of those people who have the misfortune of being molested by one of those most mournful illnesses."[27] This "truth," they continued, had been demonstrated by the testimony of Doctor Giovanni Targioni Tozzetti. Targioni Tozzetti had examined Antonio Corsini during his second hospital admission in 1758. The doctor "judged it expedient," the two administrators reported,

> that [Corsini] be transferred to enjoy the country air under the care and vigilance of some wise person, so that, with the help of a regulated cure, he might be freed from the false ideas and the melancholic fixations from which he is oppressed.[28]

The two heads of hospital pointed out that this solution was well within Corsini's reach since his estate was substantial enough that he could be maintained "with safety outside of the hospital." They proposed to the government that Corsini's estate administrator assume his care in accord with Doctor Targioni Tozzetti's recommendations. In turn, Targioni Tozzetti would regularly assess and report on "the state of [Corsini's] health" to the grand duchy's court of wards (the Magistrato dei Pupilli).[29] He did so until he determined that Corsini was well enough to be completely released from Santa Dorotea's oversight a few months later.

This section tackles the perspective of doctors in Santa Dorotea's employ. The researcher coming to these documents for the first time might assume that a hospital physician's first thoughts were to his patients and to the theory and practice of medicine that might cure them. Yet, hospital records show that Santa Dorotea's doctors worked within a larger institutional and administrative framework. Targioni Tozzetti, for example, served at least three masters – the administrators of Santa Dorotea, the government, and the court of wards.

Let's take each of these in turn. For Santa Dorotea's administrators, as we have observed, once patients were admitted, their job was to get them discharged as quickly as new patients came in. This strategy avoided overcrowding, but it also allowed them greater flexibility in containing costs by shaping the patient population in accord with sources of patient funding. The government was more preoccupied with public order. Its goal was to prevent men and women like Corsini from ending up in criminal courts and prisons. The Pupilli was a civil court established in the late fourteenth century. It was designed to provide guardianship to minors, widows, and, early on in its existence, the mentally incompetent.[30] In his capacity as a physician, Targioni Tozzetti worked with each of these agencies to find a care solution for Corsini that would be acceptable to family, hospital, magistracy, and state. His medical assessments were shaped in no small part by his allegiance to the institutional web in which he worked.

But who was Giovanni Targioni Tozzetti? Here was another character I had to explore. Further research revealed that Targioni Tozzetti was one of Italy's leading intellectual lights. His obituary of 1783 appeared in Tuscany's major literary journal – for which Targioni Tozzetti had been what we might call the science editor. That obituary filled in key knowledge gaps. I learned Targioni Tozzetti's contemporaries considered him "one of the greatest luminaries of Tuscan literature" for his great depth and breadth of erudition in practical medicine – his primary profession – and in botany, and natural history.[31] Targioni Tozzetti was very well-connected. Over the course of his life, he was admitted to and jointly founded some of Tuscany's most prestigious scholarly academies, wrote voluminously on medicine, botany, infectious disease, and agronomy, and held some of the city's most coveted posts.

After getting an advanced degree in medicine from Pisa, Targioni Tozzetti settled into a position at Santa Maria Nuova, Florence's oldest and most distinguished acute care hospital for the poor. Later, he served as a doctor for the state. In this role, he was a member director of the Medical College – the region's licensing board, as well as a consultant to the grand duchy's Board of Health.[32] It was in his capacity as a physician for the state that Targioni Tozzetti came to find himself in his late 40s consulting on cases of alleged insanity for the Magistrato de' Pupilli and Santa Dorotea.

Targioni Tozzetti's education, connections, and career put him at the forefront of Italian medicine, natural philosophy, and public health policy. The modern researcher might be surprised then to learn that the medicine he practiced was highly conservative. I knew this because, from previous research, I was familiar with contemporary medical culture. It remained anchored in a medical tradition medieval and early modern Europeans had inherited from ancient Greece. Briefly, this medical tradition held that human bodies were composed of humors whose good or bad "temperaments" promoted health or caused illness. Unlike the modern biomedical paradigm, which sees sickness or wellness as two opposite and objective physical states, Greek medicine conceived of health along an ever-shifting scale of greater or lesser equilibrium, the latter constituting wellness, the former sickness.[33]Without going into detail, the objective of medical treatment was to maintain and restore this equilibrium.

Like any disease, the cause of insanity was generally thought to be a bodily imbalance or corruption of bodily fluids that had adversely affected brain function. All the diseases mentioned in Santa Dorotea's admission and discharge records like *mania*, *melancholia*, *frenesia*, *demenza*, *delirium* and accompanying symptoms like fixed or false ideas or fantasies were caused either by head injuries or by humoral imbalances or corruptions. Therapeutics for these illnesses were no different than those for other diseases.

Like other Italian hospitals, Santa Dorotea aimed to heal the bodies *and* souls of insane men and women. The hospital's founding statutes required that a priest and at least two medical practitioners – a physician (*medico*) and a surgeon (*cerusico*) – be among the permanent staff. Statutes required that the hospital's board elect "a priest of good life and customs," who would receive a monthly salary, an apartment in the hospital to live in, and use of the kitchen and oven at hospital expense. His responsibilities included monitoring the patient population daily and reporting his observations to the chief officer of operations, celebrating daily mass in the hospital's chapel, and administering spiritual aid to those insane men and women who could receive it.[34] A doctor and surgeon were also part of the permanent staff though they did not reside on premises. Statutes instead required that they come as needed for which the doctor was paid annually, the surgeon monthly. Both were to be men of good standing. Their responsibilities included, "examining those persons lacking in mind," monitoring their conditions, and always coming to the hospital when there was need.[35]

If Santa Dorotea's priests offered spiritual care to patient souls, the hospital's medical personnel helped restore bodily equilibrium. The notes of Santa Dorotea's first salaried physician, Niccolò Buonaiuti, confirm this strategy. As he saw it, the governing board's aim was not merely to improve the physical accommodations and the bodily treatment of the insane, but to make every effort at restoring to them the most noble part of their souls, namely the intellect. To cure a person of madness was, in his words, "tantamount to saving a soul from damnation."[36] And so, Buonaiuti believed that every effort should be made to cure madness even those types that were considered incurable. In accord with long-standing Mediterranean tradition, Buonaiuti believed that diet was a key part of treatment, but an individual diet designed to accommodate each patient's constitution was impractical. He outlined rather a middle way (*strada di mezzo*) that considered the fact that patients at Santa Dorotea led largely sedentary lives with little exertion or motion and included people of different complexion, age, and sex.[37]

In addition to diet, hospital records tell us that the hospital environment was also an important part of healing. Targioni Tozzetti emphasized the connection between health and environment in his own scholarship. In 1761, he published an expansive two-volume work called *Consideration on the Causes and Remedies of Unhealthiness of the Air in the Valdinievole*. This treatise explored in detail the relationship between poor environmental conditions and diseases, such as malaria.[38] The importance of salubrious air as treatment for certain ailments undergirds his "prescription" that Antonio Corsini, once stabilized, leaves Santa Dorotea to enjoy "the country air."

Targioni Tozzetti and his colleague's assessments of Santa Dorotea's patients also served Martelli's administrative concerns about space and money. Antonio Corsini's wealth gave him access to premium services in hospital as well as what we might call out-patient services under the supervision of the hospital's physicians. Santa Dorotea's directors could use this treatment option to alleviate overcrowding. But what of the poor Antonio Bianconi whose "frenzies" brought him twice to the hospital at the request of his wife? His poverty meant that his care would have to be fully subsidized by Florence's other hospitals. That care served only his most basic needs. In fact, he was the type of patient administrators like Martelli tended to think of first when they were looking to free up space. Nine months after his first admission, Bianconi appeared in a letter Martelli wrote to the Regency Council about the hospital's population. "The number of sick people having increased to 47," he began, "we have charged the ordinary physician with taking great care in seeing if there are any [patients] capable of being released to unburden from the weight of their maintenance Santa Dorotea as much as the other hospitals of Florence…" The ordinary physician in this case was Antonio Lulli. After examining all 47 patients, he identified two for release. Antonio Bianconi was one of them. Based on Lulli's evaluation, Martelli assured the grand ducal government that these two men could be consigned to their respective homes "without any danger" to themselves or to "the public quiet."[39]

Bianconi would last nine months before being readmitted as a raving mad man (*pazzo furioso*) and for suffering the same frenzies (*frenesie*) that brought him to the hospital the first time. The goal again was "to be cured there of his sickness." But, on the evening of June 3rd, a month after his second admission, Antonio Bianconi died in Santa Dorotea. The secretary recorded no cause of death just as he had not recorded the condition Bianconi had been in upon readmission. The only other detail reported was that on the day after his death, Bianconi was buried in the hospital's parish plot.[40]

There is no way of knowing why Bianconi died and Corsini did not. There is no way of knowing whether Corsini continued to thrive outside of the hospital even though he would not be admitted a third time. But Santa Dorotea's records do demonstrate that wealthy patients could afford a higher standard of care and had access to in-patient and out-patient care options. Given that one of the hospital's principles of separation was by class, it is also likely that wealthier patients enjoyed better rooms in which, like Corsini, they might even enjoy their own furnishings. Targioni Tozzetti's deployment of his therapeutic tools was profoundly influenced by the wealth and status of individual patients and the material needs of the hospital rather than solely the medical theory that undergirds them.

Patient Voices, Family Politics

The last part of this chapter briefly explores what hospital records do not tell us, the family dramas they do not record. In the case of the two Antonios, I had to read for the silences as much as for the voices. Antonio Corsini leaves a long and detailed case in the records of Tuscany's court of wards, the Magistrato de' Pupilli, a civil arena in which families were able to negotiate long-term care solutions for mentally incompetent relatives.[41] In fact, the initial medical testimonies on Corsini's condition conducted by his physician in Prato and Antonio Lulli are missing from Santa Dorotea's records and have instead been preserved in the Pupilli's records. This happenstance underscores the challenges hospital historians face in trying to recreate patient backstories. Sometimes records are moved to places where researchers least expect to find them. One of the voices these records restore, which hospital records tend to silence, is that of Antonio Corsini himself. He comes forward to speak about his condition and his situation on his own terms and on his own behalf. These documents from the Pupilli better inform our understanding of his admission and discharge process.

In December 1756, when Giuseppe Nardi wrote to the grand ducal government, he made "two parallel requests."[42] He asked both that his cousin Antonio Corsini be admitted to Santa Dorotea and that the Magistrato Supremo, a court for petitioners seeking direct grand ducal arbitration, grants Nardi guardianship of Corsini's estate. The explicit justification for each petition was Corsini's insanity. Corsini's state of mind was less of an issue than the matter of who would control his patrimony. He was admitted immediately to the hospital, but the civil portion of his case dragged on in court for months. In the end, the Pupilli claimed jurisdiction over the case and objected to Nardi as the curator of Corsini's estate.

Corsini's physician from Prato and Antonio Lulli, Santa Dorotea's salaried physician, were called by the court to assess Corsini's condition. Both agreed that he was insane. Corsini's physician gave a particularly detailed report. Corsini, he said, had suffered about six months with "melancholic delirium without fever." He labored too with "a grave fear and profound sadness caused by mournful thoughts and the imaginary dangers that his altered fantasy represents in his mind, which together with obstinate fixation become the continual occupation of his spirit."[43] Corsini dismissed his physician's advice. Instead, he kept to himself, remained indifferent to domestic affairs, and refused to eat. The situation became so dire that he had to be force fed "so that he would not perish."[44]

Antonio Lulli's testimony was much shorter. He simply said that Corsini was "demented and incapable of attending to his own interests given the considerable depravation [*depravazione*] of the mind."[45] The difference in detail does not diminish Lulli's expertise or thoroughness. Rather, it says something again about the hospital's managerial culture that privileged economic over medical information. Lulli and Targioni Tozzeti were asked simply to decide whether a person qualified for admission or discharge. Hospital administrators trusted their expertise, accepting simple yes or no answers. The more important information from the hospital's point of view was who would pay for care. Corsini's physician, by contrast, was testifying before a court on whether Corsini's condition warranted his losing the legal right to dispose of his property as he saw fit. The court seems to have needed greater detail about the nature of his incompetence to determine whether and for how long he might require a legal guardian. Santa Dorotea's salaried physicians also based their decisions on one interview. Corsini's physician, by contrast, had treated him for half a year.

Corsini recovered not at home, but in hospital. In March 1757, Lulli and Antonio Sani, Santa Dorotea's salaried surgeon, recommended Corsini's discharge.[46] They acknowledged that he had come to the hospital suffering "mental alienations and disturbances of his fantasy originated by anguishes of the soul," but that he was greatly improved and could expect a full recovery.[47] The case was more complicated than that. While in hospital, Corsini had written a plea to the Pupilli himself, arguing that he was healthy enough to have some say in the appointment of his estate administrator. He did not deny that he suffered from bouts of insanity. In fact, he blamed his periodic afflictions on his caretaker, Giuseppe Nardi. Nardi, he said, was the son of his former guardian, Domenico, whom Corsini never trusted. Corsini's parents died when he was still a minor. Domenico, who had married his paternal aunt, assumed legal guardianship of the orphaned teenager. But the Nardis continued to intervene in Corsini's affairs even after he had reached the age of majority. Corsini claimed that Domenico had denied him the fruits of his estate, refused to give account of his administration, and even persuaded Corsini to sign contracts he did not understand that put him in debt.[48] Corsini argued that it was these circumstances in which he found himself defenseless against the predations of grasping relatives that caused him such mental anguish.[49] Admission to Santa Dorotea gave Corsini the distance from the Nardis he needed to get well enough for discharge. He would break down again the following year warranting another stay in hospital. But after he improved again, the Pupilli did not release him back into the hands of the Nardis. Instead, they chose a third party as his estate administrator. His trail grows cold thereafter, but he did not return to Santa Dorotea and the Nardis made no further claims on his patrimony.

Conclusion: No Money, No Mission

Hospital records are rich, voluminous, and layered historical sources. They offer the researcher many different entry points into the life and history of hospitals from the original mission statements and statutes drafted by visionary founders to the day-in-day-out keeping of the institution's books. Each document type has a story to tell and each speaks with a different inflection. Founding documents for example often unfold as triumphant narratives excoriating the poor conditions the hospital's founders aimed to redress. They tend to be aspirational rather than reflective of a hospital's daily operation. Hospital statutes can have a similar accent since they define in ideal terms hospital policy, governance, and personnel. Hospital-related government decrees can sound overwrought by their focus on crisis.

The hospital's daily reality was messier. Hospitals often failed to meet the lofty goals of founders and magistrates. The minutes of governing boards can begin to break this triumphalist façade by revealing the types of challenges hospitals faced in their daily operations. One of the themes that beat a steady rhythm at Santa Dorotea, year in, year out, was the concern over how to pay for the hospital's mission of care over the long term. Like many of Europe's hospitals, Santa Dorotea was an expensive institution to run. It needed a steady funding stream, which was not easy to create or maintain. And so, administrators undertook interesting experiments in fee structures and institutional investment. In fact, by far the greatest percentage of Santa Dorotea's records are devoted to hospital finance, including general income and expenditure, investments, patient fees, building maintenance and renovation costs, and "payroll".

This chapter has focused primarily on admission and discharge letters. These types of records offer an especially powerful lens onto hospital operations because they are a point of intersection in which the interests of hospital administrators, state authorities, physicians, and patients collided and collaborated to make care arrangements for sick men and women. We see these interests come alive in the cases of the two Antonios. We begin to understand what prompted Domenico Colombi to write to Niccolò Martelli on the day in December 1756. As minister of criminal justice, he aimed to remove threats to public order. When brought complaints about the behavior of allegedly mad persons, Colombi was bound by law to entrust them to the superintendent of Santa Dorotea.

Martelli's logic and goals were different. As the superintendent of a chronically cash-strapped institution, he had to see patients as financial liabilities even while acknowledging that the hospital existed to serve them. The hospital simply could not accommodate everyone all the time, but it could, through careful accounting and administration, accommodate most patients some the time. Martelli inherited and reproduced an institutional logic centered on financial sustainability. From his administrative perspective, the two Antonios were a perfect admission unit. The wealthy Signore Corsini could pay extremely high fees. His fees of 42 lire a month were among the highest received from any patient over the course of its entire history. The poor Antonio Bianconi could not pay his way, but his fees would be covered by subsidies from Florence's four major hospitals. Among Martelli's concerns in the complicated admission process was how each patient would affect Santa Dorotea's overall budget and whether he could balance fee-paying patients against the poor who would require subsidy. One might assume that the power of the state always trumped the perceived needs of an administrator. It was the other way around. Santa Dorotea's admission records show that Auditore Fiscale's concern for public order tended to play second fiddle to the hospital's financial concerns.

Concern for the hospital's bottom line also shaped the role physicians played at Santa Dorotea. In fact, one of the most curious things for a modern researcher is that the greatest medical detail we confront appears in the records of a civil court rather than those of a hospital. We are left with many questions about the relationship between patients and doctors at Santa Dorotea. Physicians were the hospital's chief gatekeepers. They determined which people qualified for admission and at what point patients could be discharged. Records indicate that physicians made those determinations based on interviews that they conducted first upon admission and then regularly thereafter. But without any specific admission protocols, we can only imagine how those interviews unfolded. Even if hospital physicians deemed a patient worthy of admission, it was not until funding sources were confirmed that they were permitted entry. And the hospital's need for money and space meant that physicians were pressured to "find" patients who were not necessarily "cured" but were healthy enough to be released.

The perspectives of families and patients are harder to capture in early modern hospital records. The cases of the two Antonios show the extent to which hospital records shroud the contexts behind a patient's admission. Court evidence relates a long and complex family drama that affected Corsini's mental health. Without comparable evidence, we have no such insight into the life of the poor Antonio Bianconi.

Overall, Santa Dorotea's records communicate more about the institution's managerial culture than they do about the nature of premodern European medicine. Still, they are a sharp lens on the history of hospitals and health care provisioning in premodern Europe. They not only show that hospital services involved and extended to the entire socio-economic spectrum but also show that wealth mattered. The rich could afford premium care while the poor had to make do with whatever the hospital provided them. But in all cases, no money, no mission proved repeatedly to be the hospital's dominant management philosophy and the philosophy that most shaped patient care and experience.

Notes

1 *ASF*, Santa Dorotea dei Pazzerelli (SD) 2, *Motupropri, Rescritti, ed altri Documenti appartenti allo Spedale di Santa Dorotea*, no. 40.
2 Ibid.
3 *ASF*, SD 3, *Motupropri*, no. 11: "…per esser ricaduto nelle solita sui fissazioni."
4 Ibid.: "a prender aria."

5 Ibid.: "Che sia permesso al supplicante di lui economo di cavarlo qualche volta, per condurlo a prendere l'aria e per fare sperimento se sin stabile il ristabilmento di detto maniaco."

6 *ASF*, SD, *Motupropri*, 44: "a goder l'aria di compagna sotto la custodia e vigilanza di qualche persona savia accio coll'aiuto d'una regolata cura si procurasse di liberarlo dalle false idee e dalle fissazioni malinchoniche delle quali è oppresso."

7 The website of the Archivio di Stato of Florence provides an *Inventario Sommario* or "Summary Inventory" of the Santa Dorotea *fondo* or collection. See, https://www.archiviodistato.firenze.it/asfi/fileadmin/risorse/allegati_inventari_on_line/n150_sdorotea.pdf. Accessed 10 August 2021.

8 ASF, SD 35, *Libro Registro di Malati A*, 45.

9 *ASF*, SD 35, *Libro Registro di Malati*, 46: "Antonio Bianconi di Firenze ricevuto questo di 7 Dicembre a ore 7 = d[opo] m[ezzo] g[iorno] per esser mantenuto e curato a spese degli spedali a forma del benigno rescritto di SMC di 4 stante."

10 For the important role, hospitals and other charitable institutions played in the economic history of medieval and early modern Europe, see Anne Borsay, "Cash and Conscience: Financing the General Hospital at Bath, 1738–1750," *Social History of Medicine* 4:2 (August, 1991): 207–29; Nicholas Terpstra, *Lay Confraternities and Civic Religion in Renaissance Bologna* (Cambridge: Cambridge University Press, 1995); Matthew Thomas Sneider, "Charity and Property: The Patrimonies of Bolognese Hospitals," (PhD Dissertation, May 2004).

11 R. Burr Litchfield, *Emergence of a Bureaucracy: The Florentine Patricians, 1530–1790* (Princeton, NJ: Princeton University Press, 1986), 95 and 101.

12 *ASF*, SD 42, *Istrumenti Ricordi*, fol. 1v.

13 The history of Santa Dorotea's founding is recorded at the beginning of ASF, SD 42, called *Instrumenti e Ricordi*. The extracts cited here can be found on 1v: primieramente che in detta casa si possino rivecer tutti quelli che sono di non sana mente chiamati volgarmente pazzi…secondo, che si possa ricevere tanto maschi quanto femmine, sia ecclesiastici come secolari, e non solamente della città e dominio fiorentino ma anco qualsivoglia altro luogo e dominio…" 3r: "Già è noto a V.A. il negozio proposto sino in vita dal padre Alberto leoni carmelitano da Mantova di fondar in questa città una casa per ricevervi quelli che patiscono di non sana mente e pazzerelli…si volse allor sentire l'Auditor Fiscale e Provveditore delle Stinche dove ora si dà ricetto a detti infelici, che ambedue risposero non aver alcuna difficultà in lasciar fondar questa opera e consegnar loro detta gente, perchè per la strettezza del luogo di dete carcere e per altre ragioni stava là tanto male che era impossibile che non migliorasse mettendosi in altra casa dove non fussi altra occupazione che della cura di questi miserabili." A copy of these documents can be found in *ASF*, RD 341, 508r–21r.

14 *ASF*, SD 42, *Istrumenti Ricordi*, fol. 2r.

15 Mary Fissell, *Patients, Power, and the Poor in Eighteenth-Century Bristol* (Cambridge: Cambridge University Press, 1991).

16 See, Lindsay Granshaw and Roy Porter, eds., *The Hospital in History* (London: Routledge, 1989); Philip Gavitt, *Charity and Children in Renaissance Florence: The Ospedale degli Innocenti, 1410–1536* (Ann Arbor: University of Michigan Press, 1990); Jonathan Barry and Colin Jones, *Medicine and Charity before the Welfare State* (London: Routledge, 1991); Sandra Cavallo, *Charity and Power in Early Modern Italy: Benefactors and Their Motives in Turin, 1541–1789* (Cambridge: Cambridge University Press, 1995); Carole Rawcliffe, *The Hospitals of Medieval Norwich* (Norwich: Centre of East Anglian Studies, University of East Anglia, 1995); Peregrine Horden and Richard Smith, eds., *The Locus of Care: Families, Communities, Institutions, and the Provision of Welfare Since Antiquity* (London: Routledge, 1998); Nicholas Terpstra, *Abandoned Children of the Italian Renaissance: Orphan Care in Florence and* Bologna (Baltimore, MD: Johns Hopkins University Press, 2005); Idem., *Cultures of Charity:*

Women, Politics, and the Reform of Poor Relief in Renaissance Italy (Cambridge, MA: Harvard University Press, 2013).

17 See, John Arrizabalaga, John Henderson, and Roger French, eds., *The Great Pox: The French Disease in Renaissance Europe* (New Haven, CT: Yale University Press, 1997); Jane L. Stevens Crawshaw, *Plague Hospitals: Public Health for the City in Early Modern Venice* (Burlington, VT: Ashgate, 2012); Cristian Berco, *From Body to Community: Venereal Disease and Society in Baroque Spain* (Toronto: University of Toronto Press, 2016); John Henderson, *Florence Under Siege: Surviving Plague in an Early Modern City* (New Haven, CT: Yale University Press, 2019).
18 *ASF*, SD 42, *Istrumenti Ricordi*, fol. 2r.
19 On the Nove, see, R. Burr Litchfield, *Emergence of a Bureaucracy,* 110–14. For this discussion in the November decree, see, *ASF*, RD 341, fols. 525rv–526rv.
20 *ASF*, RD 341, fol. 525v.
21 A brief description of this note to the grand ducal government appears in the index of ASF, SD 3 at no. 41. It is from this description that we learn the flood hit on November 30. A full copy of the letter appears under the number 41 in the register and is dated December 12, 1758.
22 ASF, SD 3, *Motupropri*, no. 41.
23 Ibid.
24 Ibid.
25 Ibid.
26 *ASF*, SD 3, *Motupropri*, no. 41.
27 *ASF*, SD 3, *Motupropri*, 44.
28 Ibid.
29 Ibid.
30 See, Elizabeth W. Mellyn, *Mad Tuscans and their Families: A History of Mental Disorder in Early Modern Italy* (Philadelphia: University of Pennsylvania Press, 2014) and Mariana Labarca, *Itineraries and Languages of Madness in the Early Modern World: Family Experience, Legal Practice, and Medical Knowledge in Eighteenth-Century Tuscany* (London and New York: Routledge, 2021). Both works draw broadly on the Pupilli, Mellyn for the period between the fourteenth and seventeenth centuries and Labarca for the eighteenth century.
31 *Novelle Letterarie,* 7 (Florence, 14 February 1783).
32 See, Giovanni Targioni Tozzetti, *Relazioni forensic: Ambiente, igiene e sanità nella Firenze dei Lorena*, ed. Susanna Pelle (Florence: Casa Editrice Le Lettere, 1998).
33 See Katharine Park, *Doctors and Medicine in Early Renaissance Florence* (Princeton, NJ: Princeton University Press, 1985) and Aaron Antonovsky, *Health, Stress, and Coping* (San Francisco, CA: Jossy-Bass Publishers, 1979).
34 *ASF*, SD 23, *Memorie*, nos. 5 and 6.
35 *ASF*, SD 25, nos. 5 and 6.
36 Ibid.: "…il principale scopo di questi signori non fosse solo il migliorare l'abitazione e trattamenti delo corpo ma di fare ogni sforzo per restituir loro la più nobili parte di lor medesimi cioè a dire l'intelletto; Opera cristiana e superiore a quella che possa gia mai fare niuno in terra perche si potrebbe dare il caso di liberare un anima dall'inferno poiche se è vero che quando uno impazza perda il merito, o l'demerito chi non vede che se quel ale era in stato di dannazione togliendoli con la mente anco il luogo di far penitenza, resta privo affatto della speranza di salvarsi e se per mezzo e de rimedi e diligenza che in torno ad esso si potessero usare egli recuperasse la sanità della mente avrebbe campo col pentirsi di fare acquisto della salute dell'anima…"
37 *ASF*, RD 341, fol. 519: "…ma gli consideri come huomini che abbino a vivere senza fatica, senza toto e menare una vita sedentaria cioè priva d'ogni sorte d'esercizio."
38 See, Pasta, *Dizionario biografico degli Italiani.*
39 *ASF*, SD 2, *Motupropri*, no. 77. The two men recommended for discharge were Antonio Bianconi and Liborio Fantechi who was admitted on May 18, 1757.

40 *ASF*, SD 35, *Libro Registro di Malati*, fol, 46.
41 Mariana Labarca has written at length on Corsini's case in her superb new book *Itineraries of Madness*. I have based a great deal of this final part on her treatment of that case in Chapter 5, 195–99.
42 Labarca, *Itineraries of Madness*, 195.
43 Cited in Labarca, *Itineraries of Madness*, 196.
44 Ibid., 196.
45 Ibid., 196.
46 This testimony is preserved in the records of the Pupilli at ASF, Magistrato dei Pupilli avanti il Principato, *Memoriali*, F. 2304, no. 87.
47 Labarca, *Itineraries of Madness*, 197.
48 Ibid., 198.
49 Ibid., 198.

Bibliography

Archival Sources in the Archivio di Stato of Florence (cited as ASF)

Magistrato dei Pupilli avanti il Principato.
Regio Diritto (cited as RD).
Santa Dorotea dei Pazzerelli (cited as SD).

Printed Primary Sources

Novelle Letterarie, 7 (Florence, 14 February 1783).
Targioni Tozzetti, Giovanni. *Relazioni forensic: Ambiente, igiene e sanità nella Firenze dei Lorena*, edited by Susanna Pelle. Florence: Casa Editrice Le Lettere, 1998.

Secondary Sources

Antonovsky, Aaron. *Health, Stress, and Coping*. San Francisco, CA: Jossy-Bass Publishers, 1979.
Arrizabalaga, John, John Henderson, and Roger French, eds. *The Great Pox: The French Disease in Renaissance Europe*. New Haven, CT: Yale University Press, 1997.
Barry, Jonathan and Colin Jones. *Medicine and Charity before the Welfare State*. London: Routledge, 1991.
Berco, Cristian. *From Body to Community: Venereal Disease and Society in Baroque Spain*. Toronto: University of Toronto Press, 2016.
Borsay, Anne. "Cash and Conscience: Financing the General Hospital at Bath, 1738–1750," *Social History of Medicine* 4:2 (1991): 207–29.
Burr Litchfield, Robert. *Emergence of a Bureaucracy: The Florentine Patricians, 1530–1790*. Princeton, NJ: Princeton University Press, 1986.
Cavallo, Sandra. *Charity and Power in Early Modern Italy: Benefactors and Their Motives in Turin, 1541–1789*. Cambridge: Cambridge University Press, 1995.
Fissell, Mary E. *Patients, Power, and the Poor in Eighteenth-Century Bristol*. Cambridge: Cambridge University Press, 1991.
Gavitt, Philip. *Charity and Children in Renaissance Florence: The Ospedale degli Innocenti, 1410–1536*. Ann Arbor: University of Michigan Press, 1990.
Granshaw, Lindsay and Roy Porter, eds. *The Hospital in History*. London: Routledge, 1989.

Henderson, John. *Florence Under Siege: Surviving Plague in an Early Modern City*. New Haven, CT: Yale University Press, 2019.

Horden, Peregrine and Richard Smith, eds. *The Locus of Care: Families, Communities, Institutions, and the Provision of Welfare Since Antiquity*. London: Routledge, 1998.

Labarca, Mariana. *Itineraries and Languages of Madness in the Early Modern World: Family Experience, Legal Practice, and Medical Knowledge in Eighteenth-Century Tuscany*. London and New York: Routledge, 2021.

Mellyn, Elizabeth W. *Mad Tuscans and Their Families: A History of Mental Disorder in Early Modern Italy*. Philadelphia: University of Pennsylvania Press, 2014.

Park, Katharine. *Doctors and Medicine in Early Renaissance Florence*. Princeton, NJ: Princeton University Press, 1985.

Rawcliffe, Carole. *The Hospitals of Medieval Norwich*. Norwich: Centre of East Anglian Studies, 1995.

Sneider, Matthew Thomas. "Charity and Property: The Patrimonies of Bolognese Hospitals," (PhD Dissertation, May 2004).

Stevens Crawshaw, Jane L. *Plague Hospitals: Public Health for the City in Early Modern Venice*. Burlington, VT: Ashgate, 2012.

Terpstra, Nicholas. *Abandoned Children of the Italian Renaissance: Orphan Care in Florence and Bologna*. Baltimore, MD: Johns Hopkins University Press, 2005.

———. *Cultures of Charity: Women, Politics, and the Reform of Poor Relief in Renaissance Italy*. Cambridge, MA: Harvard University Press, 2013.

———. *Lay Confraternities and Civic Religion in Renaissance Bologna*. Cambridge: Cambridge University Press, 1995.

4 Legal Records in Early Modern Spain

Carolin Schmitz

On a summer evening in 1939, barely a few months after the Spanish Civil War had come to an end, an expulsion struck the Archbishop's Palace in Alcalá de Henares, home of the then "Archivo General Central de España." The archive, considered one of the most important ones in Spain, was a centralized site for documenting Spain's administrative activities, covering a long stretch from 1493 until the end of the nineteenth century. It stored approximately 140,000 files, filling 2,460 meters of shelves, distributed across 76 rooms.[1] These documents, however, were not the only objects hosted under the Palace's roof. During the war, the building came under military control, and the ground floor was repurposed as a warehouse, workshop, and storage space for war machinery including highly inflammable substances such as gasoline, paraffin wax, turpentine, sulfuric acid, and grenades. An ill match for the masses of paper stored one story above. That children were playing with matches nearby can be seen literally as a spark to an explosive mix.[2] Added to this was a general lack of water in Alcalá de Henares due to the draught of the summer of 1939 and a strong north wind. All these factors orchestrated fatal conditions for a fire that was impossible to stop and eventually led to the total destruction of the archive, erasing evidence of a considerate part of Spain's past.

Among the documents lost in the fire were the collected records produced by the Real Tribunal del Protomedicato (Royal Tribunal of the Protomedicato). Established in 1477, the Royal Protomedicato was the Supreme Court for regulating the practice of medicine within the Spanish monarchy. As such, it examined and gave out licenses to medical practitioners, controlled their practice via inspections, and held civil and criminal jurisdiction over the members of the medical profession. Despite facing several problems in implementing its rules, especially in the areas outside of the Crown of Castile, the Protomedicato was founded to act as a centralized royal institution that, efficient or not, produced records documenting over centuries Spanish medicine in practice.[3] This is the type of legal source "par excellence" that historians since the late 1990s have relied upon to reconstruct the social and cultural side of medicine, such as the relationship between the wide array of practitioners, the medical encounters with their patients, issues of authority, legitimacy, trust, etc.

The fire in Alcalá de Henares and similar events, such as the collapse of the Cologne archive in 2009, the biggest municipal and communal archive north of

DOI: 10.4324/9781003094876-6

the Alps,[4] remind us that the archive is a fragile place and that conservation efforts over centuries can be destroyed in matters of seconds due to natural catastrophes or human negligence. And yet, the composition of the collection itself, decisions of what to preserve, who/what is worthy of being remembered, and who/what is not, can reflect long-enduring systems of power.[5]

My work on early modern Spanish medicine started with a focus on the history of the patient.[6] Because of the destruction of the General Central Archive of Spain and with it the records of the Real Tribunal del Protomedicato, it was not possible for me to follow the paths and methods of those historians that inspired me and a whole generation of scholars interested in ordinary medical practice in early modern Europe, namely Margaret Pelling, Gianna Pomata, and David Gentilcore. They all relied on coherent sets or series of legal records produced by medical tribunals, such as the Royal College of Physicians in London, the Protomedicato of Bologna, and the Protomedicato of Naples.[7] Furthermore, my aim was to recover the accounts of sick people across the social spectrum, not just limited to the relatively small elite and literate. I wanted to know why patients would choose one practitioner over another, how they understood and interpreted their illnesses, where they sought medical help, and so on. This agenda required me to locate the often hidden accounts of overlooked individuals who either were not able to write or whose writing was not deemed relevant enough to be preserved. As a result, I went on an arduous search for legal records scattered across numerous collections and archives, which involved delving into the deep ocean of the manifold records produced by the courts of justice that made up the Spanish, or more precisely, the Castilian legal system.[8] Because aspects of health and medicine were closely entangled with various social scenarios, I approached court records of those tribunals (civil, criminal, and ecclesiastical) that most people used for common concerns, rather than in medical tribunals. My hope was that I would find accounts that were closer to the patient or user/consumer perspective. While going through diverse sets of legal records, I soon realized that these sources are not only telling us important things about the history of the patient, but bring to light information on a wide and pluralistic set of medical practitioners, their practices, their interactions with other practitioners, and their reputations, as well as an array of individuals (priests, town officials, neighbors, friends, by-passers) that configured the setup of the medical encounter or the healing experience, more broadly. It was the sources themselves that showed me the need to make the complex social and communal dimension of these encounters the next focus of my research.

Now, there are numerous benefits to sources produced by tribunals that were created specifically to control medical practice and stored in one coherent collection: all cases are guaranteed to pertain to medicine, they tend to contain demographic and serial information, and it is possible to get a sense of the medical practitioners (type, number, origin) present in one place over a period of time. However, there are also important limits: medical tribunals run by physicians were not exactly impartial but rather protective of members of their professions. As a result, as Gianna Pomata shows, few physicians (and instead lower ranked barber-surgeons) were the focus of judicial attention. Meanwhile, the physician was styled as a "protector" from unskilled and ill-intended practitioners of lower social backgrounds.[9]

On the other hand, searching for relevant records within tribunals that are scattered across the Spanish legal landscape and contained in various collections is obviously more time-consuming and can often be frustrating. But working with non-medical tribunals can be rewarding, too, as their proceedings might be less steered by the concerns of one specific professional group (physicians), and instead can provide potentially a wider perspective and broader range of interests and actors.

To sum up, the challenges I am continuing to face are a combination of logistical (these records are not all stored in one archive or collection) and analytical (they are not a cohesive set of records, nor medical in nature). In what follows I'd like to provide a toolkit for responding to the overarching question: How do we do history of medicine using non-medical legal sources? In doing so, I reflect on a range of analytical strategies that informed my own work on Spanish legal records, but which in their essence can be applied to court documents from other geographies and time periods, as well. These include how to determine the function/role of different courts in society, how different courts provide different information about medicine (choosing a court/set of records depends on what sort of information you want to study), how to avoid reading cases and depositions at face value, how to get at cultural truths rather than actual truths, and how to resolve the tension between the normal versus the unusual.

How to Find Medicine in Legal Sources

Although the legal records produced at the various courts of justice differed in terms of structure, procedure, and content, all of them speak to some degree about the perspectives and realities of both practitioners and patients. The following gives a general overview of what kind of medical information can be obtained from legal records.

Information about practitioners can be mostly gathered from their defenses or interrogations, but also indirectly via the outer perspectives provided by witnesses or by documents produced as part of the legal procedure. These could include accounts of training, treatment methods, and the composition and fabrication of medicines; a view into the competition and/or collaboration with other practitioners; and inventory of the household, which in some cases lists specific items used for medical practice. Cases also can provide information about the different roles of medical experts in the legal arena, such as surgeons and apothecaries who examined bodies and substances involved in the production of evidence, the practice and lived realities of female healers (in particular in inquisitorial records), and the involvement of women as carers and collaborators in medical practice.[10] In rare cases, records include documents owned by individuals, such as licenses, or even material objects, such as a bag of herbs stitched into the inquisitorial trial against two sisters from Cuenca in 1615. Bags such as this one, carrying plants that were empowered through a certain set of rituals, were worn close to the chest and were common objects of protection against illness and other harms.[11]

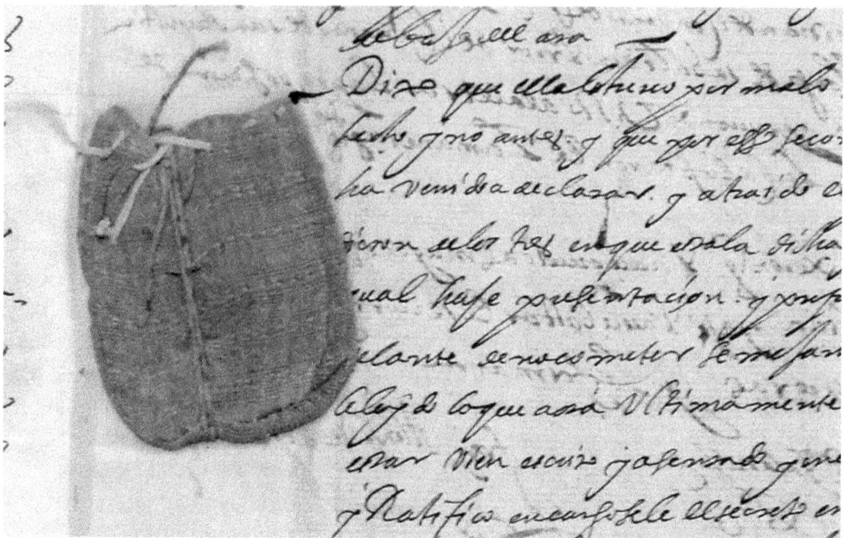

Figure 4.1 Bag with herbs stitched into inquisitorial trial record, 1615. Archivo Diocesano de Cuenca, INQUISICIÓN, Leg. 387, exp. 5498, s.f. © Obispado de Cuenca.

Accounts relevant to the patient's or sufferer's side can be retrieved mainly from the witness statements but also partly by the depositions of defendants. Together, these offer insights into exchanges between family and community members about illness and chosen therapies; how they heard about a healer's qualities or lack of skill; the effects of encounters in terms of therapeutic outcome; descriptions of treatments, including surgical procedures; assessments and actions taken before, during, and after medical encounters by family members, friends, and neighbors; the variety of spaces (taverns, inns, streets, homes) where encounters occurred; and what it meant to travel in quest of health in a largely rural society (with the help of historical maps).[12]

Legal Landscape of Spain and Characteristics of Records

No matter the cultural, geographical, or historical context, legal systems often consist of complex and overlapping hierarchies, operating on various levels. This might be confusing and tricky to navigate but it can help to have a solid understanding of the jurisdictional apparatus, knowing the competencies of different courts at different levels in theory and how jurisprudence or litigation functioned in practice. For the study of medical practice in particular, knowledge of the legal structure enables you to situate and interpret why a certain legal matter (superstitious healing practices, practicing without a license, or malpractice) is handled by one court or another, and what implications the legal conditions of a particular tribunal can have for the social lives of practitioners and patients. In the following, I discuss some of the particularities of the Castilian legal system, by way of example, to show how the different characteristics of courts provide different information about medicine, both in content and detail.

The Royal Protomedicato

With the existence of a royal tribunal specifically designed to control and oversee the practice of medicine within the Spanish monarchy, one might think that the aforementioned Tribunal of the Protomedicato would be the first and perhaps exclusive port of call where people would take their medical matters. However, this was far from the case. There are different reasons for this, but mainly it was due to the fact that the civil and penal jurisdiction it had over the members of the medical profession was limited to a defined geographic area, namely to the royal court and four leguas (about 20 km) surrounding it, and to a defined group of professionals who for most of the time included only physicians, barber-surgeons, and apothecaries. Nonetheless, it is important to account for the function of the Protomedicato as a medical regulatory board because it explains the existence of medical-related trials in other courts, as well as the Protomedicato's interconnection with those courts. Throughout the early modern period, the Protomedicato examined and licensed all medical practitioners across the Spanish peninsula. This exclusive right for examining meant that all aspiring medical practitioners, no matter from which corner of Spain and how distant from the court, had to travel to Madrid to take the exam and be granted a license by the Protomedicato. This was not very feasible in practice and as a result prompted numerous trials against those that practiced medicine without a license in civil and criminal courts on all levels. Furthermore, members of the Protomedicato also carried out inspections of apothecary shops and paid regular visits to more distant localities to ensure their regulations were implemented.[13] In addition, frequently published royal decrees did not cease to remind local communities and municipal authorities of their obligation to abide by the rules of practice established by the Protomedicato. It is therefore not surprising that other courts of justice, such as the Inquisition or civil and criminal courts, referred to the Protomedicato or cooperated with it, making its presence and demands appear interwoven with other tribunals of the Spanish legal landscape. Because of the limits in jurisdiction and also the feasibility of following the dictated rules of the Tribunal of the Protomedicato, matters related to medicine and practice ended up being taken to all sorts of courts, discussed below.

Criminal and Civil Courts

Civil and criminal courts on all levels adjudicated on regular medical practitioners as common individuals who in some way or other allegedly broke the law. Most cases involved lower ranked practitioners, such as surgeons, barbers, and bloodletters, but physicians and apothecaries appeared, as well. The offences were diverse, some specific to the profession, others concerned with general unlawful conduct.

Records in these courts provide information about breaches of professional boundaries, in most cases practicing medicine or surgery without a license, malpractice and negligence, late payments, fights, disobedience toward civil authorities, and slander and dishonorable behavior (drinking, sexual assault, etc).

Church Courts

In Spain, as in other Catholic regions, the church maintained a dense network of ordinary church courts which remain underexplored for questions of health and medicine. These diocesan or episcopal (bishop's) courts were accessible and imposed cheap trial fees, and litigated everyday issues, such as marital, financial, romantic, and spiritual disputes.[14] They also served as criminal tribunals adjudicating on infanticide and abortion cases, one of several areas for which medical practitioners, including midwives, were hired as expert witnesses. Higher ranked archbishop courts contain canonization trials of healing saints, which also involved the expertise of medical personnel.[15] Health professionals did not just appear in supporting roles but also could figure as the accused. Edward Behrend Martinez, for example, tells us about a surgeon who was prosecuted by the church court in Calahorra in 1743 "for stealing a woman's corpse so he could practice dissecting it in the local church."[16]

The Spanish Inquisition

The Tribunal of the Holy Office of the Inquisition, although an ecclesiastical tribunal, was under direct control of the Spanish monarch. It was the only institution with jurisdiction across all kingdoms of the Spanish monarchy, including the Americas.[17] With its permanently installed local tribunals, the Inquisition was preoccupied with control over the correct exercise of the Catholic faith and with suppressing heresy. It can include cases involving medical practitioners suspected of incorporating superstitious or heretical elements in their treatments, or in fact any individual engaging in unorthodox health practices. Therefore, the forms of medical practice contained in these proceedings lie primarily within what are usually called "irregular" forms of healing carried out by wise-men and wise-women, herbalists, bonesetters, or ordinary people who had not received formal credentials or official training and frequently combined empirical knowledge with (unorthodox) spiritual or magic rituals. A peculiarity of the inquisitorial records is a section contained in the first hearings of the accused called "Discurso de su vida" – literally curriculum vitae – in which the defendant was asked to provide an overview of the main steps in her/his life leading up to imprisonment. This offers a rare occasion to recover biographies of otherwise undocumented healers, including their upbringing, trajectory (mobility), and training.

The Inquisition differs in its legal procedure from the other courts (both secular and ordinary church courts) mainly due to its secret operation. This means that neither the accused nor the witnesses knew the charge they were being accused of or questioned about. As a result, the inquisitors approached witnesses and defendants with general questions, as opposed to specific questions, as in secular courts.

These open-ended questions could result in lengthy narrations filled with details that exceeded the interest of the inquisitors but prove to be vital for social historians of medicine.

To illustrate the different nature of records, dependent in which court they were produced, here are two witness testimonies, one stemming from a local criminal court, the other from a local tribunal of the Inquisition.

Figure 4.2 is a witness testimony from 1626 given by the patient Gabriel Diaz, in a trial against the barber Joan de Tolossa from Navahermosa (Toledo) who is accused of practicing surgery without a license.[18] The court record was produced by the so-called fiel del juzgado, a Toledo-based judge with jurisdiction over the Montes de Toledo, a mountainous region south of the city. A model of rural justice, this regional court adjudicated criminal and civil matters and is exceptional in conserving series of first-instance criminal causes that are held today in the Archivo Municipal de Toledo.[19]

Criminal law trial: Archivo Municipal de Toledo, AMT, C. 6213, exp. 146. Trial against Joan de Tolosa, 1626, Navahermosa. Witness: Gabriel Diaz, 46 years old.

> In the place of Navahermosa, on the said day, month and year, the said Alonso de Alfaro, in continuation of his commission, made Gabriel Diaz, neighbor of the said place, appear before him, from whom he took and received an oath by God our Lord by a sign of the cross, promising to tell the truth, and when asked about the said accusation, he said that he knows that the said Joan Alvarez de Tolossa has worked as a barber in this said place since he came to it more than a year and a half ago and he does not know if he is examined or not; and he knows this because he has seen him use and exercise it and it is public and notorious; in July of last year his urine was withheld and he went to the said Joan Alvarez to beg him for some remedy so that he could urinate because he had been unable to do so from morning till late in the evening when the sun was about to set. And the barber went to the house of this witness and with a pair of pliers he took out part of a stone that was stuck in the pipe and natural way of the urine, and seeing that he could not finish taking it out, he opened the pipe with a tool that he took out of his case, breaking it and taking out the rest of the said stone, and then he urinated without any impediment whatsoever. And the barber put on the wound an egg white and tow and in 4 days he was well and healed because the wound was small. He knows that Joan Alvarez also cured Pedro Gonzalez of a very dangerous wound in the head and healed it briefly.
>
> En el lugar de Navahermosa, a días mes y año dicho, el dicho Alonso de Alfaro, en continuación de su comisión hizo parecer ante sí a Gabriel Diaz, vecino deste dicho lugar del qual tomó y recivió juramento por dios nuestro Señor por una señal de cruz prometió dezir la verdad y preguntado por la dicha acusasión, dixo que save que el dicho Joan Alvarez de Tolossa hace officio de varvero en este dicho lugar desde que vino a el que [h]abrá más de año y medio e no save si está examinado o no; y lo save por se le [h]aver

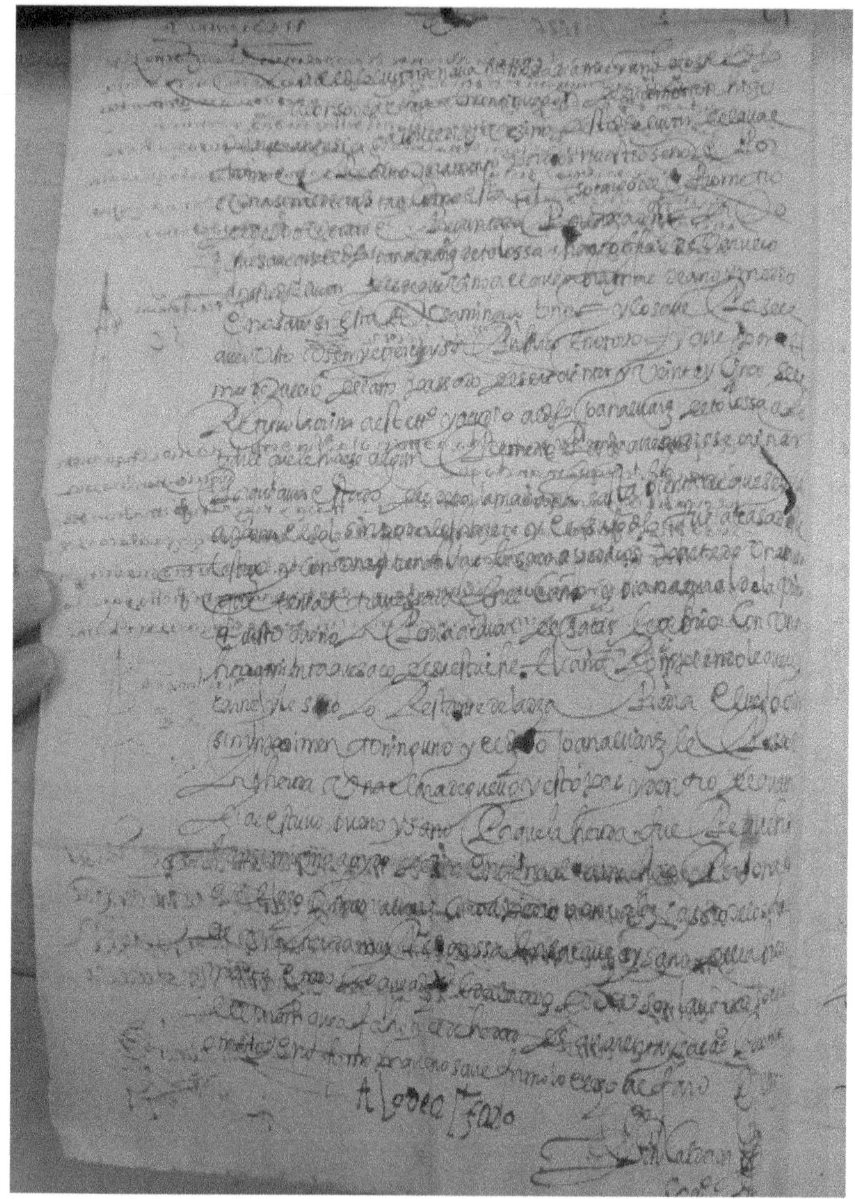

Figure 4.2 Witness testimony by Gabriel Diaz. Part of criminal trial against barber Joan de Tolosa, 1626, Navahermosa, Archivo Municipal de Toledo, AMT, C. 6213, exp. 146.

visto ussar y exercer y ser público y notorio; y que por el mes de julio del año passado de setecientos y veinte y cinco se le retuvo la orina a este testigo y acudió al dicho Joan Alvarez a rogarle que le hiciese algún remedio para

> que pudiese orinar porque [h]avía estado desde por la mañana hasta bien tarde que se iba a poner el sol sin poderla hacer. Y el varvero fue a casa deste testigo y con unas tenayas le sacó a pedazos parte de una piedra que tenía atravesado en el caño y via natural de la urina y visto que no podía acavar de sacar, le abrió con una herramienta que sacó de su estuche el caño rompiéndole que contienne y le sacó lo restante de la dicha piedra y luego orinó sin impedimiento ninguno. Y el varvero le puso en la herida una clara de guevo y estopas y dentro de 4 días estuvo bueno y sanó porque la herida fue pequeña. Sabe que Joan Alvarez también curó a Pedro Gonzalez de una herida muy peligrosa en la cabeza y sanó della brevemente.

This is a short witness statement, covering barely one page, and written in the third person. It is the patient himself giving testimony about the successful removal of a bladder stone performed by the unlicensed barber on trial. Despite being brief, it is a valuable account of a surgical intervention, precisely because it comes from the perspective of the patient, something we rarely get from other medical sources like casebooks. It provides otherwise difficult to obtain information, such as that the intervention took place at the patient's home rather than the barber shop, which, as we know from another witness, the barber was running in town. It is proof of the barber's dexterity and resourcefulness from the patient's point of view. We also learn about post-intervention care and the patient's explanation of his quick recovery (four days), which the patient understands to be due to the barber taking care in keeping the wound small.

Figure 4.3 is an excerpt from a longer witness testimony of a barber's wife who testified on the treatment her husband received by the healer Magdalena María Giménez in Villanueva de la Jara (Cuenca), who was accused by the Inquisition in 1695 of engaging in superstitious healing practices.[20] The trial record is part of the ample collection of original trial proceedings of the local tribunal of the Inquisition in Cuenca, stored today in the diocesan archive of the same town.

Local inquisitorial trial: Archivo Diocesano de Cuenca, Legajo 557, exp. 6950. Trial against Magdalena María Giménez, Villanueva de la Jara, 1695. Witness: María Escobar, wife of Antonio de Espinosa, barber, 40 years old.

/fol. 5r/

> Asked if she knows or presumes the cause for which she is called?
>
> She said that she presumes it will be to find out from her what happened in her house with Magdalena María, wife of Manuel Lovaz, a cutter and innkeeper /fol. 5v/ in the said town, as it seemed to this witness that what she saw done in her presence was wrong. [...] She said that her husband is suffering from a very protracted illness of tertian fever more than seven months ago in which he has been given different remedies of the [realm of] Medicine and that with none he has had improvement and that many people had told him that it was the evil eye, to which her husband told them to go with God [get out of here], that it was what his Lordship had chosen that he suffered from and that he did not have the evil eye, that it was humbug [patarata]; and

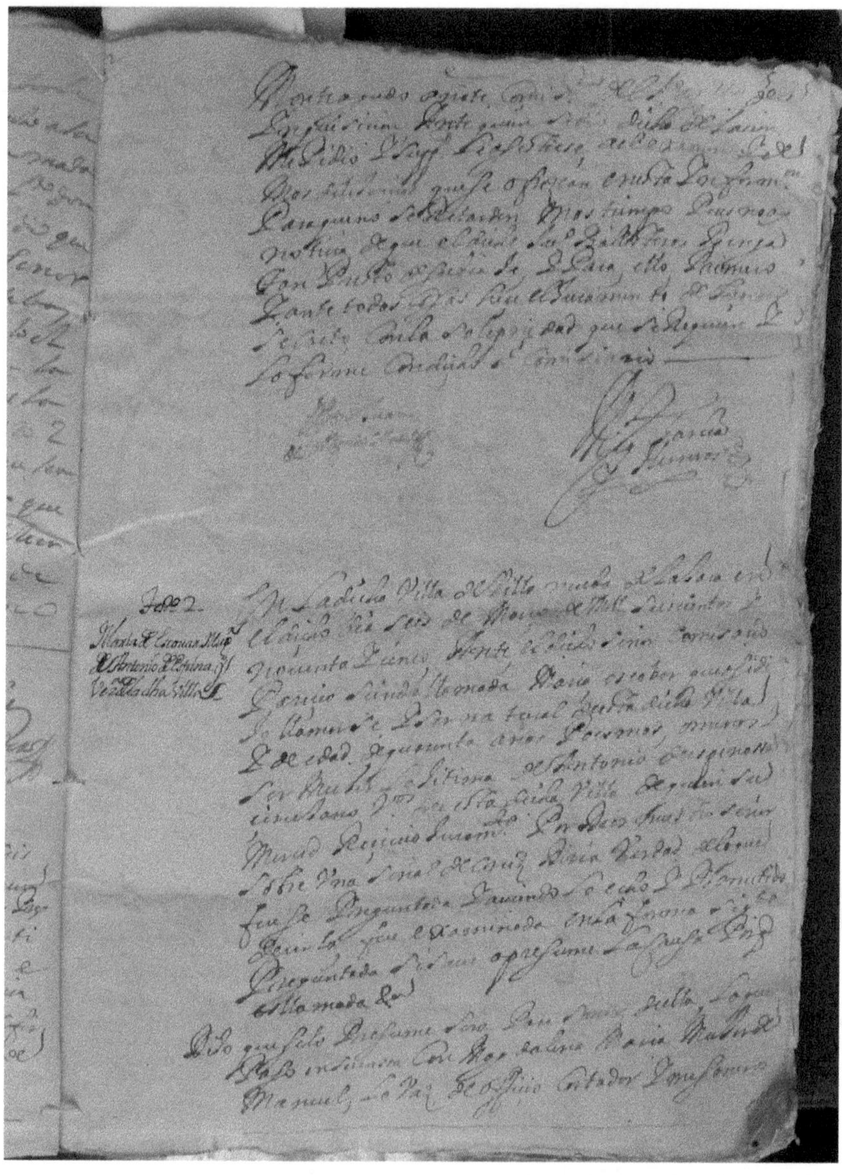

Figure 4.3 Witness testimony by María Escobar, wife of the barber Antonio de Espinosa. Part of inquisitorial trial against Magdalena María Giménez, 1695, Villanueva de la Jara, Archivo Diocesano de Cuenca, INQUISICIÓN, Leg. 557, exp. 6950. © Obispado de Cuenca.

that on one occasion a woman came in who she does not remember who she was, speaking of the protracted illness of the said husband and saying how she had told him that it was the evil eye and that he did not want to be blessed [santiguar],[21] the person said to her, 'for in the inn there is a woman who has grace for that, because a boy of Pasqual's was with a great fever [...] and as soon as he entered she [...]said, 'you have the evil eye and you have given it to me', and she blessed him, and she gave him a cloth [filled with medicinal ingredients] and the next day he was well'; and with the desire that this witness had for her husband to be well, she told him the case and persuaded him to call her and said her husband did not want to and told to this witness and Maria Espinossa, his mother, that they were going to lose in that: 'So that you may be disenchanted and find out that it is humbug [patarata], and that there is no evil eye, bring her in and you will see what happens'. /fol. 6r/ This witness asked through María Solera, wife of Pedro Donate, neighbors of this town, that she [Magdalena María, the healer] came to her house and having entered the room the said Magdalena María passed her hand on the head of the said Antonio Espinossa and said to him that it is the evil eye and well afflicted and she ordered them to bring her a dish with a little bit of water, and the said Magdalena María, having been brought the dish with the water, put her hand into a scribble candle [from where] she took out and poured into the said dish some drops [of oil], which sank to the floor of the dish, and from the said drops of oil a little serpent was formed with its head, tail, hands and feet; to which the said Magdalena María said, to the formation of the said serpent, 'See here, your mercies, the evil eye. Do you see the serpent? Well, this is the evil eye'; to which Juan de Alarcón, son of Martín de Alarcón, deceased, and María de Luna, a resident of this town, and María García Espinossa, mother of the said Antonio Espinossa were present, and it seems to her that the said María Solera, wife of the said Father Donate, was so as well; and having done all the aforementioned, she [Magdalena María, the healer] put a cloth filled with egg white, red vinegar and spirits[aguardiente] on her husband's head, which he took off as soon as she left and threw it away. And at the time of placing the cloth she said a prayer and heard her say some words in the name of the Father and of the Son and of the Holy Spirit, and of the Virgin and that she saw her doing blessings and to the water in the dish as well [...].

/fol. 5r/

Preguntada si save o presume la causa por que es llamada?

Dijo que se lo presume será para saber de ella lo que pasó en su cassa con Magdalena María, Mujer de Manuel Lovaz, de officio Cortador y mesonero / fol. 5v/ en esta dicha Villa, pues a esta testigo le pareció mal lo que vido açer en su presencia. [...] Dijo que su marido está padeciendo una enfermedad mui prolija de tercianas, más [h]a de siete meses en la qual se le [h]an [h] echo diferentes remedios de la Medicina y que con ninguno [h]a tenido mejoría y que muchas personas le [h]avían dicho que era mal de ojo, a lo qual su marido los decía que se fuesen con Dios que era lo que su Magestad era servido de que padeciese y que no [h]avía mal de ojo, que era Patarata y que en una ocasión entró una mujer que no se acuerda quien era [h]ablando de la prolija enfermedad del dicho su marido y diciendo como le [h]avía dicho que era mal de ojo y que no quería que lo santiguaran, le dijo la persona, 'pues en el mesón ay una mujer que tiene gracia para eso, porque un muchacho de Pasqual estava con una grande calentura y lo hicieron y así como entró se le enpeçó a abrir la boca y dijo, 'tu traes mal de ojo y a mí me lo [h]as pegado', y lo santiguó, y le echó una estopada y a otro día estava bueno', y con el deseo que esta testigo tenía de que su marido estubiese bueno, le contó el caso y le persuadió a que la llamara y dicho su marido no quería y les dijo a las instancias que le aciere[¿] esta testigo y María Espinossa su madre diciéndole que yva[iba] a perder en eso: 'Pues para que vmd se desengañen y sepan que es pa- /fol. 6r/ tarata y que no [h]ay mal de ojo traíganla y verán lo que sucede', y esta testigo solicitó por medio de María Solera, mujer de Pedro Donate, vecinos desta Villa, que fuera a su casa como con efecto fue y [h]aviendo entrado en el aposento la dicha Magdalena María le pasó la mano en la caveça al dicho Antonio Espinossa y le dijo 'y como que es mal de ojo y vien araygado' y mandó que la trajeren un plato con una poca de agua y la dicha Magdalena María, [h]aviendo traido el plato con el agua, entró la mano en un candel de garavato[garabato] y [h]aviendole entrado en el açeyte sacó y echó en el dicho plato unas gotas, las quales se [h]undieron al suelo del plato y se formó de las dichas gotas de açeyte una sierpecilla con su caveça, cola, manos y pies, a lo qual dijo la dicha Magdalena María, a la formación de la dicha sierpe 'Vean aquí vm. el mal de ojo. Ven Vm. la sierpe? Pues este es el mal de ojo' = a lo qual se [h]allaron presentes Juan de Alarcón, hijo de Martín de Alarcón, difunto y María de Luna, vecina de esta Villa, María García Espinossa, madre del dicho Antonio Espinossa, y le parece que tan vien estava la dicha María Solera, mujer del dicho Padre Donate, y [h]aviendo [h]echo todo lo referido le echó al dicho su marido la susodicha una estopada de clara de guebo, vinagre rosado y aguardiente en la caveça, el qual se lo quitó luego que se fue y la tiró: Y que al tiempo del ponerla, reçava y le oía decir algunas palabras en el nombre del Padre y del hijo y del espiritu santo, y de la virjen y que veía [h]açer Bendiciones y al agua del plato tan vien [...].

The open-ended question employed in the inquisitorial trial ("if she knows or presumes the cause for which she is called?") led his wife to enter a lengthy narration of the event, covering over five pages, including contextual information about how they discovered the healer, who mediated and initiated the encounter, the differing attitudes toward spiritual forms of healing and belief in the evil eye within one family, the various sites for the healer's practice (inn, domestic spaces), the exact sequences of the ritual, and who was present. Not just the barber himself but also each of the other individuals mentioned in this testimony were called to testify and gave similarly long and dense descriptions of the event, which are in most parts nearly identical to the barber's wife's version of the story.

It was not just the competency of the courts, but also their rank within the legal hierarchy that gave shape to the information and level of detail contained in each type of testimony. On the lower scale, municipal and local tribunals often served as the first instance and are characteristic for containing the original witness testimonies in full length, more detailed information on the circumstances of the initial accusation, and the hearings of the accused, which is where most of the specifics on medicine and health are found. However, many of these original court records have been lost or were never stored.[22] The immediacy and richness of details of local or first instance is often absent in the trial proceedings of higher instances, which instead relied on summaries of the arguments for distant judges to make their verdicts, sometimes years down the line. This also applies to inquisitorial records: of the numerous local tribunals, only those of Cuenca, Toledo, and Canarias have preserved most of their original trial records. For the other tribunals, to a great extent, only the annual summaries (las relaciones de causas) have survived. While the latter can offer important hints of information, they lack the rich details of the original trial proceedings. Ironically, some of the appeal courts, such as the Real Chancillerías,[23] often include litigations (or copies thereof) that occurred at various previous stages and levels, making it possible to reconstruct how the parties litigated up to the highest authority. This also means that in reconstructing the pathway of litigation in a reverse direction, it is sometimes possible to gain access to otherwise lost first-instance court proceedings that occurred at the lowest, local level.

Limitations and Problems with Legal Records and How to Overcome Them

If handled and approached with caution, reading the proceedings can feel like a journey into an intimate network of relatives, neighbors, friends, and villagers or parishioners who shared spaces and experiences in their quest for health. To make sense of these relations and connections to each other and the medical practices that were performed is part of the analytical work of using these sources.

One of the greatest values of legal records is that they make it possible to read the words of those who otherwise left no written words behind: commoners, working men and women, servants, and shepherds. However, what we read is not exactly "their" words, but words that were mediated and transmitted through various factors. It is important to be aware that many elements could influence and determine the depositions presented to the court, such as the intimidating and coercive situation of the interrogation, the different interests behind a complaint or a testimony, or the existence of several voices in the transcribed testimonies – the witnesses themselves, interrogators' guidelines, and the notaries' filters that could give (linguistic) form and coherence to an oral account.[24] Scribes sometimes used formulaic language or condensed or omitted details when recording testimony. At times, the particular form of speech (dialect, speed, vocabulary, self-corrections) might be omitted from the record. Or individuals might be cautious about how to frame or present a certain situation in front of a particular court.

Rather than accessing a legal truth about a particular issue, I am interested in using legal records to get at "cultural truth."[25] First, it is important to be aware of whether depositions were produced under duress or by choice. This matters because the motives and circumstances are so diverse that it is impossible to assess the veracity of accounts, which is why we cannot read cases at face value. Second, it is difficult to resolve contradictions that arise not only between the accusers and the accused but also between different testimonies. Therefore, my approach has not been to try to ascertain the degree of "truthfulness" they contain. Instead, I have chosen to filter out the common elements and plausible data that allow me to develop a coherent reconstruction of what happened. In other words, it is not "reality" that I aim to reveal, but the probability and likelihood of having carried out a given health practice in a given place and at a given historical moment. This probability increases progressively with the repetition of similar cases. The previous source excerpt of the evil eye is a good example of this. I have no interest in ascertaining whether the surgeon or his wife actually believed in the existence of the evil eye, or even in the healing powers of the woman healer, or whether she presented a serpent as the evil eye to her audience. What is relevant for the social history of medicine is the likelihood of the event at all and the circumstantial details that allow us to sketch a picture of what an encounter between a female healer, an ill surgeon, and his family would have looked like.

Another challenge is that these sources were produced through conflicts, which make it tricky to distinguish the exceptional from the normal.[26] Is what we read, for example, about a female bonesetter's use of dragon's blood to make a topical remedy called a plaster an unusual or common practice? [27] In other words, is this an experience shared by a few or by many? In following the approach of other scholars who have worked with judicial records, I tend to contextualize specific cases with external, often printed sources.[28] In particular, when it comes to understanding the principle behind a certain medical practice or technique, individualized remedies such as pills or plasters, or assessing the commonality of ingredients, reading contemporary printed medical and surgical texts can be immensely helpful. As for the bonesetter's case, a look into surgical literature of the time suggests that dragon's blood was not as unorthodox as it sounds, but a type of red resin from the Drago tree (Dracaena), a common ingredient in plasters that helped bring dislocated joints back into place.[29]

But referring to print is not always possible, especially when it comes to patients' behaviors or irregular practices that do not fit within the canon of official medicine. Let us take for example the practice of bringing a lock of a patient's hair to a healer to be blessed or diagnosed. In this case, I resort to gathering as many similar case studies as possible, which allows me to develop a sense of the commonality of the practice. This particular method of medicine-by-proxy, I have found within eight different places in the inquisitorial records, widely dispersed over the region of Cuenca between 1630 and 1746.[30] In this way, even without the possibility to contextualize certain behaviors using external sources, collecting similar cases can elucidate the relationship between the "exceptional" and the "normal" within the same type of source.

Accessing Handwritten Legal Records and Logistics of Archival Work

In general, working with witness testimonies involves lots of reading and often extraneous, irrelevant information. Once you have detected a useful case, the first step is to make the handwriting legible by transcribing as much of it as possible or necessary. Statements can have changing handwriting, depending on scribes and regional differences or changes over time (they tend to be more tidy toward the latter part of the seventeenth century). The second step is (re-)organizing the file, as sometimes the file itself is not sorted chronologically. This is a particular challenge of records from appeal courts or higher courts containing various stages of a trial. Sorting the case according to the chronology of events, or, when more cases are combined, to establish which document was produced in which court of justice at which time, is an important step to disentangle the complexities of an overlapping court system. It is not always clear whether the structure of the court record reflects the natural compilation of papers, or if it is a result of moving archives in politically challenged situations (after the abolition of the Inquisition), or an archivist's attempt to structure the documents.

The third step is to map out the information. Because some individuals are repeatedly mentioned in statements and witnesses are mentioned by other witnesses in their testimonies, it is crucial to understand the connections between everyone involved. This can be achieved by creating hand-drawn mind maps that visually represent and sort the interconnected information in the testimonies. This step of the process shares elements of detective's work and it is exciting to see the interrelated map evolve and come together.

When it comes to the actual logistics of working in an archive, the way the archive has cataloged their records is vital to accessing documents. Cataloging is an ongoing activity, producing differing results and formats that range from online databases to internal digital catalogs to published books and even outdated but still existent catalog cards in wooden drawers. An important piece is the descriptions of records in catalogs. Especially when searching for medical practitioners, it is extremely helpful when the profession of those involved in a lawsuit is mentioned. But this is not always the case, and often it can be a long road to assembling a set of relevant records.

If you are working on Spanish records, a good place to start is the Portal of Archivos Españoles (PARES). This is an extensive network of public archives, including descriptions and digitized images of records, that is free to access. In addition to PARES, many of the archives holding legal records, such as the Chancillería de Valladolid and Granada, have their own databases, sometimes accessible online, other times only via the archives' internal computers. In any case, always contact the archive in advance to inquire about modes of operating (available databases, working hours, how many records can you order at once/during the day, reproduction policy and if fees apply for taking pictures).

Your chosen set of records will determine the research questions and approach, which can be highly dependent on accessibility and practicality. Yet, even more than the level of cataloging and digitization, the personal involvement of archivists can make visits to the archive not just pleasant but extraordinary and memorable. Let me close with a personal anecdote. A few minutes before 11 am, the archivist of the Archivo Diocesano de Cuenca, a priest named Don Marcelino who occasionally smoked next to the window, made his daily announcement that it was time for the "almuerzo" (extended coffee break), entrusting the archive to the visitors staying behind for 45 minutes. Others (including myself) followed the invitation to coffee, where we chatted over research interests, particular cases, and personal matters, which facilitated the exchange of references to legal cases and ultimately access to the sources. The sources are relevant, but so are the people running the archive and the personal connections established between other visiting scholars within the reading rooms and outside of it, which can sometimes be the starting point for long-lasting scholarly friendships.

Notes

1 Rafael Fraguas, Cinco siglos de desmemoria | Madrid | EL PAÍS (elpais.com), El Archivo Central, que guardaba miles de documentos, ardió en el palacio arzobispal de Alcalá hace 70 años, 11 August 2009. See also, Luis Palop and María Carrillo Tundidor (eds.), *De Palacio a Casa de los Arqueólogos. Pasado y futuro del Palacio Arzobispal de Alcalá de Henares* (Madrid: Comunidad de Madrid, 2019).

2 Manuel Romero Tallafigo, "Archivo General Central de Alcalá de Henares (1939) y el del Reino de Nápoles (1943). Los grandes archivos pueden morir," *Boletín ANABAD LXVI* 2 (2016): 201–26.

3 María Luz López Terrada, "The Control of Medical Practice under the Spanish Monarchy during the Sixteenth and Seventeenth Centuries," in Víctor Navarro Brotóns and William Eamon (eds.), *Más allá de la Leyenda Negra: España y la Revolución Científica* (Valencia: Universitat de Valencia, 2007), pp. 283–94; María Soledad Campos Díez, *El Real Tribunal del Protomedicato castellano, siglos XIV–XIX* (Cuenca: Ediciones de la Universidad Castilla-La Mancha, 1999).

4 "Why did the Cologne city archive collapse?" Interview with Bettina Schmidt-Czaia, *The Guardian*, 27 March 2009. https://www.theguardian.com/world/2009/mar/27/germany-cologne.

5 Michel-Rolph Trouillot, *Silencing the Past: Power and the Production of History* (Boston: Beacon Press, 1995).

6 Carolin Schmitz, *Los enfermos en la España barroca y el pluralismo médico. Espacios, estrategias, actitudes* (Madrid: Consejo Superior de Investigaciones Científicas, 2018).

7 Margaret Pelling, *Medical Conflicts in Early Modern London: Patronage, Physicians, and Irregular Practitioners 1550–1640* (Oxford: Clarendon Press, 2003); Gianna Pomata, *Contracting a Cure. Patients, Healers and the Law in Early Modern Bologna* (Baltimore, MD: The Johns Hopkins University Press, 1998); David Gentilcore, *Healers and Healing in Early Modern Italy* (Manchester: Manchester University Press, 1998).

8 Important differences marked the two crowns that compounded the Spanish monarchy – the Crown of Castile and the Crown of Aragon – even beyond the political centralization culminating in the *Decreto de Nueva Planta* (1713). As the complexities involved also impacted greatly the way how the control of medical practice was organized, I decided to first focus on the more populous Crown of Castile. López Terrada, "The Control of Medical Practice." For recent research on legal records from the Crown of Aragon, see Carmel Ferragud and Mariluz López Terrada, "Despejando las

sospechas. Informes medicos en los tribunales de justicia de la comarca de la Ribera del Júcar (ss. XVI y XVII)," *Dynamis*, 38, 1 (2018): 65–86.

9 Pomata, *Contracting a Cure.*

10 Carolin Schmitz and María Luz López Terrada, "Healing across Ideological Boundaries in Late Seventeenth-Century Madrid," in Margaret E. Boyle and Sarah E. Owens (eds.), *Health and Healing in the Early Modern Iberian World: A Gendered Perspective* (Toronto: Toronto University Press, 2021), pp. 21–51.

11 Inquisitorial trial against Juana y Juliana, daughters of Catalina López, Cuenca, 1615. Archivo Diocesano de Cuenca, Leg. 387, exp. 5498. Schmitz, *Los enfermos*, pp. 208–10.

12 Carolin Schmitz, "Travelling for Health: Local and Regional Mobility of Patients in Early Modern Rural Spain," Paul Nelles and Rosa Salzberg (eds.), *Connected Mobilities in the Early Modern World: The Practice and Experience of Movement* (Amsterdam: Amsterdam University Press, 2023), pp. 87–110.

13 Outside the Crown of Castilia, these inspections, however, were met increasingly with backlashes from local authorities, prompted by the unwillingness to tolerate the interference of a royal (Castilian) institution.

14 Edward Behrend-Martinez, "Episcopal Courts in Iberia, Italy and Latin America," in Charles H. Parker and Gretchen Starr-LeBeau (eds.*), Judging Faith, Punishing Sin: Inquisitions and Consistories in the Early Modern World* (Cambridge: Cambridge University Press, 2017), pp. 77–88. With regard to annulment of marriage due to health reasons (impotence), see Edward Behrend-Martinez, *Unfit for Marriage: Impotent Spouses on Trial in the Basque Region of Spain 1650–1750* (Reno: University of Nevada Press, 2007).

15 Laura Guinot, *Mujeres y Santidad: Sanadoras por mediación divina. Un estudio desde la microhistoria (siglos XVII y XVIII)* (Granada: Comares Editorial, 2021).

16 Behrend-Martinez, "Episcopal Courts," p. 81. The archival reference of the case is Archivo Catedralicio y Diocesano de Calahorra, Legajo 23/25–21, Treviño, 1743.

17 Henry Kamen, *The Spanish Inquisition: A Historical Revision*. Fourth Edition (New Haven, CT: Yale University Press, 2014); Francisco Bethencourt, *The Inquisition. A Global History, 1478–1834* (Cambridge: Cambridge University Press, 2009).

18 Schmitz, *Los enfermos*, 97–102.

19 Alfredo Rodríguez González, *Justicia y criminalidad en Toledo y sus Montes en la Edad Moderna* (Toledo: Consorcio de Toledo, Ayuntamiento, 2009).

20 Schmitz, *Los enfermos*, pp. 114–17.

21 "Santiguar, to Bless, properly as a Priest, a Bishop, or a Father, and making a sign of the Cross. But there are also cheating old Women, and Knavish Fellows, who pretend to have particular Blessings to cure sick People, and those impose upon the Ignorant". John Stevens, *A New Spanish and English Dictionary. Collected from the Best Spanish Authors Both Ancient and Modern [...]*(London: George Sawbridge, 1706), p. 349, 3.

22 Richard L. Kagan, *Lawsuits and Litigants in Castile, 1500–1700* (Chapel Hill: The University of North Carolina Press, 1981).

23 The *Real Chancillerías* were royal appeal courts, one based in Valladolid and the other in Granada, representing geographical division of the Crown of Castile in a northern and southern district.

24 Elizabeth Cohen, "She Said, He Said: Situated Oralities in Judicial Records from Early Modern Rome," *Journal of Early Modern History* 16 (2012): 403–30.

25 I am developing here the idea put forward by Louise Nyholm Kallestrup: "The construction of the accused and the accusation were closely linked to ideas of how certain individuals or groups behaved. When denouncing a person, an accuser may have made up stories about the suspect, but these stories were necessarily full of cultural truths; they needed to be plausible in order to convince the judge." Louise Nyholm Kallestrup, *Agents of Witchcraft in Early Modern Italy and Denmark* (Basingstoke: Palgrave, 2015), p. 8.

26 On the exceptional normal see Carlo Ginzburg, "Micro-History: Two or Three Things That I Know About It," *Critical Inquiry* 20 (1993): 33.
27 The bonesetter Mariana Pérez was practicing on the road between Burgos and Cuenca in the 1650s, ADC, Leg. 496, exp. 6592.
28 Cathy McClive, *Menstruation and Procreation in Early Modern France* (Farnham and Burlington: Ashgate 2015), pp. 15–17.
29 Andrés Tamayo, *Tratados breves de Algebra y Garrotillo. Por el Licenciado Andrés de Tamayo, Médico y Cirujano, hijo del Licenciado Tamayo, Cirujano de su Magestad* (Madrid, 1621), 16v, reprinted in Juan Calvo's famous *Primera y segunda parte de la Cirugía universal* (Valencia, 1690).
30 Schmitz, "Travelling for Health," p. 93.

Bibliography

Behrend-Martinez, Edward, "Episcopal Courts in Iberia, Italy and Latin America." In *Judging Faith, Punishing Sin: Inquisitions and Consistories in the Early Modern World*, edited by Charles H. Parker and Gretchen Starr-LeBeau, 77–88. Cambridge: Cambridge University Press, 2017.

Behrend-Martinez, Edward, *Unfit for Marriage: Impotent Spouses on Trial in the Basque Region of Spain 1650–1750*. Reno: University of Nevada Press, 2007.

Bethencourt, Francisco. *The Inquisition. A Global History, 1478–1834*. Cambridge and New York: Cambridge University Press, 2009.

Calvo, Juan. *Primera y segunda parte de la Cirugía universal*. Valencia, 1690.

Campos Díez, María Soledad. *El Real Tribunal del Protomedicato castellano, siglos XIV–XIX*. Cuenca: Ediciones de la Universidad Castilla-La Mancha, 1999.

Cohen, Elizabeth. "She Said, He Said: Situated Oralities in Judicial Records from Early Modern Rome." *Journal of Early Modern History*, 16 (2012): 403–30.

Ferragud, Carmel and Mariluz López Terrada. "Despejando las sospechas. Informes médicos en los tribunales de justicia de la comarca de la Ribera del Júcar (ss. XVI y XVII)." *Dynamis* 38 (2018): 65–86.

Fraguas, Rafael. "Cinco siglos de desmemoria." *El País*, August 11, 2009, www.elpais.com. [accessed: January 15, 2023].

Gentilcore, David. *Healers and Healing in Early Modern Italy*. Manchester: Manchester University Press, 1998.

Ginzburg, Carlo. "Micro-History: Two or Three Things That I Know About It." *Critical Inquiry* 20 (1993): 33.

Guinot, Laura. *Mujeres y Santidad: Sanadoras por mediación divina. Un estudio desde la microhistoria (siglos XVII y XVIII)*. Granada: Comares Editorial, 2021.

Kagan, Richard L. *Lawsuits and Litigants in Castile, 1500–1700*. Chapel Hill: The University of North Carolina Press, 1981.

Kallestrup, Louise Nyholm. *Agents of Witchcraft in Early Modern Italy and Denmark*. Basingstoke: Palgrave, 2015.

Kamen, Henry. *The Spanish Inquisition: A Historical Revision*. Fourth Edition. New Haven, CT: Yale University Press, 2014.

López Terrada, María Luz. "The Control of Medical Practice under the Spanish Monarchy during the Sixteenth and Seventeenth Centuries." In *Más allá de la Leyenda Negra: España y la Revolución Científica*, edited by Víctor Navarro Brotóns and William Eamon, 283–94. Valencia: Universitat de Valencia, 2007.

McClive, Cathy. *Menstruation and Procreation in Early Modern France*. Farnham: Ashgate, 2015.

Palop, Luis and María Carrillo Tundidor, eds. *De Palacio a Casa de los Arqueólogos. Pasado y futuro del Palacio Arzobispal de Alcalá de Henares*. Madrid: Comunidad de Madrid, 2019.

Pelling, Margaret. *Medical Conflicts in Early Modern London: Patronage, Physicians, and Irregular Practitioners 1550–1640*. Oxford: Clarendon Press, 2003.

Pomata, Gianna. *Contracting a Cure. Patients, Healers and the Law in Early Modern Bologna*. Baltimore, MD: Johns Hopkins University Press, 1998.

Rodríguez González, Alfredo. *Justicia y criminalidad en Toledo y sus Montes en la Edad Moderna*. Toledo: Consorcio de Toledo, Ayuntamiento, 2009.

Romero Tallafigo, Manuel. "Archivo General Central de Alcalá de Henares (1939) y el del Reino de Nápoles (1943). Los grandes archivos pueden morir." *Boletín ANABAD* 2 (2016): 201–26.

Schmitz, Carolin. *Los enfermos en la España barroca y el pluralismo médico. Espacios, estrategias, actitudes*. Madrid: Consejo Superior de Investigaciones Científicas, 2018.

Schmitz, Carolin. "Travelling for Health: Local and Regional Mobility of Patients in Early Modern Rural Spain." In *Connected Mobilities in the Early Modern World: The Practice and Experience of Movement*, edited by Paul Nelles and Rosa Salzberg, 87–110. Amsterdam: Amsterdam University Press, 2023.

Schmitz, Carolin and María Luz López Terrada. "Healing across Ideological Boundaries in Late Seventeenth-Century Madrid." In *Health and Healing in the Early Modern Iberian World: A Gendered Perspective*, edited by Margaret E. Boyle and Sarah E. Owens, 21–51. Toronto: Toronto University Press, 2021).

Stevens, John. *A New Spanish and English Dictionary. Collected from the Best Spanish Authors Both Ancient and Modern* […]. London: George Sawbridge, 1706.

Tamayo, Andrés. *Tratados breves de Algebra y Garrotillo. Por el Licenciado Andrés de Tamayo, Médico y Cirujano, hijo del Licenciado Tamayo, Cirujano de su Magestad*. Madrid, 1621.

Trouillot, Michel-Rolph. *Silencing the Past. Power and the Production of History*. Boston, MA: Beacon Press, 1995.

5 Brotherhoods, Poor Relief, and Health Care

Laurinda Abreu

Around 30–50 percent of the total population of Europe needed external relief to survive hunger and disease in the early modern period. Some of these poor people received help from brotherhoods, associations set up in the Middle Ages along the lines of trade corporations, craft associations, or guilds. Most brotherhoods were confraternities operating under the aegis of the Church, although there were many that chose the tutelage of central government. Their main purpose was to dispense charity in the form of mutual support, both spiritual support for all brothers and material support for those in temporary or permanent difficulties, including the family of any brother who died. Nonmembers who were poor or sick as well as pilgrims and travelers might also benefit from occasional aid, especially from brotherhoods that owned hospitals, which were mostly little more than hostels that could provide them with accommodation (for two or three nights), meals, and medical care from a bloodletter or surgeon or, more rarely, a physician. Brotherhoods were highly popular in Western Christian culture. For many people, brotherhoods were the most important source of support at times of necessity, and some tried to maximize this aid by joining several. In Catholic communities, the brotherhood movement has survived to the present day with aims not very dissimilar to those that prevailed when they were first created.

There are abundant sources concerning poor relief in Europe and in those parts of the world affected by European colonization that provide information about early modern medicine, medical training, and healing practices. Historians use these kinds of sources to capture the experiences of the poor and also those of the social and political elites. The socioeconomic upheavals that assailed the West from the mid-fourteenth century led prosperous individuals and governments to take an interest in poor relief. The wealthy saw in the widespread social and health-care problems new opportunities to assert their positions in society and in politics, whereas rulers – especially from the late fifteenth century onward in the context of early modern state formation – realized that the people could be useful for consolidating their power and so began to attend to them as a matter of governance. Given the social importance of brotherhoods and the wealth that many of them had acquired – which they administered almost entirely as they saw fit – they were naturally targeted by measures adopted both by the local elites and by central government. By the period in question, it is almost only through their eyes that the poor

DOI: 10.4324/9781003094876-7

are presented to researchers. Thus, the available sources do not capture firsthand accounts by the poor themselves, but rather statements mediated by the clerks and scribes working for the elites. Consequently, historians must use them with great care. This chapter offers strategies for such research, focusing in particular on certain civil brotherhoods run by local authorities under crown tutelage in Portugal during the early modern period: the *misericórdia* brotherhoods.

Portugal had had a stable monarchy since the end of the fourteenth century and its economy was sustained by the wealth from its overseas empire in Africa, Asia, and America, which it began to build early in the fifteenth century. In the 1490s, the country embarked on a process of political centralization and administrative reorganization, including in the area of health and poor relief. Having lagged behind in hospital reform, which some Italian cities, England, and France had carried out long before, Portugal then took the lead by simultaneously restructuring medical training (especially empirical training), hospitals, and poor relief.[1] The *misericordia* brotherhoods, whose aims were shaped by the Christian doctrine of the seven spiritual and seven corporal works of mercy (based on Matthew 25:34–36), were at the heart of many of these reform policies.

The first *misericórdia* was founded in Lisbon in August 1498. By 1521, another 76 had sprung up, and by the end of the eighteenth century there were 317 in Portugal and 77 in its empire. In the mother country, the crown gave them a near-monopoly in poor relief delivery and hospital management. Together with municipal councils, the *misericórdias* were the main employers of officially recognized healers such as physicians, surgeons, and apothecaries. The crown also gave the *misericórdias* attributes that distinguished them from other brotherhoods: their relief efforts were to focus on the community and not their own members; in their membership, governing bodies, and management, there should be a balanced representation of different social groups, from members of the highest social strata to craftsmen; and they should all base their by-laws on the rules of the Lisbon *Misericórdia's* statute (*Compromisso* – "commitment" – in Portuguese), four versions of which were used until the nineteenth century: the 1498 manuscript version and the three printed editions of 1516, 1577, and 1618.

Therefore, to understand the poor relief sources, it is also important to examine the influences and roles of the government in Portugal, as is the case anywhere. *Misericórdias* were created in the context of a renewal of charitable activity, which across Europe sought to respond more effectively to increasing poverty and destitution. Together with measures adopted by some Italian cities, the secular *misericórdia* model may have inspired Juan Luis Vives (1492–1540) and his work *De subventione pauperum* (*On Assistance to the Poor*, 1526), which guided the changes in the way relief was delivered as introduced by both Catholic and Protestant leaders in Europe during the sixteenth century. Vives advocated that relief provision should be organized centrally and run by secular authorities, and it should be rational in that its recipients be subject to careful selection. These were principles that the *misericórdias* had been implementing since 1498.

In practice, poor relief reforms tended to be carried out by the central government regardless of the country's religious orientation, even in cases where the

Church played a prominent role in them, as in Italian cities and France. The poor were selected on the basis of a large number of eligibility criteria that defined the deserving poor; begging and vagrancy were condemned and controlled. Some features were more specific to Protestant states such as England: in particular, they rejected the salvific aims of charity and generally they based the organization of poor relief on the parishes and funded it principally from taxes – in contrast to Catholic lands, where poor relief continued to depend primarily on charitable donations. Overall, relief and healthcare provision gave rise to fairly similar source material all over early modern Europe.

Like other brotherhoods, the *misericórdias* began keeping records of their most significant acts without much concern for narrative or for the completeness of the information provided. A single register was often used to record the dates of brothers' admissions and deaths, the sums defrayed on religious celebrations and relief, decisions on asset management, and other details. This changed in 1577, when in the new edition of the Lisbon *Misericórdia's* statute, the crown required the institution to keep separate books for recording its most important activities ("On the books that by obligation there shall be in the Casa da Misericórdia"); namely, books for the admission of brothers, for the poor who were aided, for royal provisions, for elections, for wills, for the rules governing services and/or functions (chapel, dispensary, hospital, etc.), and for the most important documents received and/or issued by the brotherhood.

The measures introduced by the 1577 statute to modernize and bureaucratize the *misericórdias'* internal affairs increased the amount of documentation that they were required to produce.[2] There were two main reasons for this. First, it was in line with the increased relief responsibilities that they were being given, especially as a result of their annexation of hospitals, which the crown had been systematically handing over to them since 1564,[3] together with the abandoned children that the hospitals had in their charge. Second, it was aimed at enabling the *misericórdias* to keep better control of their wealth, which at the time was growing exponentially due to the incorporation of the hospitals' assets and the receipt of pious donations with salvific aims associated with the cult of Purgatory (these were encouraged by the Council of Trent [1545–1563] and channeled toward the *misericórdias* by the Portuguese crown, given that these brotherhoods had their own churches or chapels).

All these information streams can be followed in the *misericórdias'* archives, some of them continuously over hundreds of years. A survey that I conducted in the documentation of more than 300 of these institutions showed that the brotherhoods usually complied – either to the letter or with some creativity – with the crown's 1577 requirements for the production and organization of information, not least because they knew that they could be visited by the royal auditors at any moment.[4] As the daily activities of the *misericórdias* became more complex, so the documents produced tended to become more specialized. This happened, for example, with the asset books, which started to be split into registers for different categories of information, such as sources and inventories of properties, claims (suits at law against debtors or the heirs of donors who refused to fulfill the terms of their relatives' wills), types of income and expenses, and so on. The records of the various forms of relief provided were also subdivided into separate books for the sick cared for in hospitals, persons given relief at home ("outdoor relief"), women provided with marriage dowries, prisoners, foundlings, Christian captives to be ransomed, women in cloistered retreats, funerals for the poor, and other such activities. When, as often happened, the *misericórdias* also ran their own pharmacies, the information available may extend to the production and use of medicaments.

Another category of documents in the *misericordias'* archives that deserves attention involves material that testifies to their relations with the crown and with the Catholic Church. Sources relating to the former are almost always plentiful and diverse, attesting to the close association between the *misericórdias* and the crown, deriving in part from the rare privilege that these brotherhoods enjoyed of being able to communicate directly with the king. They include laws of general application or applicable only, in particular, cases; matters that passed through the royal chancelleries; and matters enacted by letter, order, or provision. The most important of these documents, because of what they represented both legally and symbolically, were the institution's by-laws, the rules which governed its internal affairs and its relations with the outside world. After drawing up its by-laws, each *misericórdia* had to send them for approval to the monarch, who would add his signature and seal both to confirm the institution's association with royal power and to validate the by-laws as consistent with the original document (the statute of the Lisbon *Misericórdia*).[5] Usually, they were kept under the greatest care and protection in the brotherhood's coffers.

In contrast, documents of a religious nature are only found in significant quantities in two subject areas: religious ceremonies performed on the principal dates in the liturgical year, and the celebration of masses for souls in Purgatory, as required by pious bequests that the institutions had received, together with documents attesting to their (frequently bad) relationships with the chaplains who officiated in these masses.

Depending of course on their extent and state of preservation, *misericórdia* archives generally include a wide variety of documents, almost always in unbroken series up to the present day, with information on perceptions of poverty and social exclusion, types of relief work, healing practices, and health care provided by a specific society. Since these sources also provide a glimpse into the social composition of the area and its material and religious life, they offer researchers who ask the right questions a comprehensive understanding of the society in question. For the history of medicine, health, and healing, two are particularly relevant. The first consists of regulatory documents, including the brotherhoods' statutes and the by-laws of their hospitals, both ultimately stemming from the crown, while the second is the source material resulting from the way these rules were put into practice in the hospitals and in outdoor relief.

One approach to analyzing these by-laws and statutes involves examining how they reveal political attitudes toward medical knowledge and the expansion of healthcare provision for the poor. For example, during the Middle Ages, sickness was seen by society as the antechamber to death, and visiting the sick was considered one of the seven corporal works of mercy that all Christians were expected to observe. The statutes of medieval brotherhoods included the duty of performing this charitable act ("visit the sick") and often specified that their members should stay with sick brothers through their final breaths and funeral rites. In the Lisbon *Misericórdia's* first statute of August 1498, however, the formulation of this act was expanded to read "visit and treat the sick." The version of 1516 rendered this passage with a further change, stating emphatically that "the second [work of mercy] is to treat the sick." Although subtle, such revisions alert the historian to the possibility that they may reflect people's changing perceptions of the healing power of medicine. This conjecture finds support in a closer reading of the 1498 and 1516 statutes. While they both retained the idea that it was obligatory for the brothers to visit the sick every month to bring them spiritual consolation and material relief, they also stipulated that the brotherhood's physician (who was to take part in these visits) should use the visits to identify patients who needed hospital treatment and have them admitted, with the *misericórdia* administrator's agreement. With regard to this line of interpretation, it is particularly significant that the king himself decided to include in the 1516 statute the privilege he had granted to the Lisbon *Misericórdia* in November 1498, which required the city's hospitals to take in patients referred to them by the *Misericórdia* and to keep them "for as long as may be necessary for their health and to give them everything necessary for their sicknesses."[6] The inclusion of this privilege showed that it was to be considered a rule and was therefore applicable to all the other *misericórdias*, since they drew up their own by-laws based on the Lisbon *Misericórdia's* statute, as mentioned previously. It also showed that the king now saw hospitals as being more than mere hostels (the model that was still predominant).[7] Rather, he had come to regard them as places with medical, healing functions that should be used for healthcare purposes. This new attitude was immediately set out in the new hospital by-laws.

These subtle changes in language should inform the way historians examine the new hospital by-laws, especially those of the first early modern Portuguese hospital, Todos os Santos (All Saints') Hospital in Lisbon. Modeled on Santa Maria Nuova Hospital in Florence, its construction began in 1492; in 1504, it received its first by-laws, which gave pride of place to its medical aims and healthcare practitioners. Among many other aspects, the document included guidelines on admitting patients and how those who did not require hospitalization should be attended to; a description of the duties to be performed by each practitioner; the procedures to be followed in the twice daily clinical rounds to examine the hospitalized patients; and the care to be taken with patients' diets and the cleanliness of patients, wards, and clothing. Although most healthcare practitioners – surgeons, apothecaries, bloodletters, leechers, midwives, bonesetters, tooth-pullers, and others – were trained empirically, as was common at the time, only academically trained physicians had the authority to make decisions about patient care.[8] In 1514, the king ordered that these same by-laws be adopted by all hospitals that had no by-laws of their own (which was most of them, according to a survey carried out around that time), from the new "big hospitals" that the crown was setting up in the main towns and cities, to smaller, local hospitals, albeit adapted to their more limited resources.[9]

To gain a broader view of the approach that the political authorities took in dealing with the field of medicine, historians need to look at other documents: the first Chief Physician's Statute (*regimento do físico-mor*), issued in 1515 (and, with a few minor changes introduced in 1521, still in force until the early nineteenth century); and the guidelines that from the late 1530s shaped the reform of the medical curriculum taught at the University of Coimbra (the only university in the country at that time), in an attempt to make its faculty of medicine more attractive. This process was triggered by King Manuel I's decision – building on measures initiated by his predecessors – to grant the chief physician powers to recognize medical degrees obtained abroad, make surgeons equivalent to physicians (under specific conditions), oversee the training of apothecaries, and control doctor–patient relations. These new powers turned him into a major competitor of the university, leading it to accuse him of "fabricating" physicians from uneducated, ignorant surgeons. Their rivalry resulted in lengthy lawsuits that ran in the courts throughout the early modern period.[10] The researcher should therefore be careful to interpret the *misericórdia* statutes and hospital by-laws in light of the stormy relationship between the medical authorities, as revealed by the documents that regulated their activities.

Once in possession of this context, which reveals incipient centralizing policies in the field of poor relief and health care, the historian must then problematize it in light of what is already known for other parts of Europe, particularly France and England, where studies of this kind are more developed. When dealing with Portugal, it is important to determine to what extent the royal dicta were implemented. Researchers have to be aware that, despite their importance, normative sources cannot be read uncritically. Whether they were actually put into practice depended on unforeseeable circumstances, both material and human. At a time when written culture was not accessible to all, how the *misericórdia* statutes and hospital by-laws were interpreted and complied with could depend on how literate the brotherhoods' clerks and administrative officers were. It could also depend on the sums they had available for their poor relief and healthcare activities, as well as on the interests of whoever was in charge of these institutions, as well as their families and protégés. In fact, these are the topics for which there is most evidence in contemporary documents. Even in the poorest archives, researchers are often able to find enough information to reconstruct the ways in which the relations between recipients and distributors of relief were organized and regulated.

In contrast to the paperwork portraying the social relations between donors and recipients, the documentation on sickness and treatment is scarcer and less informative. Only toward the end of the eighteenth century did records of Portuguese hospitals and outdoor relief start to regularly include typologies of disease and methods of diagnosis and treatment. Until then, most records relating to the sick and poor gave only their name, parents' names, place of birth, and marital status. Therefore, the researcher has to search for sources that complement the documentation produced directly by the hospitals and outdoor relief. Recommended sources are the *misericórdias'* minutes (records of management decisions) and ledgers of expenses. Although each of these document types can be studied separately, they yield much richer information if analyzed together. The minutes, for example, may reveal the relations between academic and empirical healthcare practitioners, with an assessment of each one's performance. The ledgers of expenses show the salaries corresponding to each type of training (academic and empirical) and also the costs associated with the treatments utilized by each group.

One of the most relevant topics and, perhaps, one of the least obvious to a new researcher concerns the problematic (when applied to the remote past) concept of medicalization. A glance at the ledgers shows that the largest expenditure went toward acquiring foodstuffs: chickens, eggs, and grain for outdoor relief and different kinds of meat, eggs, wine, bread, and sweetmeats for the hospitals. Meanwhile, the minutes show the importance that the *misericórdia* administrators attached to the contracts made with their suppliers, as they give details of clauses specifying not only the price but also the quality of the meat, bread, and milk being purchased. The researcher should be careful not to take such information at face value or to interpret it merely as performing the third work of mercy ("feed the hungry"). Using food as a medicament was common practice in Hippocratic–Galenic medicine, and in this case the richness of the diet usually given to hospital patients may also point to a definition of sickness that included physical exhaustion, which might result from a variety of causes, including hard labor, as Colin Jones and others have argued.[11] Moreover, such a high-calorie diet would help counteract the debilitating effects of the most common treatments, such as bloodletting, purgatives, and emetics.

Yet more information can be extracted by cross-referencing the four types of documentation – records of outdoor relief, hospital records, minutes of meetings, and ledgers of expenses – and combining qualitative and quantitative methods. The profiles of hospital patients and recipients of poor relief, for example, can only be reconstructed using this methodology. Hospital care and outdoor relief have most often been studied quantitatively using a wide variety of indicators, which have revealed cycles, fluctuations, structures, and discontinuities in numbers of beneficiaries, start and end dates of the care received, the average length of time of a particular service, the gender of those involved, and other parameters. However, just using statistical, graphic, or other tools to read such data creates traps for the unwary that can distort findings. Trends in variables taken out of context and without regard for the purposes for which they were produced have little to say about the people involved, their lives, their family situations, or their social trajectories.[12]

The advantages of multidimensional analysis are demonstrated in research that I conducted using two nominal databases listing hospital patients in two cities in southern Portugal: Évora, which had an agricultural economy, in the seventeenth and eighteenth centuries; and Setúbal, a salt-making and fishing town, in the late eighteenth century. Although the patient records did not include occupations, most patients were non-residents and sought hospital care during the working season, especially during the slack times between the more labor-intensive jobs on the farms or salt pans. They disappeared when the work was finished, only to return in subsequent years when they repeated the same pattern of behavior, sometimes for decades. The conclusion could safely be drawn that they were migrant workers who looked to the hospitals for support that they could not find in the community because they had no social ties. This gave more substance to another conclusion derived from an analysis of local residents who sought hospital care in the same period. Their hospital admissions occurred all year long and did not track the seasonal rhythms of work, and they had far higher death rates than the non-residents, particularly in the case of women.[13] Altogether, the information points to the fact that local residents only went to the hospital when they were seriously ill or even *in extremis*, and they went to seek specialist medical care.[14]

When the same methods are used to study outdoor relief, it is found that such relief was reserved almost exclusively for the local poor, predominantly lone women, widows, and those with dependent children, and/or the sick or people with some kind of physical or age-related disability.[15] They all had access to healthcare practitioners who worked at the hospital but provided medical relief at people's homes on specific days. This relief could include nursing and medication as well as prescribed foodstuffs, as mentioned above.[16] While most of the poor people helped by the *misericórdias* were given relief only irregularly, there were cases of families that received it every month. It proved possible to track some of these over several generations, and a trend was seen of women marrying at a younger age and household members having more children. This may have been due to several factors: they could get medical care more promptly (which also applied to adults and had an impact on their ability to work and contribute to the household economy); their better diet reduced infant mortality; and they did not need to resort to abandoning their newborns.[17] This study additionally revealed that members of the local elite also asked for outdoor relief, alleging debt problems, an inability to live according to their social status, or a lack of money to provide their children with dowries for marriage or life in a convent. Unlike the previous group, they were almost always given relief in the form of cash allowances – large sums, sometimes also over generations.[18] According to the social logic of the *ancien régime*, it was as important to prevent the poor from falling into destitution as it was to stop the elite from sliding down the social ladder.

This method of combining qualitative and quantitative approaches also helps the researcher see research questions that might otherwise be missed. One of the most stimulating questions relates to the decisions made by hospital administrators: why would they allow all patients to benefit from their hospital's resources free of charge if the law stated that those who could afford their treatment should pay for it? The research revealed that the hospital administrators – who were the governing elites of the *misericórdias* and often the municipal council – owned most of the land, the fishing boats, and the salt pans. By throwing open their hospital doors gratis to everybody, including migrant workers, they were ensuring that the labor they needed remained available (these workers had no need to return home), the workers could hold on to their wages rather than spend them on board and lodging, and the local economies were kept running. Equally, by keeping workers in the hospitals during their down time between jobs, they could to some extent avoid disorder and violence in the streets.[19]

This conclusion also leads the researcher to use these sources to account for other matters that at first glance lie outside the field of health care and poor relief.

An example is the social composition of the *misericórdia* brotherhoods, how their governing bodies were put together and how they acquired their power. To investigate these topics, the researcher has to go back to the by-laws and to the royal order requiring the *misericórdias* to maintain a balance of nobles and other social groups in their membership. Since most local areas did not have enough nobles to make up the required 50 percent, the crown allowed them to grant equivalent status to members of locally respected trades, such as goldsmiths or merchants. The *misericórdias'* ability to produce new social categories was soon noticed by poorer villages and smaller towns, which hastened to petition the king for a *misericórdia* to be founded in their lands. In some way, charitable brotherhoods by their very nature had the ability to ennoble local people, at a time when social mobility was limited. This was a particularly valuable benefit, because the laws of the kingdom stipulated that local council seats could only be filled by the "best in the land." For individuals from the lower strata, getting into the *misericórdia* could be the culmination of an arduous *cursus honorum* that usually began in the socially less well-regarded brotherhoods and continued step by step up the fraternal hierarchy, gathering social capital on the way that would help the aspirant secure a place in the most elitist of all brotherhoods: the *misericórdias*. Once installed in their governing bodies and then also managing to be elected as municipal councilors, these men would find a way to move around from one institution to another and so build up powerful client networks; these would then help them to impose their values and interests on their communities and use the institutions' assets for their own ends. In short, the choices they made regarding the distribution of health care and poor relief in the hospitals cannot be dissociated from their own social trajectory. It is also noteworthy that even *misericórdias* with very limited archives kept registers of the admission of brothers and elections to their governing bodies, suggesting that they were especially careful to preserve these volumes. Ultimately, they acted as a kind of pedigree for those who had no other titles or honors.

Another of the numerous topics that these sources can shed light on is the relationship between brotherhoods (*misericórdia* brotherhoods and others) and the Church. The religious world view and the values of Christianity permeate the discourse of relief institutions in both Catholic and Protestant countries until the eighteenth century. However, historians also have demonstrated that poor relief institutions tended to be governed more by reason than by faith. In Portugal, this rational attitude in brotherhoods that worked with poor relief – particularly the *misericórdias* – extended to the use of funds allocated for the celebration of masses for souls in Purgatory. Almost all the *misericórdia* archives have document trails resulting from the steps that the brotherhoods and the crown took together to obtain the pope's approval for these funds to be transferred to the hospitals. If the application was well organized and the reasons put forward by the brotherhoods were convincing, the pope generally had no qualms about accepting the argument that taking care of the living did as much good for the souls of the dead as singing masses and that the living were more in need than the dead. In Todos os Santos Hospital, such money paid for around 30 percent of the hospital's expenses until the eighteenth century.[20] A comparative study covering Catholic Europe could help to delimit the extent of this still poorly known device, which might cast doubt on many preconceived ideas about the role played by religion in relief institutions.

In conclusion, archive material on the *misericórdias* and their hospitals enables researchers to reconstruct histories that are at once shared, since they were molded by the same general guidelines, and unique, in that they tell the specific story recorded over the centuries of each locality where a *misericórdia* was founded. The fact that many *misericórdias'* archives hold series of documents covering several centuries opens up a vast range of possibilities for long-term comparative studies at various scales, from microhistory to the major themes of economic and social history and, because of their role in shaping and reshaping the local elites, political history as well. They also allow comparisons to be made within and between rural and urban areas, coastal and inland regions, the north and south of the country, motherland and empire, and, within the empire, the distinctive features of diverse localities.[21] In the specific field of health care and poor relief, it is possible, for instance, to address the evolution of the concept of the deserving poor, how brotherhoods' governing elites prioritized the various forms of poor relief and medical care, the number of hospitals in existence at local, regional, and national levels, the number and type of healthcare practitioners, the services provided in the hospitals and through outdoor relief, and how they developed, the social profile of the poor and/or sick, and countless other topics.[22]

Notes

1 The author is grateful to Christopher J. Tribe for translating this essay. The translation was financed by Portuguese national funds through the Foundation for Science and Technology, under project UIDB/00057/2020, CIDEHUS/Universidade de Évora. For the Portuguese poor relief reform, see, among many others, Laurinda Abreu, *The Political and Social Dynamics of Poverty, Poor Relief and Health Care in Early-Modern Portugal* (London and New York: Routledge, 2016).

2 See Ângela Barreto Xavier, José Pedro Paiva, "Introdução," in *Portugaliae Monumenta Misericordiarum (PMM)*, vol. 4, José Pedro Paiva and Ângela Barreto Xavier (eds.) (Lisboa: Universidade Católica Portuguesa/União das Misericórdias Portuguesas, 2005), 7–30.

3 This annexation, which the crown conducted in 1564, went against the decisions of the Council of Trent, at which the episcopacy was encouraged to strengthen its hold over hospitals. Prisoners were particularly badly affected by the annexation: the crown acknowledged that prisons were both a political problem – it was not easy for the king's justices to penetrate the complex world of people who controlled prisons – and a social and public health problem. Prisons were indeed filthy and rife with scurvy, rheumatism, edema, and all kinds of epidemics, so they were veritable tombs for the poor, who were the only ones magistrates left to languish there. *Misericórdias* represented their only hope for a meal, medical care, and a court appeal, and these benefits were cut drastically after the hospitals started to play a major role in the *misericórdias'* lives.

4 Laurinda Abreu, "Processos de integração de normas e práticas nos campos da assistência e da saúde (Portugal, séculos XVI–XVIII)," in *Ciência e Poder na primeira Idade Global*, Amélia Polónia, Fabiano Bracht, Gisele da Conceição, and Monique Palma (eds.) (Porto: Universidade do Porto, Faculdade de Letras, 2016), 19–39.

5 It was only once its by-laws had been approved that the *misericórdia* existed in law and could enjoy the many benefits accruing to brotherhoods under royal protection, especially those that provided the material and administrative conditions in which they could operate. While the crown might approve occasional adaptations, it would not allow changes that distorted the fundamentals of the Lisbon statute.

6 *PMM*, vol. 3, 386.

7 The king revealed his new understanding of the role of hospitals a few days after his coronation in December 1495, in the by-laws for the Espírito Santo Hospital in Montemor-o-Novo, a small town in southern Portugal. This document foreshadows some of the rules later set out in the 1504 Todos os Santos statute. Laurinda Abreu, "Oferta e regulação em saúde: o legado de D. Manuel I (1495–1521)," in *As sete obras de misericórdia corporais. Santas Casas de Misericórdia, sécs. XVI–XVIII*, Maria Marta Lobo de Araújo (ed.) (Braga: Santa Casa da Misericórdia de Braga, 2018), 35–57.

8 Guenter B. Risse, "Before the Clinic Was 'Born': Methodological Perspectives in Hospital History," in *Institutions of Confinement: Hospitals, Asylums, and Prisons in Western Europe and North America, 1500–1950*, Norbert Finzsch and Robert Jütte (eds.) (New York: Cambridge University Press, 1996), 75–96.

9 Abreu, "Oferta e regulação em saúde."

10 This complex situation is examined by Laurinda Abreu in "Tensions between the Físico-Mor and the University of Coimbra: The Accreditation of Medical Practitioners in Ancien-Regime Portugal," *Social History of Medicine* 31 (2018): 231–57.

11 As late as 1779, the statute for the Setúbal hospital still declared that diet was the primary remedy in treatment. Colin Jones, *The Charitable Imperative: Hospitals and Nursing in Ancien Régime and Revolutionary France* (London and New York: Routledge, 1989).

12 Laurinda Abreu, *The Political and Social Dynamics of Poverty*, 206, footnote 81.

13 The situation was different in the migrant workers' places of origin. Unsurprisingly, women there outnumbered men in hospital admissions.

14 Abreu, *The Political and Social Dynamics of Poverty*, 209–18.

15 As was common throughout Europe, and not only in Catholic countries. See Timothy Wales, "Poverty, Poor Relief, and the Life Cycle," in *Land, Kinship and Life Cycle*, Richard Smith (ed.) (Cambridge: Cambridge University Press, 1984), 351–404.

16 It is important to distinguish this kind of medical relief, which was aimed at a limited number of individuals, from the support that the municipalities provided (in principle) to a broader social spectrum, which the crown organized from 1568 onward (Abreu, *The Political and Social Dynamics of Poverty*, 90–104). For the situation elsewhere, see, for example, Steven King, P*overty and Welfare, 1700–1850: A Regional Perspective* (Manchester: Manchester University Press, 2000); and Steven King and Alannah Tomkins (eds.), *The Poor in England, 1700–1850: An Economy of Makeshifts* (Manchester: Manchester University Press, 2003).

17 There is abundant literature on this subject in the case of England. See for example the works listed by Steven King in "Pauvreté et assistance. La politique locale de la mortalité dans l'Angleterre des XVIIIe et XIXe siècles," *Annales. Histoire, Sciences Sociales* 61, 1 (2006): 31–62.

18 Rute Pardal, *Práticas de caridade e assistência em Évora (1650–1750)* (Lisboa: Colibri, 2015).

19 Abreu, *The Political and Social Dynamics of Poverty*, 206–18.

20 Rute Ramos, *O Hospital de Todos os Santos: História, Memória e Património Arquivístico (sécs. XVI–XVIII)* (Lisboa: Colibri, 2022).

21 Laurinda Abreu, "Health Care and the Spread of Medical Knowledge in the Portuguese Empire, Particularly the Estado da Índia (Sixteenth to Eighteenth Centuries)," *Medical History* 64, 4 (2020): 449–66; Joanna Innes, "The Regulation of Charity and the Rise of the State," in *The Routledge History of Poverty, c.1450–1800*, David Hitchcock and

Julia McClure (eds.) (London: Routledge, 2020), 3–20; Philippe Sassier, *Du bon usage des pauvres. Histoire d'un thème politique (XVIe–XXe siècle)* (Paris: Fayard, 1990).

22 This is an important point, since the number of poor people who had access to formal relief is known to have been incomparably smaller than the number of the needy. Among the many works by scholars who have examined this question, see the introduction by John Henderson and Richard Wall to *Poor Women and Children in the European Past* (London: Routledge, 1994); Marco Van Leeuwen, "Logic of Charity: Poor Relief in Preindustrial Europe," *Journal of Interdisciplinary History* 24 (1994): 589–613.

Bibliography

Abreu, Laurinda, "Health Care and the Spread of Medical Knowledge in the Portuguese Empire, Particularly the Estado da Índia (Sixteenth to Eighteenth Centuries)." *Medical History* 64 (2020): 449–66.

Abreu, Laurinda. "Oferta e regulação em saúde: o legado de D. Manuel I (1495–1521)." In *As sete obras de misericórdia corporais. Santas Casas de Misericórdia, sécs. XVI–XVIII*, edited by Maria Marta Lobo de Araújo, 35–57. Braga: Santa Casa da Misericórdia de Braga, 2018.

Abreu, Laurinda. *The Political and Social Dynamics of Poverty, Poor Relief and Health Care in Early-Modern Portugal*. London and New York: Routledge, 2016.

Abreu, Laurinda. "Processos de integração de normas e práticas nos campos da assistência e da saúde (Portugal, séculos XVI–XVIII)." In *Ciência e Poder na primeira Idade Global*, edited by Amélia Polónia, Fabiano Bracht, Gisele da Conceição, and Monique Palma, 19–39. Porto: Universidade do Porto, Faculdade de Letras, 2016.

Abreu, Laurinda. "Tensions between the Físico-Mor and the University of Coimbra: The Accreditation of Medical Practitioners in Ancien-Regime Portugal." *Social History of Medicine* 31 (2018): 231–57.

Henderson, John and Richard Wall. *Poor Women and Children in the European Past*. London: Routledge, 1994.

Innes, Joanna. "The Regulation of Charity and the Rise of the State." In *The Routledge History of Poverty, c.1450–1800*, edited by David Hitchcock and Julia McClure, 3–20. London: Routledge, 2020.

Jones, Colin. *The Charitable Imperative: Hospitals and Nursing in Ancien Régime and Revolutionary France*. London and New York: Routledge, 1989.

King, Steven. "Pauvreté et assistance. La politique locale de la mortalité dans l'Angleterre des XVIIIe et XIXe siècles." *Annales. Histoire, Sciences Sociales* 61 (2006): 31–62.

King, Steven. *Poverty and Welfare, 1700–1850: A Regional Perspective*. Manchester: Manchester University Press, 2000.

King, Steven and Alannah Tomkins, eds. *The Poor in England, 1700–1850: An Economy of Makeshifts*. Manchester: Manchester University Press, 2003.

Pardal, Rute. *Práticas de caridade e assistência em Évora (1650–1750)*. Lisboa: Colibri, 2015.

Ramos, Rute. *O Hospital de Todos os Santos: História, Memória e Património Arquivístico (sécs. XVI–XVIII)*. Lisboa: Colibri, 2022.

Risse, Guenter B. "Before the Clinic Was 'Born': Methodological Perspectives in Hospital History." In *Institutions of Confinement: Hospitals, Asylums, and Prisons in Western Europe and North America, 1500–1950*, edited by Norbert Finzsch and Robert Jütte, 75–96. Cambridge: Cambridge University Press, 1996.

Sassier, Philippe. *Du bon usage des pauvres. Histoire d'un thème politique (XVIe–XXe siècle)*. Paris: Fayard, 1990.

Van Leeuwen, Marco. "Logic of Charity: Poor Relief in Preindustrial Europe." *Journal of Interdisciplinary History* 24 (1994): 589–613.

Wales, Timothy. "Poverty, Poor Relief, and the Life Cycle." In *Land, Kinship and Life Cycle*, edited by Richard Smith, 351–404. Cambridge: Cambridge University Press, 1984.

Xavier, Ângela Barreto and José Pedro Paiva, "Introdução." In *Portugaliae Monumenta Misericordiarum (PMM)*, vol. 4, edited by José Pedro Paiva and Ângela Barreto Xavier, 7–30. Lisboa: Universidade Católica Portuguesa/União das Misericórdias Portuguesas, 2005.

Part II

Medical Writing

6 Medical Casebooks

Lauren Kassell

Introduction: Lady Curson's Case

On Thursday, September 3, 1618, Lady Curson, a gentlewoman from a prominent English family who was in her mid-thirties, had borne numerous children, run a sizeable household, and sometimes practiced medicine, sent a letter and a urine sample to her favorite astrologer-physician. She had consulted him regularly for more than a decade, sometimes about herself, sometimes for others. Her questions were usually about health. She worried about her pregnancies and had digestive troubles. Occasionally she asked about financial matters. On this day, she was suffering from a fever.

The astrologer-physician was Richard Napier, a clergyman in Buckinghamshire with a thriving medical practice. We know about Lady Curson's consultation with him because he wrote it down in his casebook. He recorded her name, the village where she lived, and age, plus the date and time, 7:40 pm, that her message arrived. Then he drew a "horoscope," namely a grid that represented the heavens divided into 12 sections called "houses" onto which he plotted the positions, as seen from the Earth, of the five known planets and the Sun and Moon for that moment. He also noted the planetary positions for the day of the previous month when she had taken to bed. Such calculations were at the heart of "horary" astrology, which was particularly prevalent in seventeenth-century England (Figure 6.1).[1]

Most medical practitioners in medieval and early modern Europe would have agreed that the human body was a microcosm that was connected to the universe, the macrocosm, and that the movements of the planets could accordingly be used to predict the course of a disease. But for Napier, and other practitioners of horary astrology, the moment, literally the hour, that things occurred, was of paramount significance. Whatever a physician might observe from the outward signs of a patient's appearance and behavior or deduce about the internal workings of her body from the qualities of her urine and other excrements, these were of secondary significance for the horary astrologer. Likewise, what the patient and those around her said about her condition was not as important as what was signaled in the stars.

Or so Napier had been taught by his mentor, Simon Forman, a London astrologer as famous for his expert judgments as he was notorious for his arrogant disregard of local medical authorities. For Forman, who had little formal education, knowledge

DOI: 10.4324/9781003094876-9

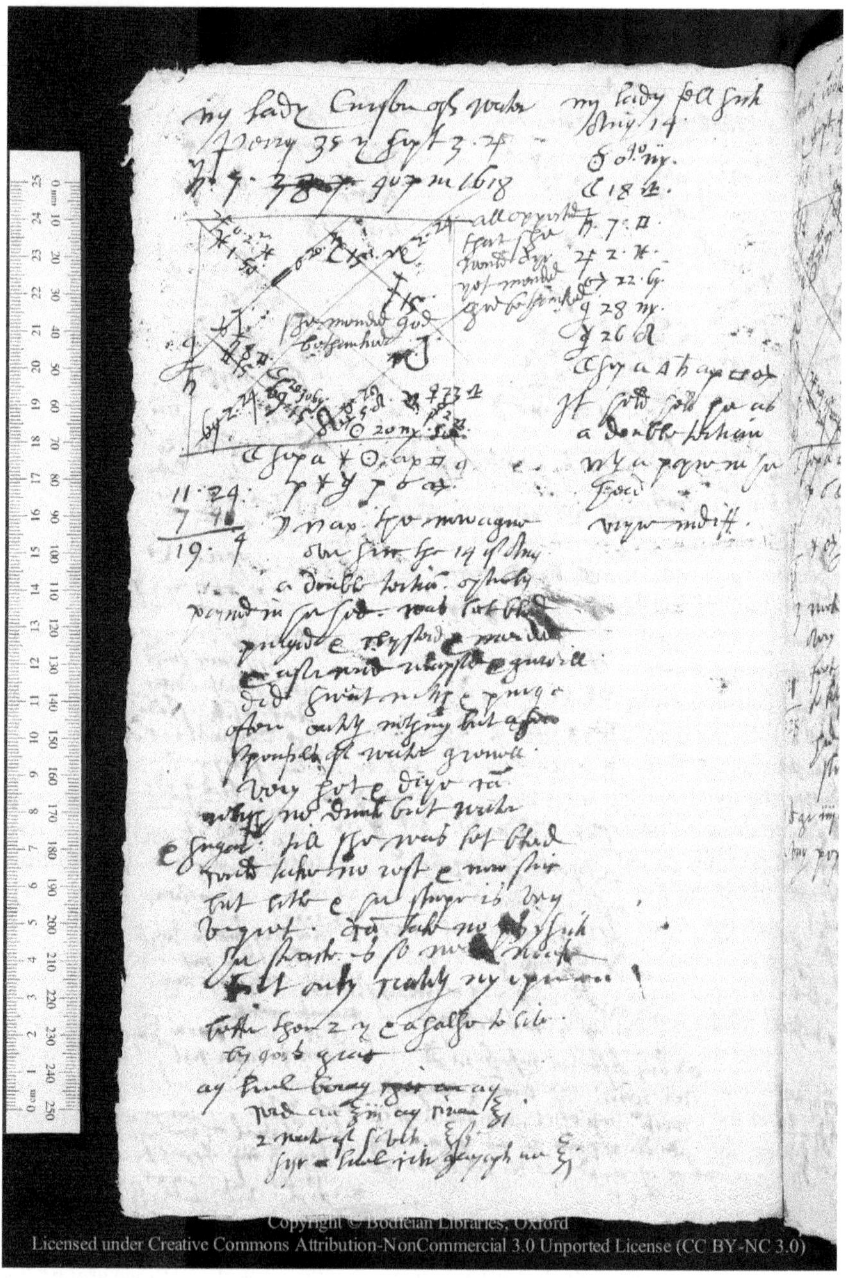

Copyright © Bodleian Libraries, Oxford
Licensed under Creative Commons Attribution-NonCommercial 3.0 Unported License (CC BY-NC 3.0)

Figure 6.1 [M]y lady Curson of water Perry 35 y sept 3. ♃ h. 7. 38 p 40 pm 1618
[In chart] She mended, God be thanked.
[Right of chart] All expected that she would dye yet mended God be thanked.

Moon Cauda draconis ap[plying]. The new ague. Ever since the 14 of Aug. a doubled tertian extremely pained in her head. Was let blood, purged and clystered and mended & afterward relapsed & grew ill. did sweat much and purge often eateth nothing but a few spoonfulls of water grewell. Very hot and dry can relish no drink but water and sugar. Till she was let blood could take no rest and now since but little and her sleep is very unquiet. Can take no physic her stomach is so wea[blot] weak but only craveth my opinion. Better than two years and a half to live by God's grace.

Aqua luel?? borage [deletion] aqua cord[ialis?] an (ounces)iij aqua cinam[oni] (ounces)j two water of s? vitr(??) (ounces)(semis) [i.e. half an ounce]. syr[up] [deletion] luel?? citr gayagh(?) an (ounces)j

[column break; CASE47441]
my lady fell sick Aug. 14.
sun 0. \40/ Virgo.
moon 18 Libra.
Saturn 7 square.
Jupiter 2 Pisces.
Mars 22 Cancer.
Venus 28 Virgo.
Mercury 26 Leo.
Moon sep[aratur] a trine Saturn ap[plicans] square Mars [Moon is separating from trine with Saturn, applying to square with Mars].

It held held [sic] her as a double tertian with a pain in her head urine indiff.

Bodleian Library, Oxford, MS Ashmole 230, f. 20v, https://cudl.lib.cam.ac.uk/view/MS-ASHMOLE-00230/48, copyright Bodleian Libraries

of astrological medicine was ancient and God-given. Thousands of pages of his writings remain extant. These include numerous manuals of astrological medicine, along with works on alchemy, various forms of magic, history, day-by-day and fabulous accounts of his own life, and, in the model that Napier would follow, records of his medical consultations, which we now call "casebooks." Perhaps Napier consulted one of Forman's guides to astrology, or another manual, to understand the cause of her fever and predict whether the illness would prove fatal.

Despite Forman's insistence that the patient's words and urine were but "tokens" of her will to be healed, Napier copied the content of Lady Curson's now-lost letter into his casebook. In short, she had suffered from a recurring fever and headache for three weeks. She had been let blood and purged upwards and downwards. She was hot and dry, could not eat or drink, and slept little. She – in Napier's account of her words – "Can take no physic her stomach is so wea[blot] weak but only craveth my opinion." He predicted, though we do not know whether he told her this, that she would live for more than two and half years. He considered her decumbiture, that is the planetary positions when she had first become ill on August 14. He inspected her urine, sent with the letter, and found it "indifferent." And he prescribed various waters, cordials, and syrups. Later, he noted, in the middle and to the right of the chart, "All expected that she would dye yet [she] mended God be thanked."[2]

Lady Curson's case documents a typical early modern medical encounter. The patient consulted the practitioner, in this instance in writing. She had consulted other practitioners before him and asked Napier for his "opinion," specifying that she did not want medicine. He assessed everything from the qualities of her urine to what she reported about her health to the effects of the planetary motions on her body. And, despite her request for no physic, he prescribed gentle, strengthening remedies. What makes this encounter unusual is that Napier wrote it down, parsing her words and in some cases including whole phrases into his casebook. Cases like this one provide rare evidence about constructions of medical knowledge and experiences of health, disease, and medicine in the past. Casebooks, together with complementary sources like Forman's guide, make it possible to study the histories of regimes of health and healing that are inflected, through writing and experience, with normative assumptions about gender, social status, and other forms of difference.

Casebooks were serial collections of cases, a form of writing that was entwined with the ways in which medical encounters were conducted and which itself has a history. Lady Curson's case is one of around 70,000 that Richard Napier recorded from the late 1590s, when he began practicing as an astrologer, until his death in 1634. This chapter considers the ways in which casebooks can be studied as evidence for experiences of health and disease otherwise lost to the historical record, as products of medical encounters in which practitioners and patients negotiated commensurate and competing understandings, as testaments to the changing ways in which natural knowledge was made, and as artifacts that demonstrate how documents have been produced and preserved. Napier's casebooks will be our loadstar throughout, and it is with them that we will begin. Then we will turn to the broader history of "casebooks," itself a label of convenience to refer to a type of medical writing in the seventeenth century, rather than a conventional genre invoked at the time. Throughout we will ask how best to study these records and what they actually record, and in conclusion we will turn to their apparent promise to provide evidence of everyday experiences of health and healing in the past.

Richard Napier's Casebooks

Richard Napier was a clergyman in Buckinghamshire who became a prominent medical practitioner through a combination of self-study and tutelage under a mentor. He styled himself as a physician, though this label was officially reserved for men who had studied medicine at university and been licensed to practice. His casebooks span nearly four decades and fill 60 hefty volumes. They are one of the largest surviving sets of private medical records, complete except for a missing volume covering a period of nine months in 1613–1614.

Following the methods of his mentor, Simon Forman, Napier's consultations took a standard form. Napier asked the patient's name, age, and sometimes occupation or address. Where the querent was not the patient, or multiple people were present, the doctor noted their relationships and whether the patient consented to the consultation. Then the patient or his or her representative posed a question, thereby investing the practitioner with the authority to make somatic and social judgments. These encounters could take place in person, by proxy, or, as in the case of Lady Curson, in writing. Occasionally Napier attended wealthy clients at home, but patients usually came to his house or sent messengers. Then, as he had done for Lady Curson, Napier drew a horoscope, also known as a chart or figure, dividing the celestial sphere into 12 zodiac houses, one for each of the celestial signs, and plotting the locations of the planets within them at the significant moment, usually when the question was asked or the message arrived. Thereafter the records become less systematic. An entry might contain a judgment based on the horoscope, other sorts of evidence gleaned from the patient's words or appearance, the quality of the urine, or the doctor's observations. Unlike most physicians, Napier did not feel the pulse and seems not to have used touch to examine his patients. Some cases include remedies and payments. When Napier added follow-up details, often from third parties, we glimpse communication beyond the encounter.

Writing these notes was central to the way in which Napier conducted the consultation, in part because he needed to work with a pen in hand in order to calculate the astrological figures, in part because he chose to keep account of his consultations. Some other practitioners also recorded notes when they met with their patients, though, as we will see, these notes were seldom preserved. The result is that Napier's casebooks – like Forman's, of which only six years survive – are rich yet written in fragmented phrases in a messy script. They are often ambiguous about whether a patient articulated a complaint or the astrologer-physician, like other doctors, discerned it from the stars or other signs, such as the color, smell, and taste of the patient's urine, the strength and speed of the pulse, and the complexion of the skin. All of these diagnostic techniques were part of learned medicine, and all of them were contested at some stage or another. Horary astrology, as practiced by Napier, was frequently dismissed as marketplace quackery that appealed to women and foolish people. At best it was arbitrary, at worst it was deterministic. Regardless of the techniques that a practitioner used, in early modern "bedside medicine" patients and practitioners negotiated narratives of illness and readings of signs, drawing on epistemologies more shared than competing.[3] In Napier's casebooks, only fragments of these encounters survive, not full case histories. They document the everyday experiences of illness and health, amongst other topics, of more than 60,000 people. Three-quarters of them consulted Napier only once, evidence of the piecemeal approach to medicine at this time. Even the cases of regular clients remain dispersed, not consolidated into a narrative. For instance, Lady Curson, with whom we began, was involved with more than a hundred cases between 1606 and her death in 1619, often as a patient and querent, sometimes as a third party.[4]

In short, Napier's casebooks are systematic, extensive, arcane, messy, and more like lists than narratives. They were rough notes, not intended to be read let alone studied. Historians, as we will see in the next section, have approached them with a variety of quantitative and qualitative methods.

Studies of Richard Napier's Casebooks

Napier's casebooks survived but, whether through happenstance or design, the papers of most doctors did not. Robert Pierce, a prominent Bath physician working several decades after Napier, shows us a glimpse of his messy study when he noted, in a published collection of cases, that he had assembled them "in looking up my old scater'd Papers, of many Years standing." Pierce's published book remains, but, to my knowledge, his scattered papers do not. Similarly, Nicholas Culpeper, the author of numerous English medical books who also practiced astrological-physic, apologized to his reader for only including one example of particular decumbiture, a horoscope for the moment a person became ill or, literally took to bed, even though he had many to hand, because "I want time to insert them, or if I did not, I would not blot paper with them."[5] Again, Culpeper's printed works survive, but his manuscripts do not.

When Napier died, he left his books and papers, which included Forman's casebooks, to his nephew, Sir Richard Napier (1607–1676), to whom he had taught astrology. Sir Richard added his own cases and passed the expanded collection to his son, Thomas Napier (b. 1646), who then sold it to Elias Ashmole (1617–1692) when Sir Richard died. Ashmole collected British antiquities, including numerous books and manuscripts on occult topics. He had the casebooks of Forman and the two Napiers bound into 66 volumes. Most of them contain more than 500 folio pages and cover a single year. Ashmole donated his collections to the University of Oxford in 1677 and founded the Ashmolean Museum there in 1683. In the 1840s, William Black was commissioned to catalogue the Ashmole manuscripts – an indispensable finding aid – and in 1860 the collection of books and manuscripts, including the casebooks, was moved to the Bodleian Library, where they continue to be housed today.[6]

In the 1970s, social and cultural historians began to mine the Forman and Napier casebooks for information about everyday life in early modern England. In *Religion and the Decline of Magic* (1971), Keith Thomas calendared the numbers of consultations held by Forman, Napier, and other English astrologers to argue that droves of people turned to them to cope with the uncertainties of life in early modern England. A. L. Rowse's prurient *Simon Forman: Sex and Society in Shakespeare's Age* (1974) described the romantic, pecuniary, and political antics of Forman and the Londoners who consulted him, sometimes relying on misreadings of the manuscripts. Following Rowse, literary scholars have identified notable figures amongst Forman's clientele and used his casebooks to add color to Shakespeare's poorly documented life. Emilia Lanier, the accomplished poet who was for a time mistakenly identified as the Bard's Dark Lady, consulted Forman about her health and fortune and became intimate with him (quite how intimate is unclear).[7]

Following Thomas's approach, Michael MacDonald focused on the cases of madness in Napier's casebooks. His landmark study combined innovative computational techniques with subtle discursive analysis to demonstrate how, in an era before mental illness was medicalized and its sufferers institutionalized, the astrologer helped his patients and their families to make sense of social and psychological uncertainties. Ronald Sawyer's doctoral dissertation, written under MacDonald's direction, used his sampling methods and profiled Napier's medical practice as a whole.[8] Through the 1980s, historians used other early modern casebooks to write histories of experiences of illness and healing, but none of them drew on collections as extensive or complete as Forman's and Napier's.[9] At the same time, Forman's and Napier's casebooks provided choice examples for social historians, especially those concerned with gender. As social history gave way to cultural history, Forman's and Napier's casebooks attested to the workings of early modern bodies.[10]

I began studying Forman's casebooks in the 1990s. In dialogue with Thomas and MacDonald, I read Forman's guide to astrology alongside his casebooks to argue that he used the language of the stars to cultivate the trust of his patients. I developed this argument within a broader study of Forman's work as an astrologer-physician.[11] The systematic (though messy) nature of Forman's and Napier's casebooks, and their massive scale, prompted me to set up a digital humanities project, called the Casebooks Project, to produce a digital edition of their records. Just as MacDonald had used cutting-edge computational methods in the 1980s, so the Casebooks Project used cutting-edge digital tools in 2010. Our work was motivated by social and anthropological trends in the history of medicine and prompted by Margaret Pelling's attention to everyday medical practice, Roy Porter's call for the recovery of lost voices, and Barbara Duden's historicization of the "natural" body. It used computers to recover the voices of ordinary people, the "human contents" of the past.[12] We aimed to capture, through a digital edition of the astrologer-physicians' casebooks, the encounters that produced these records and the qualities of the records themselves. In addition to the digital edition, we produced a series of ancillary outputs to support, improve, and communicate our work. We were a team of seven, funded by the Wellcome Trust from 2008 to 2018. At the outset, I had thought that digital tools would provide a means of mastering the evidence in this unwieldy archive. Instead, we found that working with digital technologies raised as many questions about historical evidence as it answered. I reflected on this work in a pair of articles. I also attempted to situate Forman's and Napier's casebooks within a broader history of record keeping practices in early modern England.[13]

In parallel with our work, and in some cases drawing on it, social and cultural historians of medicine and gender have returned to questions about patients and drawn examples from a range of practitioners.[14] As the Casebooks Project released more cases and refined our search facilities, Forman's and Napier's records began to feature in new studies of the classic topics of melancholy, reproduction, and gendered bodies. Historians continue to use Forman's and Napier's casebooks to study a range of topics that include, and also go beyond, clinical encounters, including disease categories, childbirth, emotions, devotional practices, and work.[15]

Napier's records have been mined for evidence of the everyday lives of ordinary and extraordinary people in early modern England. They have invited quantitative analysis and rewarded readings of their cases against and along the grain. They have shaped how the history of medicine, particularly the history of medical encounters in early modern Europe, has been written, as we will see in the concluding section. First, we need to reflect on the nature of casebooks as historical documents.

What Are Casebooks?

Napier's records are unusually extensive, but they are not unique. Many medical practitioners in early modern Europe habitually recorded their cases day by day, year by year. These serial records were sometimes called diaries, collections of cures and observations, or practice books. In the mid-eighteenth century, they came to be called casebooks, borrowing the term from legal records. I inherited this term from previous scholars of Forman's and Napier's casebooks, though some scholars prefer to refer to this form of writing as practice journals.[16] Whatever the terminology, since the 1980s, as part of the same trend that led historians to study Napier's and Forman's records, studies have read doctors' notebooks for evidence of everyday medical practices, patient experiences of health and illness, and forms of medical knowledge. In this section, we will consider how and why doctors developed this new form of writing. In the next and final section, we will return Napier's records and the kinds of histories that they have been used to write.

Doctors across Europe developed practices of recording details of their consultations in the 1500s, motivated, depending on their training and the context in which they worked, by an increasing interest in particular instances in nature, a self-consciousness about the ancient foundations of medicine, and familiarity with new forms of written accounting. Reconstructing this history from extant documents, like Napier's casebooks, is challenging because so few examples survive and, when they do, their contents are usually limited to registers of names and prescriptions, perhaps with notes of payment or a few details of the cases. For instance, Hartmann Schedel recorded the names and prescriptions for his patients drawn from across the social spectrum in Nördlingen and Amberg around 1500. Several decades later, Georg Palm recorded his day-to-day practice as a municipal physician in Nuremberg for 25 years, and his contemporary Johannes Magenbuch recorded cases of the Nuremberg elite. Hiob Finzel, a physician active in the small towns of Weimar and Zwickau, recorded more than 10,000 consultations in the form of short notes over almost 25 years, from 1565 to 1589. Other examples of sixteenth-century learned casebooks include Francesco Partini's notebook, in Latin and Italian, written from at least 1536 up to 1567. It contains 80 cases, some written by Partini himself, others by different physicians on his request, all addressed to the highest members of the aristocracy from Trent and Tyrol and to the members of the imperial family's entourage. Further north, Georg Handsch only recorded the cases of those patients that he deemed in some way particularly noteworthy. In the middle of the seventeenth century, Georg Hieronymus Welsch, physician and scholar from Augsburg, collected consilium from numerous physicians.[17] Scarce records survive. Others are known to be lost. For instance, Gemma Frisius, the Dutch mathematician and physician who had studied in Leuven in the 1520s and then taught there until his death in 1555, reputedly kept a pair of notebooks, one of observations about the stars and weather, the other for medicine. Similarly, his compatriot and contemporary Pieter van Foreest noted that he began recording medical cases when he turned his attention from heavenly observations to microcosmical (earthly) ones – though some of van Foreest's cases are preserved in his printed observations.[18]

While some European physicians recorded cases in registers or account books, others modeled their cases on those of ancient physicians, most notably Hippocrates, the "father of medicine," and Galen, the second-century Greek physician who worked in the courts of imperial Rome and systematized the Hippocratic writings. Hippocratic texts, such as the widely circulated *Epidemics*, contained hundreds of case histories. Galen, in contrast, did not collect cases. Instead, he used them as examples in the texts, such as *Methodus medendi*, that became staples for teaching rational medicine in medieval European universities. Medieval scholars often included cases, in the form of examples, in the margins of their works. Thousands of European manuscripts remain extant, the earliest in Latin then also in vernacular languages, from the twelfth through seventeenth centuries that include *experimenta* singly, then later gathered into collections as particular instances of observed and experienced knowledge – cases – moved from the margins to the center of texts.

This brings us to a mode of recording cases known as *consilia*. A *consilium* was a consultation, often framed as a response to a question, theological, legal, or medical. Dating from Republican Rome, and reemerging in northern Italy around 1200, medical consilia would become the building blocks of elaborate regimen to preserve health, treatises on disease, or collections of didactic works. A consilium typically began by naming the patient and narrating the history of the disease to date, including opinions on it by other authorities. The second part was a regimen to prevent illness or restore health and a treatment, often listing multiple remedies and sometimes borrowing the argumentative style of legal cases. Consilia concluded with a summary describing the outcome. By the end of the fourteenth century, collections of consilia were commonplace in Bologna and would soon be found in neighboring universities. Physicians ordered their collections, following other genres of practical medicine, by disease from head to toe. By the fifteenth century, astrologers – many of whom were medical men – were following this example to make collections of horoscopes, again combining details with prescriptions to improve health, avoid danger, and obtain riches.

These developments were facilitated by a shift in the relationship between memory and written records that began in the eleventh century. Fragmentary evidence of links between medieval scholarly practices and bureaucratic innovations can be seen in memoranda of medical and astrological cases from the decades around 1400. A century later, novel habits of account keeping and interests in testimonials and natural particulars converged at bedsides, consulting rooms, and doctors' desks, framed as an imperative to improve medicine.

Some doctors' records focused on treatments and payments, others on narratives of diseases and cures, often written from rough notes or memory at the end of the day. Practices were local, with teachings emanating from the universities with the movements of students and the transmission of texts. For instance, professors at Ferrara and Padua in the 1540s encouraged their students to record case histories. In his teachings at hospital bedsides at the University of Padua in c. 1540–1551, Giovanni Battista da Monte, as reported by his students, set out how a doctor was to use his senses to understand particular cases. Da Monte was teaching a kind of medicine appropriate to private consultations with the nobility, as opposed to poor people in hospitals, in which, as Jerome Bylebyl notes, a "patient's way of life, if not his body, was more open to examination." His students collected his consilia and published them, first in an edition in 1554, then expanded to include 434 cases in a 1583 work by Joannes Crato.[19] Just as Crato saw the Padua professor as an innovator in the way in which he conducted consultations and recorded cases, so others of the era looked for novelty in the way in which consultations were conducted.

Occasionally doctors reflected on the place of writing cases in their practices. From the late sixteenth century, they increasingly stressed their debt to Hippocrates, as noted above, when describing the patterns of good medical practice. For instance, in 1573, Francois Valleriola, professor of medicine in Turin, noted,

> [Hippocrates] wrote on tablets all that he saw occurring in the sick person, and narrated the complete *historia* of the disease and what happened to the sick each day, each hour, each moment, giving specifically the name of each person ....[20]

A few decades later, Francis Bacon echoed earlier scholars when he lamented that physicians had lost "the ancient and serious diligence of Hippocrates, which used to set down a narrative of the special cases of his patients, and how they proceeded, and how they were judged by recovery or death." In 1654, Nicholas Culpeper, the English astrologer and medical reformer, translated a work by the German medical reformer Simeon Partlicius, which included an elaboration on ideas attributed to Hippocrates about the duties of a physician. Partlicius's list of the doctor's duties concluded with guidelines on how to order practice. He should keep a "Catalogue of Authors," a "Diary," a list of notable "observations," cultivate a herb garden, and record "his best Experiments in such an order that he may know redily how to find them." Each day should begin with remembering what he did the day before. In the afternoon, he should gather simples, study medical books, and visit his patients. In the evening, he should reflect on what he did during the day, perhaps updating his diary, and "commit something to memory."[21]

As doctors had begun systematically to record cases, medical professors harnessed print to extend their case-based methods of teaching from face-to-face meetings with their pupils to the nascent Republic of Letters. For instance, Amatus Lusitanus, a Jewish physician living in Italy, published 700 cases, a hundred at a time between 1551 and 1566. His *Centuriae curationum* (Hundreds of Treatments) established a new genre. Other collections were eclectic by design: Johan Schenck von Grefenberg's *Observationes medicinae, rarae, novae, admirabiles et monstrosae* (1585–1597), the most significant late sixteenth-century collection, combined observationes from ancient and medieval texts, his network of correspondents, and his own practice. Producing observationes was an epistolary and bibliographical exercise, an instance of the drive to collect that shaped sixteenth- and seventeenth-century inquiry. By 1700, around a hundred authors had published collections of cases like these, typically ordered from head-to-toe or according to disease category and sometimes combined with cases from other, historical practitioners.[22] At the same time, individual cases became staples of the new periodicals published by Europe's learned societies. Collections of cases continued to be produced through the eighteenth century, some following old head-to-toe orders, others ordered by diseases. Thus, despite innovative technologies – physical examinations, quantitative testing, postmortem investigations – doctors relied on a vast medical library, reaching back through the centuries, to classify diseases. Medical knowledge was produced through the study of published cases, old and new.[23]

By the time Napier began practicing medicine in the late 1590s, it had become reasonably common for doctors to record their cases, either as complete registers or notes of particular cases or some combination. But the resulting manuscripts are usually lost: only a dozen or so have been located from before 1600, and several hundred from 1700, ranging from fragments of a few cases to many thousands. More work needs to be done to establish existing numbers from the following century. From extant casebooks, extractions from them as individual or collected cases in printed works, and prescriptive literature (often called deontological texts), we know that casebooks followed conventions – recording name, date, age, complaint, its cause, and perhaps a prescription or payment – but varied from practitioner to practitioner. Some were like account books, written at the time of the encounter. Astrological records, of which Napier's are an example, typically took this form. Others were written when a doctor returned to his study after a day of visiting patients; they are akin to journals and diaries.[24] Like these ego-documents, they have been subject to the whims of preserving and archiving personal papers. Because Napier's casebooks have been preserved, so too have thousands of conversations between patients and practitioners that would otherwise be lost to the historical record.

Conclusions: Casebooks and Histories of Patients

With the turn to the patient in the 1980s, casebooks, like letters, diaries, and other ego-documents, promised a bottom-up view of illness and healing. For sociologically and anthropologically minded historians, the problem with the patient's voice is not simply that it is lost, but that it is always a discursive construct. For many years, however, histories of the patient either focused on medical practice, sidestepping the silent patient as an unknowable construct, or uncritically unearthed the sufferer from the archives.[25] The books by MacDonald and Duden, mentioned above, provided models for how casebooks and the related genre of medical observations could be used to write fresh histories of medicine. MacDonald's study centered on the records of madness in Napier's casebooks. Duden's centered on the multi-volume observations on the diseases of women by Johann Storch, an early eighteenth-century German physician. While Napier's casebooks were formulaic and chronologically ordered, Storch's presented a synoptic view of the women's cases, juxtaposing the events that the women recounted to him with stories from other sources. Duden recovered a form of medical encounter in which illness and women's bodies were socially located, known to the women and accessible to the doctor through their spoken words and bodily signs. As Duden comments on

MacDonald's work, it shows "the presence of a body internally undivided and externally unbounded," a precursor to "[t]he 'body' as a discrete object of social control." Storch and Napier, though working almost a century and hundreds of miles apart, similarly documented an era before the "natural body" had taken shape. This was a moment in history when, to extrapolate Duden's argument, a doctor's writing could be embodied.[26]

In 1992, Guenter Risse and John Harley Warner challenged historians of medicine to make full use of patient records to study the dynamics of medical practice and, where possible, to recover patients' voices mediated through practitioners' pens. They began with Erwin Ackerknecht's 1967 call for "behaviorist" studies of medical therapeutics, through case histories, and noted that it had taken two decades for such work to take root. They defined the variety of documents, both personal and institutional, that constitute medical records: case histories, clinical charts, patient notes. They mentioned the existence of medical records from the sixteenth and seventeenth centuries, including Napier's, but their discussion centered on the late eighteenth century onwards. They noted that these records are rich with quantitative and qualitative material and cautioned that they should not be read as clear, objective chronicles, or unmediated accounts of patient experiences. Case histories, they stressed, were narratives, written within analytic frameworks that were themselves politically, ideologically, and personally specific. With these provisos, they detailed the opportunities for using medical records to study the histories of medical practice, the demographics of disease, social and cultural differences and healing, and the relation between medical practices and scientific ideas. Warner revisited the topic in 1999, reiterating the link between an interest in patient records and the more general trends amongst historians to study practice, to attend to narrative, and to identify new historical sources, and he urged historians to consider the form that such records take as part of the project of studying their contents.[27] Casebooks, like other medical records, have a history.

Casebooks document medical encounters and potentially record patient voices, but they do not necessarily contain narratives of illness. Medical records range in form from lists of repeated categories of data to various sorts of narratives. As bundles of data, they can be readily quantified, providing apparently objective statistics about patient demographics and categories of disease. Casebooks and computing, Risse and Warner noted, have long been associated. Their quintessential historian, in the persona of MacDonald, risked being buried under mountains of computer printouts. As a pioneer of historical computing, he used punched notecards, knitting needles, and a mainframe computer to calculate data from a sample of 2,000 cases of patients suffering from forms of mental disorders. His student, Ronald Sawyer, followed him, studying the disease profile of Napier's medical practice as a whole through sampling successive months in successive years, e.g. January 1601 and February 1602.[28] Napier's casebooks contain countable data, and they record narrative sequences, often expressed in terms of causal events. These records were framed within conventions of writing narratives and collecting data.

Napier's casebooks provide an example of the challenges and opportunities of using this sort of record to write histories of health and medicine. First cases and casebooks need to be located, either as archived manuscripts, in printed books, or in digitized or databased versions of these texts.[29] If they are subjected to quantitative analysis, one must be careful about whether the data represents a practitioners' practice in full or selections from it together with additional cases. They can be studied as written documents, both in terms of their form (manuscript or print) and their generic conventions (account books or observations, for instance). If they contain discursive material, however brief, they will reward careful, perhaps even associative reading, often alongside other sorts of ego-documents like letters and dairies or prescriptive writings like medical manuals or self-help books. If you find yourself confronting a case or a casebook, try to make sense of what the record itself, in its physical form, tells you about how and why it was produced; ask what every word means, even if you think you already know; and imagine what was happening beyond the page, the things that, for one reason or another, were not written down.

I chose to begin this chapter with Lady Curson's consultation with Napier in September 1618 because it represents a typical entry in his casebooks, and showcases the power of the digital edition to identify her as one of his most frequent clients and to home in on this particular, somewhat unusual encounter. She demonstrates her own prowess as a healer, and he records her self-diagnosis, perhaps even her own words. Early modern medical casebooks document everyday experiences and have the potential to disrupt standard accounts of how health and healing worked in the past.

Notes

1 Lauren Kassell, Michael Hawkins, Robert Ralley, John Young, Joanne Edge, Janet Yvonne Martin-Portugues, and Natalie Kaoukji, eds., "CASE47440," *The Casebooks of Simon Forman and Richard Napier, 1596–1634: A Digital Edition*, https://casebooks.lib.cam.ac.uk/cases/CASE47440. See also CASE47441, a decumbiture for August 14 written on the same page. Michael MacDonald, "The Career of Astrological Medicine in England," in *Religio Medici: Medicine and Religion in Seventeenth-Century England*, ed. Ole Grell and Andrew Cunningham (Aldershot: Ashgate), 62–90. This chapter draws on a substantial amount of scholarship that, for reasons of space, is not all cited here. Readers can consult the secondary sources below for additional details and context, as well as Lauren Kassell, Michael Hawkins, Robert Ralley, and John Young, "Further Reading," A Critical Introduction to the Casebooks of Simon Forman and Richard Napier, 1596–1634, https://casebooks.lib.cam.ac.uk/astrological-medicine/further-reading. References to supplementary material on the *Casebooks* website are hereafter cited as "Kassell, et al. (eds.), *Casebooks Digital Edition*" followed by the url to the specific section of the site.

2 On urine as tokens, see Lauren Kassell, *Medicine and Magic in Elizabethan London: Simon Forman, Astrologer, Alchemist and Physician* (Oxford: Oxford University Press, 2005), 138. Her escape was temporary: in another entry, Napier noted that she died a year later.

3 See, for instance, Claudia Stein, "The Meaning of Signs: Diagnosing the French Pox in Early Modern Augsburg," *Bulletin of the History of Medicine* 80 (2006): 617–48; Olivia Weisser, "Boils, Pushes and Wheals: Reading Bumps on the Body in Early Modern England," *Social History of Medicine* 22 (2009): 321–39.

4 Kassell et al. (eds.), "Magdalen Dormer [Curson] [Young Lady Curson] (PERSON22807)," *Casebooks Digital Edition*, https://casebooks.lib.cam.ac.uk/cases/PERSON22807.

5 Robert Pierce, *Memoirs of Bath: Or, observations in three and forty years practice* (Bristol, 1697), Preface, sig. C2v; Nicholas Culpeper, *Semiotica Uranica: Or an Astrological Judgment of Diseases from the Decumbiture of the Sick* (London, 1651), 58.

6 "Reading the Casebooks" in Kassell, et al. (eds.), *Casebooks Digital Edition*, https://casebooks.lib.cam.ac.uk/reading-the-casebooks/the-manuscripts/about-the-volumes; William Black, A Descriptive, Analytical and Critical Catalogue of the Manuscripts Bequeathed unto the University of Oxford by Elias Ashmole (Oxford: Oxford University Press, 1845).

7 Keith Thomas, *Religion and the Decline of Magic: Studies in Popular Beliefs in Sixteenth- and Seventeenth-Century England* (London: Weidenfeld & Nicholson, 1971); A. L. Rowse, *Simon Forman: Sex and Society in Shakespeare's Age* (London: Weidenfeld & Nicolson, 1974). For examples of literary studies, see James Shapiro, *1599: A Year in the Life of William Shakespeare* (London: Faber and Faber 2005); Charles Nicholl, *The Lodger: Shakespeare on Silver Street* (London: Allen Lane, 2007). On Lanier, see "Meet the Patients," in Kassell, et al. (eds.), *Casebooks Digital Edition*, https://casebooks.lib.cam.ac.uk/using-the-casebooks/meet-the-patients/emilia-lanier.

8 Michael MacDonald, *Mystical Bedlam: Madness, Anxiety, and Healing in Seventeenth-Century England* (Cambridge: Cambridge University Press, 1981); Ronald Sawyer, "Patients, Healers and Disease in the Southeast Midlands, 1597–1634," PhD diss., University of Wisconsin, 1986.

9 See especially Lucinda McCray Beier, *Sufferers and Healers: The Experience of Illness in Seventeenth-Century England* (London: Routledge, 1987); Katherine Williams, "Hysteria in Seventeenth-Century Case Records and Unpublished Manuscripts," *History of Psychiatry* 1 (1990): 383–401.

10 They feature, for instance, in Patricia Crawford, "Attitudes to Menstruation in Seventeenth-Century England," *Past & Present* 91 (1981): 47–73; Martin Ingram, "Ridings, Rough Music and the Reform of Popular Culture in Early Modern England," *Past & Present* 105 (1984): 79–113; Anthony Fletcher, *Gender, Sex and Subordination in England 1500–1800* (New Haven, CT: Yale University Press, 1995); Linda Pollock, "Childbearing and Female Bonding in Early Modern England," *Social History* 22 (1997): 286–306. On cultural histories/bodies, see Ulinka Rublack, "Fluxes: The Early Modern Body and the Emotions," *History Workshop Journal* 53 (2000): 1–16; Laura Gowing, *Common Bodies: Women, Touch and Power in Seventeenth-Century England* (New Haven, CT: Yale University Press, 2003); Lesel Dawson, *Lovesickness and Gender in Early Modern English Literatur*e (Oxford: Oxford University Press, 2008).

11 Lauren Kassell, "How to Read Simon Forman's Casebooks: Medicine, Astrology and Gender in Elizabethan London," *Social History of Medicine* 12 (1999): 3–18; Kassell, *Medicine and Magic*. My work was written in parallel with Barbara Traister, *The Notorious Astrological Physician of London: Works and Days of Simon Forman* (Chicago, IL: University of Chicago Press, 2001).

12 Kassell, et al. (eds.), *Casebooks Digital Edition*, https://casebooks.lib.cam.ac.uk. Margaret Pelling, *The Common Lot: Sickness, Medical Occupations, and the Urban Poor in Early Modern England* (London: Routledge, 2016); Roy Porter, "The Patient's View: Doing Medical History from Below," Theory and Society 14 (1985): 175–98; Roy Porter, "The Patient in England, c. 1660–c. 1800," in Medicine in Society, ed. Andrew Wear (Cambridge: Cambridge University Press, 1992), 91–118; Barbara Duden, *The Woman Beneath the Skin: A Doctor's Patients in Eighteenth-Century Germany*, trans. Thomas Dunlap (Cambridge, MA: Harvard University Press, 1991 [1987]). Tim Hitchcock, "Academic History Writing and Its Disconnects," *Journal of Digital Humanities* 1 (2011); Tim Hitchcock, "Big Data for Dead People," historyonics.blogspot.co.uk, December 9, 2013.

13 Lauren Kassell, "Paper Technologies, Digital Technologies: Working with Early Modern Medical Records," in *The Edinburgh Companion to the Critical Medical Humanities*,

ed. Anne Whitehead, Angela Woods, Sarah Atkinson, Jane Macnaughton, and Jennifer Richards (Edinburgh: Edinburgh University Press, 2016), 120–35; Lauren Kassell, "Inscribed, Coded, Archived: Digitizing Early Modern Medical Casebooks," *Journal for the History of Knowledge* 2 (2021): 1–18; Lauren Kassell, "Casebooks in Early Modern England: Astrology, Medicine and Written Records," *Bulletin of the History of Medicine* 88 (2014): 595–625.

14 For instance, Weisser, "Boils, Pushes and Wheals"; Wendy Churchill, *Female Patients in Early Modern Britain: Gender, Diagnosis, and Treatment* (Farnham: Ashgate, 2012); Boyd Brogan, "The Masque and the Matrix: Alice Egerton, Richard Napier and Suffocation of the Mother," *Milton Studies* 55 (2014): 3–52; Ofer Hadass, *Religion, and Magic in Early Stuart England: Richard Napier's Medical Practice* (University Park: Penn State University Press, 2018).

15 For a few of many examples, see Erin Sullivan, *Beyond Melancholy: Sadness and Selfhood in Early Modern England* (Oxford: Oxford University Press, 2016); Daphna Oren-Magidor, "Literate Laywomen, Male Medical Practitioners and the Treatment of Fertility Problems in Early Modern England," *Social History of Medicine* 29 (2016): 290–310; Katherine Foxhall, *Migraine: A History* (Baltimore, MD: Johns Hopkins University Press, 2019); Leah Astbury, "When a Woman Hates Her Husband: Love, Sex, and Fruitful Marriages in Early Modern England," *Gender & History* 32 (2020): 523–41; Philippa Carter, "Childbirth, 'Madness', and Bodies in History," *History Workshop Journal* 91 (2021): 29–50.

16 Martin Dinges, Kay Peter Jankrift, Sabine Schlegelmilch, and Michael Stolberg, eds., Medical Practice, 1600–1900: Physicians and their Patients, trans. Margot Saar (Leiden: Brill, 2015); Kassell, "Casebooks in Early Modern England."

17 These examples and more can be found in Michael Stolberg, "Empiricism in Sixteenth-Century Medical Practice: The Notebooks of Georg Handsch," Early Science and Medicine 18 (2013): 487–516; Michael Stolberg, "A Sixteenth-Century Physician and His Patients: The Practice Journal of Hiob Finzel, 1565–1589," Social History of Medicine 32 (2019): 221–40; Michael Stolberg, *Learned Physicians and Everyday Medical Practice in the Renaissance*, trans. Logan Kennedy and Leonhard Unglaub (Berlin: De Gruyter, 2021); Alessandra Quaranta, "The *Consilia* by Learned Physicians Pietro Andrea Mattioli and Francesco Partini: Dialectic Relations between Doctrine, Empirical Knowledge and Use of the Senses in Sixteenth-Century Europe," *Social History of Medicine* 35 (2022): 20–48. For a survey centered on English examples, see Kassell, "Casebooks in Early Modern England."

18 This paragraph, and much of this section, draws on Lauren Kassell, "Cases," in *Information: A Historical Companion*, ed. Ann Blair, Paul Duguid, Anja Goeing, and Anthony Grafton (Princeton, NJ: Princeton University Press, 2021), 358–65.

19 Jerome Bylebyl, "The Manifest and the Hidden in the Renaissance Clinic," in Medicine and the Five Senses, ed. W. F. Bynum and Roy Porter (Cambridge: Cambridge University Press, 1993), 40–60, on p. 60; see also Monica Calabrito, "Curing Melancholia in Sixteenth-Century Medical Consilia Between Theory and Practice," *Medicina nei secoli arte e scienza* 24 (2012): 627–64; Stein, "The Meaning of Signs"; Quaranta, "The *Consilia.*"

20 Quoted from Gianna Pomata, "Praxis Historialis: The Uses of Historia in Early Modern Medicine," in *Historia: Empiricism and Erudition in Early Modern* Europe, ed. Gianna Pomata and Nancy Siraisi (Boston: MIT Press, 2005), 105–46, on p. 129. See also Brian Nance, "Wondrous Experience as Text: Valleriola and the *Observationes medicinales,*" in *Textual Healing: Essays on Medieval and Early Modern* Medicine, ed. Elizabeth Jane Furdell (Leiden: Brill, 2005), 101–17.

21 Francis Bacon, *The Advancement of Learning* (London, 1605), book 2.X.4; Simeon Partlicius, *A New Method of Phisick*, trans. Nicholas Culpeper (London, 1654), 107.

22 On observations, see essays by Gianna Pomata, especially "Sharing Cases: The *Observationes* in Early Modern Medicine," Early Science and Medicine 15 (2010): 193–236 and "Observation Rising: Birth of an Epistemic Genre, 1500–1650," in *Histories of Scientific Observation*, ed. Lorraine Daston and Elizabeth Lunbeck (Chicago, IL: University of Chicago Press, 2011), 45–80. For a list of early modern printed medical observations, see Pomata, "Sharing Cases," Appendix, 232–36. For printed English medical observations, see the 226 titles tagged as such in Mary E. Fissell and Elaine Leong, eds., *Reading Early Medicine (beta)*: https://reademed.mpiwg-berlin.mpg.de/search?simple_search=observations&type=All. See also their selection of works centered on cases: https://reademed.mpiwg-berlin.mpg.de/books/genre/542/cases.

23 Volker Hess and J. Andrew Mendelsohn, "Case and Series: Medical Knowledge and Paper Technology, 1600–1900," History of Science 48 (2010): 287–314; J. Andrew Mendelsohn, "Empiricism in the Library: Medicine's Case Histories," in *Science in the Archives: Pasts, Presents, Futures*, ed. Lorraine Daston (Chicago, IL: University of Chicago Press, 2017), 85–109.

24 See, for instance, Dinges et al., *Medical Practice*; Kassell, "Casebooks in Early Modern England"; Stolberg, *Learned Physicians*.

25 Flurin Condrau, "The Patient's View Meets the Clinical Gaze," Social History of Medicine 20 (2007): 525–40.

26 Duden, *Woman Beneath the Skin*, 11. Duden makes a particular claim about the exceptional nature of Storch's writing on p. 69.

27 Guenter B. Risse and John Harley Warner, "Reconstructing Clinical Activities: Patient Records in Medical History," *Social History of Medicine* 5 (1992): 183–205; John Harley Warner, "The Uses of Patient Records by Historians – Patterns, Possibilities and Perplexities," *Health & History* 1 (1999): 101–11.

28 Sawyer, "Patients, Healers and Disease," 468 ff.

29 To date, only the casebooks of Forman, Napier, and their associates have been produced as digital editions. For digitized manuscripts, see George Bate, "Medical Casebook," in *Wiley Digital Archives: The Royal College of Physicians – Part II*: http://WDAgo.com/s/23119b0b. See also the digital edition of *The Consultation Letters of Dr William Cullen (1710–1790)*: https://www.cullenproject.ac.uk/.

Bibliography

Primary Sources

Bacon, Francis. *The Advancement of Learning.* London, 1605, book 2.X.4.

Bate, George. "Medical Casebook." In *Wiley Digital Archives: The Royal College of Physicians – Part II:* http://WDAgo.com/s/23119b0b.

The Casebooks of Simon Forman and Richard Napier, 1596–1634: A Digital Edition: https://casebooks.lib.cam.ac.uk. Edited by Lauren Kassell, Michael Hawkins, Robert Ralley, John Young, Joanne Edge, Janet Yvonne Martin-Portugues, and Natalie Kaoukji.

The Consultation Letters of Dr William Cullen (1710–1790): https://www.cullenproject.ac.uk/.

Culpeper, Nicholas. *Semiotica Uranica: Or an Astrological Judgment of Diseases from the Decumbiture of the Sick.* London, 1651.

Partlicius, Simeon. *A New Method of Phisick*, trans. Nicholas Culpeper. London, 1654.

Pierce, Robert. *Memoirs of Bath: Or, observations in three and forty years practice.* Bristol, 1697.

Reading Early Medicine (beta): https://reademed.mpiwg-berlin.mpg.de/search?simple_search=observations&type=All. Edited by Mary E. Fissell and Elaine Leong.

Secondary Sources

Astbury, Leah. "When a Woman Hates Her Husband: Love, Sex, and Fruitful Marriages in Early Modern England." *Gender & History* 32 (2020): 523–41.

Black, William. A Descriptive, Analytical and Critical Catalogue of the Manuscripts Bequeathed unto the University of Oxford by Elias Ashmole. Oxford: Oxford University Press, 1845.

Brogan, Boyd. "The Masque and the Matrix: Alice Egerton, Richard Napier and Suffocation of the Mother." *Milton Studies* 55 (2014): 3–52.

Bylebyl, Jerome. "The Manifest and the Hidden in the Renaissance Clinic." In Medicine and the Five Senses, edited by W. F. Bynum and Roy Porter, 40–60. Cambridge: Cambridge University Press, 1993.

Calabrito, Monica. "Curing Melancholia in Sixteenth-Century Medical *Consilia* between Theory and Practice." *Medicina nei secoli arte e scienza* 24 (2012): 627–64.

Carter, Philippa. "Childbirth, 'Madness', and Bodies in History." *History Workshop Journal* 91 (2021): 29–50.

Churchill, Wendy. *Female Patients in Early Modern Britain: Gender, Diagnosis, and Treatment*. Farnham: Ashgate, 2012.

Condrau, Flurin. "The Patient's View Meets the Clinical Gaze." Social History of Medicine 20 (2007): 525–40.

Crawford, Patricia. "Attitudes to Menstruation in Seventeenth-Century England." *Past & Present* 91 (1981): 47–73.

Dawson, Lesel. *Lovesickness and Gender in Early Modern English Literatur*e. Oxford: Oxford University Press, 2008.

Dinges, Martin, Kay Peter Jankrift, Sabine Schlegelmilch, and Michael Stolberg, ed. Medical Practice, 1600–1900: Physicians and Their Patients, trans. Margot Saar. Leiden: Brill, 2015.

Duden, Barbara. *The Woman Beneath the Skin: A Doctor's Patients in Eighteenth-Century Germany*, trans. Thomas Dunlap. Cambridge, MA: Harvard University Press, 1991 [1987].

Fletcher, Anthony. *Gender, Sex and Subordination in England 1500–1800*. New Haven, CT: Yale University Press, 1995.

Foxhall, Katherine. *Migraine: A History*. Baltimore, MD: Johns Hopkins University Press, 2019.

Gowing, Laura. *Common Bodies: Women, Touch and Power in Seventeenth-Century England*. New Haven, CT: Yale University Press, 2003.

Hadass, Ofer. *Religion, and Magic in Early Stuart England: Richard Napier's Medical Practice*. University Park: Penn State University Press, 2018.

Harley Warner, John. "The Uses of Patient Records by Historians – Patterns, Possibilities and Perplexities." *Health & History* 1 (1999): 101–11.

Hess, Volker and J. Andrew Mendelsohn, "Case and Series: Medical Knowledge and Paper Technology, 1600–1900." History of Science 48 (2010): 287–314.

Hitchcock, Tim. "Academic History Writing and its Disconnects," *Journal of Digital Humanities* 1 (2011).

Hitchcock, Tim. "Big Data for Dead People" historyonics.blogspot.co.uk.

Ingram, Martin. "Ridings, Rough Music, and the Reform of Popular Culture in Early Modern England." *Past & Present* 105 (1984): 79–113.

Kassell, Lauren. "How to Read Simon Forman's Casebooks: Medicine, Astrology and Gender in Elizabethan London." *Social History of Medicine* 12 (1999): 3–18.

———. *Medicine and Magic in Elizabethan London: Simon Forman, Astrologer, Alchemist and Physician*. Oxford: Oxford University Press, 2005.

———. "Casebooks in Early Modern England: Astrology, Medicine, and Written Records." *Bulletin of the History of Medicine* 88 (2014): 595–625.

———. "Paper Technologies, Digital Technologies: Working with Early Modern Medical Records." In *The Edinburgh Companion to the Critical Medical Humanities,* edited by Anne Whitehead, Angela Woods, Sarah Atkinson, Jane Macnaughton, and Jennifer Richards, 120–35. Edinburgh: Edinburgh University Press, 2016.

———. "Cases." In *Information: A Historical Companion*, edited by Ann Blair, Paul Duguid, Anja Goeing, and Anthony Grafton, 358–65. Princeton, NJ: Princeton University Press, 2021.

———. "Inscribed, Coded, Archived: Digitizing Early Modern Medical Casebooks." *Journal for the History of Knowledge* 2 (2021): 1–18.

MacDonald, Michael. "The Career of Astrological Medicine in England." In *Religio Medici: Medicine and Religion in Seventeenth-Century England*, edited by Ole Grell and Andrew Cunningham, 62–90. Aldershot: Ashgate, 1996.

———. *Mystical Bedlam: Madness, Anxiety, and Healing in Seventeenth-Century England.* Cambridge: Cambridge University Press, 1981.

McCray Beier, Lucinda. *Sufferers and Healers: The Experience of Illness in Seventeenth-Century England.* London: Routledge, 1987.

Mendelsohn, J. Andrew. "Empiricism in the Library: Medicine's Case Histories." In *Science in the Archives: Pasts, Presents, Futures*, edited by Lorraine Daston, 85–109. Chicago, IL: University of Chicago Press, 2017.

Nance, Brian. "Wondrous Experience as Text: Valleriola and the *Observationes medicinales*." In *Textual Healing: Essays on Medieval and Early Modern Medicine*, edited by Elizabeth Jane Furdell, 101–17. Leiden: Brill, 2005.

Nicholl, Charles. *The Lodger: Shakespeare on Silver Street*. London: Allen Lane, 2007.

Oren-Magidor, Daphna. "Literate Laywomen, Male Medical Practitioners and the Treatment of Fertility Problems in Early Modern England." *Social History of Medicine* 29 (2016): 290–310.

Pelling, Margaret. *The Common Lot: Sickness, Medical Occupations, and the Urban Poor in Early Modern England.* London: Routledge, 2016.

Pollock, Linda. "Childbearing and Female Bonding in Early Modern England." *Social History,* 22 (1997): 286–306.

Pomata, Gianna. "Praxis Historialis: The Uses of Historia in Early Modern Medicine." In *Historia: Empiricism and Erudition in Early Modern Europe*, edited by Gianna Pomata and Nancy Siraisi, 105–46. Boston: MIT Press, 2005.

———. "Sharing Cases: The *Observationes* in Early Modern Medicine." Early Science and Medicine 15 (2010): 193–236.

———. "Observation Rising: Birth of an Epistemic Genre, 1500–1650." In *Histories of Scientific Observation*, edited by Lorraine Daston and Elizabeth Lunbeck, 45–80. Chicago, IL: University of Chicago Press, 2011.

Porter, Roy. "The Patient's View: Doing Medical History from Below." Theory and Society 14 (1985): 175–98.

———. "The Patient in England, c. 1660–c. 1800." In Medicine in Society, edited by Andrew Wear, 91–118. Cambridge: Cambridge University Press, 1992.

Quaranta, Alessandra. "The *Consilia* by Learned Physicians Pietro Andrea Mattioli and Francesco Partini: Dialectic Relations between Doctrine, Empirical Knowledge and Use of the Senses in Sixteenth-Century Europe." *Social History of Medicine* 35 (2022): 20–48.

Risse, Guenter B. and John Harley Warner. "Reconstructing Clinical Activities: Patient Records in Medical History." *Social History of Medicine* 5 (1992): 183–205.

Rowse, A. L. *Simon Forman: Sex and Society in Shakespeare's Age*. London: Weidenfeld & Nicolson, 1974.

Rublack, Ulinka. "Fluxes: The Early Modern Body and the Emotions." *History Workshop Journal* 53 (2000): 1–16.

Sawyer, Ronald. "Patients, Healers, and Disease in the Southeast Midlands, 1597–1634." PhD diss., University of Wisconsin, 1986.

Shapiro, James. *1599: A Year in the Life of William Shakespeare*. London: Faber and Faber 2005.

Stein, Claudia. "The Meaning of Signs: Diagnosing the French Pox in Early Modern Augsburg." *Bulletin of the History of Medicine* 80 (2006): 617–48.

Stolberg, Michael. "Empiricism in Sixteenth-Century Medical Practice: The Notebooks of Georg Handsch." Early Science and Medicine 18 (2013): 487–516.

———. "A Sixteenth-Century Physician and His Patients: The Practice Journal of Hiob Finzel, 1565–1589." Social History of Medicine 32 (2019): 221–40.

———. *Learned Physicians and Everyday Medical Practice in the Renaissance*, trans. Logan Kennedy and Leonhard Unglaub. Berlin/Boston, MA: De Gruyter, 2021.

Sullivan, Erin. *Beyond Melancholy: Sadness and Selfhood in Early Modern England*. Oxford: Oxford University Press, 2016.

Thomas, Keith. *Religion and the Decline of Magic: Studies in Popular Beliefs in Sixteenth- and Seventeenth-Century England*. London: Weidenfeld & Nicholson, 1971.

Traister, Barbara. *The Notorious Astrological Physician of London: Works and Days of Simon Forman*. Chicago, IL: University of Chicago Press, 2001.

Weisser, Olivia. "Boils, Pushes and Wheals: Reading Bumps on the Body in Early Modern England." *Social History of Medicine* 22 (2009): 321–39.

Williams, Katherine. "Hysteria in Seventeenth-Century Case Records and Unpublished Manuscripts." *History of Psychiatry* 1 (1990): 383–401.

7 Experimenting with Drugs

Alisha Rankin

> In the year 1580 on St. Jacob's Day, the illustrious, high-born prince Lord Wilhelm, Landgrave of Hesse, tested the terra sigillata, which Andreas Berthold of Oschatz provided, in Kassel, in the following manner, on dogs.[1]

So begins the intriguing description of a test conducted at the court of Landgrave Wilhelm IV of Hesse-Kassel (1532–1592), which aimed to determine whether an antidote called terra sigillata was effective against poison. This experiment can be found in a German-language manuscript containing medicinal recipes, *Cod. Pal. germ. 177*, now held in the University of Heidelberg Library (Figure 7.1). The anonymous author describes a series of tests on dogs using terra sigillata and four different poisons, including three poisonous plants – aconite, nerium, and apocynum – as well as mercury sublimate, a chemical poison. Eight unlucky dogs acted as the test subjects. In each test, one dog was given a dose of poison, followed by an equal dose of the terra sigillata, and a second dog received the same poison, often in a lower dose, but no antidote. The scribe neatly numbered the tests, recorded the description of each dog and the poison and antidote dosage it received in German, and switched to Latin for a narrative of what happened to each animal. The Latin anecdotes are remarkable both in their detail and their outcomes. They meticulously describe the paroxysms, expulsions, and other symptoms the dogs experienced and record whether the animal lived or died. In all cases, the dogs that received the terra sigillata survived, while the dogs that only received poison died.

At a basic glance, this short document raises many questions that are not immediately easy to answer. Who was Landgrave Wilhelm of Hesse, and why was he conducting poison experiments on dogs? What was terra sigillata? Why was it thought to cure poison? What did people think about the astonishing outcome of these tests? When and why did this account find its way into a recipe collection belonging to the Palatinate court? And what does it tell us about early medical experiments? This essay will try to solve these puzzles. I will build out from the manuscript, first addressing the kinds of questions and problems that the historian encounters when faced with a text of this nature. I will then broaden the scope to examine why this text can be found in a recipe collection and what significance this dog trial had in the history of medicine in late sixteenth-century Germany. As we will see, this manuscript provides a window on the nascent history of experiment

DOI: 10.4324/9781003094876-10

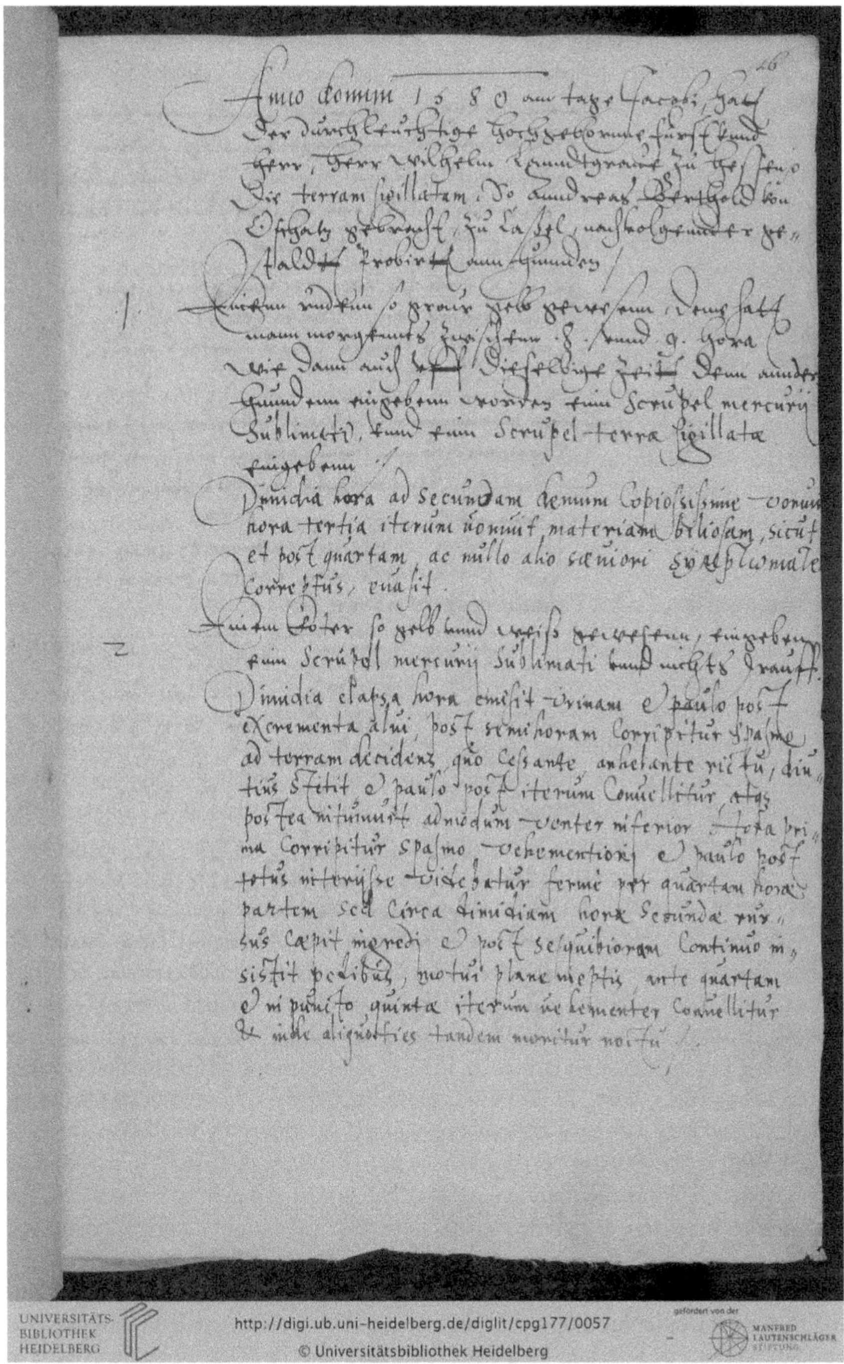

Figure 7.1 Landgrave Wilhelm's Dog Trials, dated 1580. University of Heidelberg Library.

in sixteenth-century Europe. Yet it gives us an obstructed view. There is much that this short text conceals, and only by looking elsewhere can we fully understand it. Viewing one text in isolation only gets us so far – we need to look elsewhere and compare to find the full picture.

For the historian to even begin assessing this document, the first task is to read it. Most of the recipes in *Cod. Pal. germ. 177* are in German, but this excerpt is written in both German and Latin. A researcher thus needs to have reading competency in both languages and also the ability to parse the sixteenth-century German script known as *Kurrentschrift* (a skill that takes practice, as some letters of the alphabet look quite different from their modern forms). Unlike some of the other entries in *Cod. Pal. germ 177*, this document is written in secretary hand, the handwriting taught to professional copyists, which makes it more accessible than many pages of the manuscript.[2] Yet learning to read the document is just the first step in decoding its puzzles. Once we can decipher it, the content is at once fascinating and perplexing. Both the scene described in this text and the document itself have complex histories, and both demonstrate the importance of seeking context and examining problems from all angles when analyzing manuscript materials.

The Manuscript: *Codex Palatinum germanicum 177*

Let's start with the manuscript, cataloged simply as a "Medical Manuscript Collection" (*Medizinische Sammelhandschrift*). This generic label hides a surprisingly adventurous history. *Codex Palatinum germanicum* (abbreviated as *Cod. Pal. germ.*) *177* was part of the Biblioteca Palatina, or Princely Palatine Library, a jewel among the German libraries of the Renaissance. The library was officially founded by Elector Ottheinrich of the Palatinate in the 1550s, but it drew on the holdings of past Palatine princes. It contained gems of German religion and literature, including a ninth-century illuminated gospel book and a stunning fourteenth-century masterpiece of Minnesang literature, the Codex Manesse. An early seventeenth-century visitor from Oxford, Thomas Coryat, marveled that "no Librarie of all Christendome, no not the Vatican of Rome nor Cardinall Bessarions of Venice can compare with it," although he loyally claimed that it still did not surpass the Oxford library.[3] Until the early seventeenth century, the Biblioteca Palatina was held at the Palatine castle in Heidelberg, but then disaster struck. In 1622, Catholic troops sacked Heidelberg during the Thirty Years' War. The castle was partially destroyed (you can still see the ruins today), and Pope Gregory XV quickly claimed the library for himself as spoils of war. The entire library was packed up and sent to the Vatican in 1623, supervised by Leone Allacci, the Vatican librarian. Most of the library remains in Rome today, but 848 German manuscripts returned to Heidelberg in 1816 amid complex diplomatic negotiations. These German texts are known as the *Codices Palatini germanici*.[4]

This history has direct relevance to understanding *Cod. Pal. germ. 177*. In addition to its spectacular holdings, the Biblioteca Palatina also contained thousands of workaday books of religion, medicine, literature, and law. The documents sent to the Vatican in the seventeenth century contained both bound manuscripts and loose pieces of paper. In Rome, the piles of paper were divided into book-sized chunks and bound in plain, white parchment binding. Manuscripts with this seventeenth-century Roman binding exist as bound manuscripts only because someone in Rome decided to make them so – and *Cod. Pal. germ. 177* falls into this category. The historian thus needs to proceed carefully and question the extent to which the documents in the "medical manuscript collection" originally belonged together.

In the case of *Cod. Pal. germ 177*, most of the individual entries probably did belong to one owner. In the first decade of the twenty-first century, a team of researchers carefully analyzed all of the *Codices Palatini germanici* and digitized them.[5] Nearly a third of the texts were medical, and the researchers published a special study of the medical manuscripts.[6] Using water marks (distinctive markings made in the paper production process) as well as handwriting and document analysis, the Heidelberg researchers determined that most sections of *Cod. Pal. germ. 177* were closely connected to a German princess, Duchess Elisabeth of Saxony (1552–1590), wife of Count Palatine Johann Casimir of Simmern (1543–1592).[7] The dog trials sit between two sections of medicinal recipes on which Duchess Elisabeth wrote her name. If you look closely at the dog trial description, you can see evidence of folds in the paper, suggesting that the document came to Elisabeth enclosed in a letter – as was also the case for many (although not all) of the documents in *Cod. Pal. germ. 177.*

We cannot know how many hands the dog trials passed through on their way to Duchess Elisabeth; nor can we assume that she intended these papers to be bound into a manuscript and preserved for posterity. We also don't know when the trial account was copied, or when Elisabeth received it. At the same time, this long back story fills in one piece of the puzzle. The dog trials at the castle in Kassel garnered enough interest from other German courts that the results were shared in a letter that found its way to Duchess Elisabeth. The letter's location among the plundered Heidelberg papers is also significant. In 1580, the date of the dog trials, the duchess resided in her husband's palace in Kaiserslautern. She did not move to Heidelberg until 1583, when Johann Casimir became regent of the Palatinate – which either means that this letter traveled with her to Heidelberg or that the description continued to circulate a few years after Landgrave Wilhelm's dog trials took place. Either way, their place among her papers suggests that some importance was attached to them.

At this point, however, we are left with some crucial questions. Why was this document of interest to Duchess Elisabeth? Was this test a one-off event, or was it part of a larger pattern? And how does it fit into the overall history of experiment? It's time to look beyond *Cod. Pal. germ 177* to try to uncover its context. Three names stand out immediately in the opening lines of the dog trials. The first is Landgrave Wilhelm IV of Hesse-Kassel, whose support for scientific endeavors, especially astronomy and alchemy, is well known.[8] The second is terra sigillata, the antidote being tested, and the third is Andreas Berthold of Oschatz, who provided the terra sigillata.

The German Terra Sigillata

An article by the historian Karl H. Dannenfeldt helps us with Andreas Berthold and his terra sigillata.[9] Dannenfeldt notes that terra sigillata originally referred to clay found on a particular hillside on the Greek isle of Lemnos. Once a year, in a religious ceremony, the clay was refined, formed into medallions, and stamped with the image of Diana (hence terra sigillata, or "sealed earth"). The medallions were prized as an antidote to poison and stomach complaints, lauded by Galen and mentioned in medieval Arabic and Latin texts. In Western Europe, supplies of the drug were limited and concerns about fraud abounded, especially after the Ottomans captured Lemnos in 1456. A growing interest in terra sigillata combined with concerns about Turkish control of the drug opened a space for local, European earths purported to have similar properties.[10] Around 1550, a Paracelsian physician in Silesia named Johannes Schulz (widely known as Johannes Montanus) discovered a new medicinal earth in the mountains outside the city of Striga (later Striegau and now Strezgom, Poland). This earth began to be mined and stamped with a seal containing three mountains, and it became an important part of the Strigan economy. Dannenfeldt also notes that a man named Andreas Berthold published the first treatise about the Silesian earth in 1583.[11]

With this helpful information in mind, we can turn to Andreas Berthold. A quick search on the WorldCat (First Search) database reveals that Berthold's book on terra sigillata, *Terrae sigillatae nuper in Germania repertae* (Frankfurt am Main, 1583), was originally published in Latin and translated into English in 1587.[12] The Latin version contains an appendix written by Johannes Montanus; the English version leaves off this appendix and adds a note on where to buy the drug, but is otherwise more or less true to the Latin. Berthold identifies his terra sigillata as a new, German earth with the same properties as the esteemed Lemnian terra sigillata: useful against poison, plague, the bites of venomous animals, headaches, brain inflammation, excess bleeding, head colds, intestinal complaints, burns, and wounds, among others. At the end of Berthold's description of the drug's marvelous properties are letters testifying to the terra sigillata's success – and here we find another account of Landgrave Wilhelm's dog trials! This version is nearly identical to the handwritten copy in *Cod. Pal. germ. 177*, except that the description of the dog trials is prefaced by a letter from two of the landgrave's physicians, Maritius Thaurer and Laurencius Hyperius, and his apothecary Johan Krug. The two physicians' names also appear at the bottom of the trial description, a detail that is missing from the handwritten document.[13]

The letter adds significant context to Landgrave Wilhelm's dog trials. It describes how Berthold came to the landgrave with a medicinal earth he had discovered in an old gold mine outside of Schweidnitz in Silesia. Berthold claimed that it could cure poison, plague, and various diseases. Distrustful of these marvelous claims, Landgrave Wilhelm commanded his physicians to "make a perfect tryall of the saide earth," upon which they conducted a "double proofe" on eight dogs.[14] The physicians summarized the trial's impressive results in their letter and noted that, given its overwhelming success, Berthold had requested a "letter of credite." Landgrave Wilhelm had granted the request and commanded that the letter be signed by the physicians and sealed with his privy seal, "both in the favour of the man and advancement of the truth."[15] The brief mention of Berthold in *Cod. Pal. germ. 177* thus obscures his larger role in the story of the German terra sigillata.

Indeed, the Kassel dog trials are just one of three testimonial letters describing similar experiments. The second letter comes from Count Wolfgang II of Hohenlohe (1546–1610) and attests to the success the terra sigillata in a test on a criminal condemned to death. Count Wolfgang's letter notes that Berthold's terra sigillata had been proven previously "by sundrie witnesses upon a great number of dogges, which made me also desirous to see the triall of it."[16] This remark shows that Elisabeth of Saxony was not the only person to receive an account of Landgrave Wilhelm's dog trials and that other aristocrats took the tests seriously. Count Wolfgang's test took place in Langenburg castle in January 1581, conducted by his physician, Georg Pistorius, and his apothecary, Johannes Lutzen, in front of a crowd of aristocrats and commoners. The prisoner survived a fatal dose of sublimated mercury and was banished from coming within ten miles of Langenburg. Like the letter from Landgrave Wilhelm's physicians, the letter from Count Wolfgang emphasized that he had agreed to give Berthold a written testimonial "for the furtherance and advancement of the truth" and that the letter was signed "with our seale Manuell," referring to the wax seal that was typically affixed to official communications.[17]

The final testimonial letter came from the mayor and aldermen of the town of Jülich and described a trial on dogs that took place in February 1580. In this case, a citizen of Cologne named Crisant von Cronenberg came to Jülich in Berthold's name, bringing a sample of Berthold's terra sigillata and offering to test it on two dogs in front of the town magistrates. This trial, overseen by the town surgeon Johannes Ottweiler, had a similarly impressive outcome – the dog given the terra sigillata survived, and the dog who received only poison died. Cronenberg left with "our Letters of Credence, sealed with our common Seal," which he then turned over to Berthold. In this case, the letter provides a more detailed description of the remedy itself. It consisted of earthen medallions – some red, some gray – stamped with a coat of arms portraying the sun, half moon, and five planets as well as the letters ABVO (Andreas Berthold von Oschatz). This description suggests that Berthold's earth was different from the Strigan earth that Dannenfeldt discussed, and indeed, Berthold's use of the plural "terrae sigillatae," or sealed earths, in the Latin title suggests that more than one kind of terra sigillata was in play. Specimens of terra sigillata held in the Basel Pharmacy Museum today confirm the existence of multiple types of German terra sigillata (see Figures 7.2 and 7.3).

All of this information helps us answer a few crucial questions about the document in *Cod. Pal. germ 177*. Landgrave Wilhelm's test on dogs was not an isolated event – it was part of a series of trials conducted by Andreas Berthold, whose terra sigillata was viewed as a promising new antidote. The outcome of these tests using poison was taken as a marker of overall efficacy against numerous ailments, and the results were taken seriously enough that rulers like Landgrave Wilhelm agreed to issue official testimonial letters, stamped and sealed, to Berthold. This helps explain why someone shared a handwritten description of dog trials with Duchess Elisabeth of Saxony (and, it seems, with other aristocrats at German courts).

There is strong evidence in *Cod. Pal. germ. 177* that Duchess Elisabeth remained interested in Berthold's work: a letter from Andreas Berthold himself, addressed to

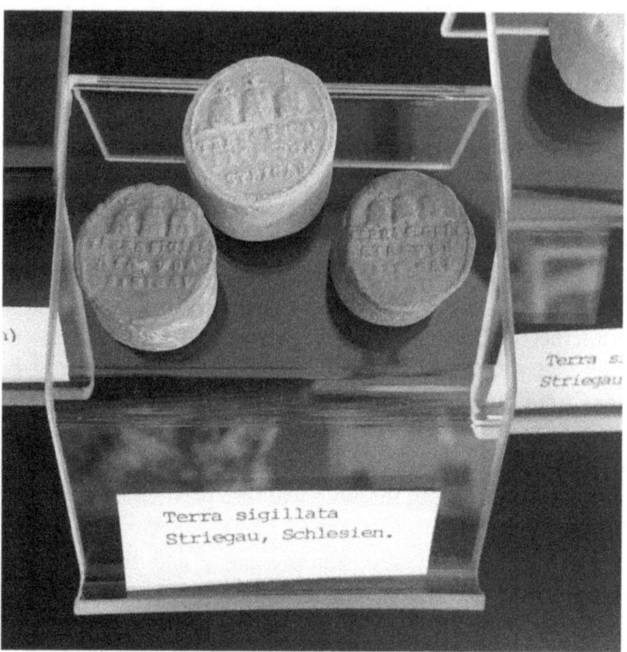
Terra sigillata
Striegau, Schlesien.

Figure 7.2 Silesian Terra sigillata from Striga, Basel Pharmacy Museum. Photo by the author.

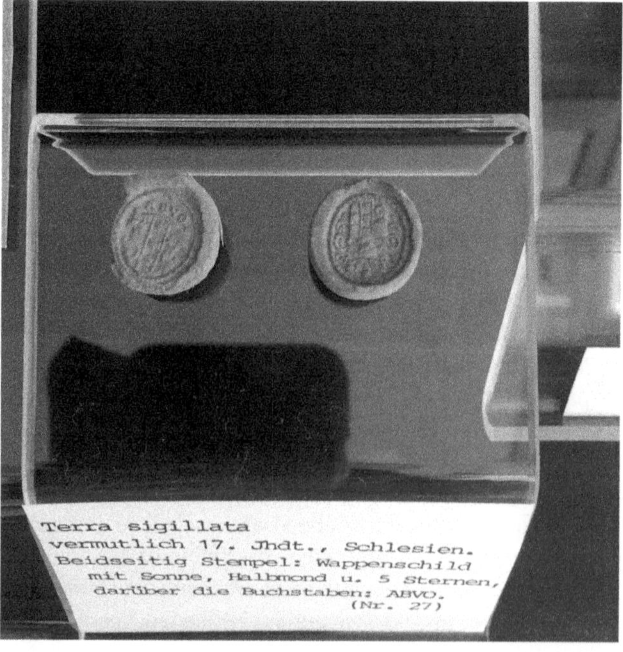
Terra sigillata
vermutlich 17. Jhdt., Schlesien.
Beidseitig Stempel: Wappenschild
mit Sonne, Halbmond u. 5 Sternen,
darüber die Buchstaben: ABVO.
(Nr. 27)

Figure 7.3 Andreas Berthold's terra sigillata, Basel Pharmacy Museum. Photo by the author.

a "Luminous high-born Duchess," can be found about 30 folios after the dog trials (Figure 7.4). The tone of the letter suggests that it was not the first time Berthold had written to the unnamed duchess (not definitively Duchess Elisabeth, but likely given the context). He notes that she "desired that I reveal to her nature's hidden secrets that I have in part discovered in fact and in trials."[18] The rest of the letter details the occult (hidden) medical properties of various materials – stones, roots, herbs, and snakeskin. It describes no actual tests, but Berthold's use of the word *Proba* (test or trial) seems to reflect an explicit request from the duchess. In short, Berthold's terra sigillata trials provoked interest in other meaningful medical tests, at least among some members of the German aristocracy.

If one starts looking further, it becomes clear that Berthold's dog trials were just the tip of the iceberg. Using poison on living subjects to test antidotes – including tests on condemned criminals – became a regular practice between 1524 and 1600. Evidence of these tests appears in various printed texts and archival documents – including the archival file for Count Wolfgang of Hohenlohe's test on the condemned thief, which reveal that the count played a far more active role in seeking to use the condemned criminal as a test subject than Berthold's official letter suggests. My book *The Poison Trials: Wonder Drugs, Experiment, and the Battle for Authority in Renaissance Science* (2021) uses these poison antidote tests as a window on evolving ideas about experiment, authority, and medical ethics. Here I would like to zero in on just the first of these issues. How do Landgrave Wilhelm's dog trials – and other tests of poison – fit into the history of experimental practices?

Early Experimentation

Experiment as we know it today did not exist in the sixteenth century. While we might think of experiment as a scientific procedure that tests a hypothesis with the aim of learning or teaching a fact (or multiple facts), the medieval understanding of experiment simply referenced something done in practice. While it could mean a test that attempted to ascertain or demonstrate something, it could also just refer to a practice done or observed through experience. From the sixteenth through eighteenth centuries, the "testing" connotation of experiment started to eclipse its other meanings. Foundational works on the history of scientific experiment by authors such as Charles Schmitt, Peter Dear, Steven Shapin, and Simon Schaffer place the major experimental "moment" in the later seventeenth century, as natural philosophers built off the foundation laid by Galileo Galilei (1564–1642) and Francis Bacon (1561–1626).[19] This scholarship has focused particularly on the mathematical and physical sciences as the catalyst for consolidating notions of experiment. There are solid linguistic and theoretical arguments for this chronology. As Schmitt has shown, the words "experiment" and "experience" were near synonyms until the seventeenth century, and other words like "trial," "proof," or "historia" could also signify experimental practices. Indeed, the author of our document merely notes that Landgrave Wilhelm "tested" (*probiertt*) the terra sigillata on dogs. Additionally, the development of experiment has tended to be discussed in tandem with anti-Aristotelian movements in the mathematical and physical sciences, in which attacks on Aristotle's geocentric cosmology and physics gained increasing support.

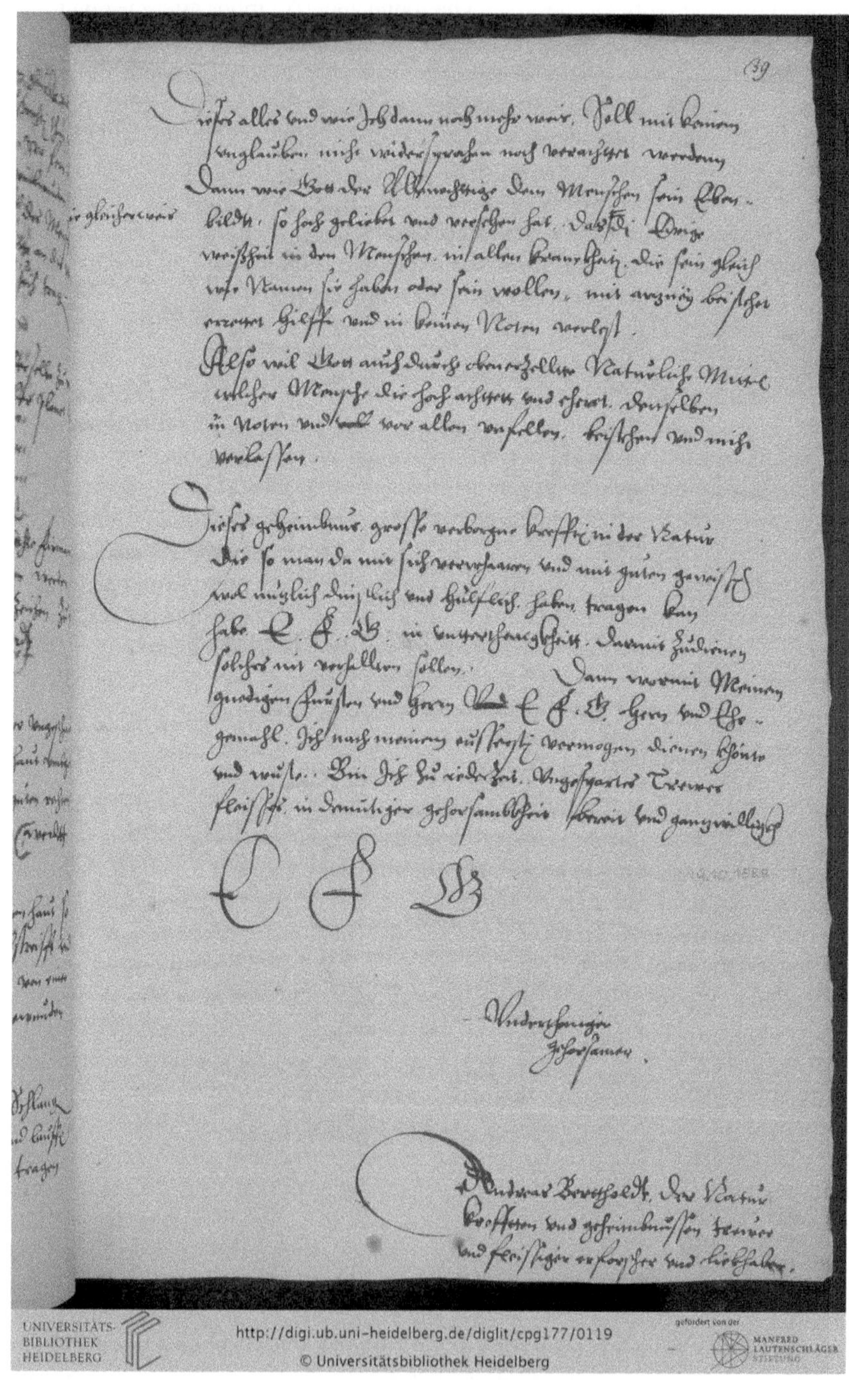

Figure 7.4 Final page of a letter from Andreas Berthold to an unnamed duchess, in Berthold's hand. University of Heidelberg Library.

Scholarly medicine followed Galen more than Aristotle, and Galen's physiology of four humors continued to dominate medical theory.[20] Medical experiments rarely aimed at overturning Galen in the same way that Galileo's experiments tried to poke holes in Aristotle's theories, although they did sometimes highlight places where Galen was wrong. For example, the famous anatomist Andreas Vesalius gleefully used his own human dissections to showcase Galen's erroneous assumptions based on animal dissections, since Galen had been unable to dissect humans. Nonetheless, Vesalius fully accepted Galen's general theoretical principles.[21] The only true theoretical threat to Galen before the seventeenth century was the iconoclastic Swiss healer Paracelsus, who derided Galenic medicine and promoted a new chemical theory of the body. Despite widespread interest in Paracelsus's medicines, his theories gained less traction, and there was little experimental protocol that pitted the Galenic and Paracelsian theories against each other.[22]

In our document, the physicians who oversaw the dog trials at Landgrave Wilhelm's court were committed Galenists, and although Andreas Berthold drew on Paracelsian ideas in his book, those theories do not appear in any of his trial descriptions. There appears to be no interest in overturning accepted dogma in this document or other poison trials. Some physicians even used tests of poison antidotes to underscore the writings of medical authorities like Galen and Avicenna.[23] This approach tended to be typical of medical experimentation. In early modern Europe, experiments rarely aimed at repudiating authorities. Instead, they tended to focus on *what worked*, rather than on specific theories. Both Galenists and Paracelsians were avid experimenters.

If one considers experimental methods rather than medical theories, however, it becomes clear that medicine played a leading role in the development of experimentation. Historians such as Michael McVaugh, Harold Cook, and Paula Findlen have pointed to numerous instances of proto-experimental practices in medieval and early modern medicine, particularly in the area of drug testing, anatomical investigations, and the study of mineral waters.[24] Evan Ragland has shown that the phrase "to make an experiment/experience/trial" was widespread among sixteenth-century learned physicians.[25] Although the language of experiment remained unspecific, the idea of a test that could be provoked deliberately (rather than just observed) was well developed by the sixteenth century.[26] Landgrave Wilhelm's dog trials fit squarely in this trend.

Even so, this experimental account demonstrates a striking thoroughness in the way the trial was conceived. The testers meticulously chose eight different dogs and four different poisons, and each poison was tested on two animals – one that received the antidote and one that did not. Both the Latin and English versions of Berthold's text describe this test as a "double proof," a term vaguely reminiscent of our modern use of a "control" group in clinical trials.[27] However, trying to find "modern" experimental ideas in early modern experiment is fraught with pitfalls. If one looks closer, one notes that the testers carefully manipulated the trial in several ways that would no longer seem relevant to us. They describe each dog's color and features and make an attempt to pair up dogs of a similar markings: for example, the first pair of dogs included a "gray-yellow male dog" and a "yellow and white mutt;" and the second and third pairs all had dark coats with white throats. While the color of a dog would likely no longer seem like a useful variable for us to consider, it is a marker of the care with which this experiment was devised. The document also notes that all of the tests took place at the same time of day, "between eight and nine in the morning," and it carefully records every symptom the dogs experienced after ingesting the poison and (for half) the antidote.[28] Although these dog trials may appear gruesome and excessively cruel to us now, they were a very carefully contrived set of tests set up with significant attention to detail, and someone recorded the results in a methodical document that was shared with other princely courts.[29]

The Dog Trials in Context

What should we make of this very strange document? How should we fit it into both the history of medicine in general and the history of experiment in particular? For one thing, it adds evidence to the notion that an interest in medical experimentation was widespread in sixteenth-century Europe. At the same time, tests of poison antidotes stand out as particularly meticulous in terms of record keeping. Most of the medical experiments in Ragland's study made only brief mention of "making a trial," without any discussion of method. Yet like Landgrave Wilhelm's dog trials, several other contemporary accounts of poison trials gave extensive detail in terms of elapsed time, symptoms, and quantities. Something about testing poison prompted a greater interest in record keeping – and that something was likely the strong interest in finding effective antidotes at princely courts. After all, Renaissance rulers lived in constant fear of being poisoned, and constant rumors of attempted and actual poisonings flew across Europe.[30]

The dog trials recorded in *Cod. Pal. germ 177* provide an early window on the increasing complexity of experimental thinking in the sixteenth century. By testing multiple poisons on dogs, Landgrave Wilhelm's physicians presaged the broader (often gruesome) use of animals in seventeenth-century medical experimentation.[31] Nevertheless, Landgrave Wilhelm's dog trials remained firmly rooted in sixteenth-century courtly conventions – they took place for the benefit of the prince's health, they focused on promising new drugs, and they quickly became incorporated into epistolary exchanges. These exchanges were not limited to men. The document almost certainly exists today because Duchess Elisabeth deemed it important.[32] Following the winding path of why she (likely) did so and how the document came to rest in Heidelberg leads to surprisingly interesting places.

Notes

1 "*Anno domini* 1580 am Tage *Jacobi* hatt der durchleuchtige hochgeborne Furst vnnd Herr, Herr Wilhelm, Landgraue zu Hessen etc., die *terram sigillatam*, So Anndreas Berthold von Oschatz gebracht, zu Kassel, nachvolgenderweise probiertt ann Hunden." Universitätsbibliothek Heidelberg, *Codex Palatinum germanicum* (hereafter *Cod. Pal. germ*) 177, fol. 16r.

2 There are many websites that offer tutorials and exercises in reading *Kurrentschrift*, such as the University of Zurich (https://www.adfontes.uzh.ch/tutorium/schriften-lesen/schriftgeschichte/fruehneuzeitliche-schrift) and the University of Vienna (https://gonline.univie.ac.at/erste-schritte-in-kurrent/lese-und-schreibuebungen), and there are even YouTube videos that teach the handwriting. The Beinecke Library at Yale University has a tutorial for reading English secretary hand (https://beinecke.library.yale.edu/article/quarantine-reading-learn-read-secretary-hand).

3 Thomas Coryat, *Coryats Crudities Hastily Gobled vp in Five Moneths Trauells in France, Sauoy, Italy, ... Some Parts of High Germany, and the Netherlands* (London: Printed by William Stansby for the author, 1611), 477–78, https://search.proquest.com/docview/2240870301.

4 Veit Probst, "Digitization at the Heidelberg University Library: The Digital Bibliotheca Palatina Project," *Digital Philology* 6, no. 2 (2017): 213–33, https://doi.org/10.1353/dph.2017.0011.

5 The digitized manuscripts can be viewed here: https://digi.ub.uni-heidelberg.de/de/bpd/virtuelle_bibliothek/codpalgerm/1xx.html. On the digitization project, see especially Probst, 213–33.

6 Matthias Miller and Karin Zimmermann, eds., *Die medizinischen Handschriften unter den Codices Palatini germanici 182–303*, 2005, http://www.ub.uni-heidelberg.de/archiv/5709. On the medical manuscripts, see also Debra L. Stoudt, "The Medical Manuscripts of the Bibliotheca Palatina," in *Manuscript Sources of Medieval Medicine: A Book of Essays*, ed. Margaret Rose Schleissner (New York: Garland, 1995), 159–81.

7 Miller and Zimmermann, *Die medizinischen Handschriften*, 420–34.

8 Bruce T. Moran, "Wilhelm IV of Hesse-Kassel: Informal Communication and the Aristocratic Context of Discovery," in *Scientific Discovery: Case Studies*, ed. Thomas Nickles (Dordrecht: D. Riedel, 1983), 67–96.

9 Karl H. Dannenfeldt, "The Introduction of a New Sixteenth-Century Drug, Terra Silesiaca," *Medical History* 28 (1984): 174–88.

10 Dannenfeldt, 174–75. Katharine Park has described the spread of a Maltese terra sigillata known as St. Paul's earth in Italy. Katharine Park, "Country Medicine in the City Marketplace: Snakehandlers as Itinerant Healers," *Renaissance Studies* 15 (2001): 104–20.

11 Dannenfeldt, "Terra Silesiaca," 176–78. For more on the relationship between Montanus and Berthold, see Alisha Rankin, *The Poison Trials: Wonder Drugs, Experiment, and the Battle for Authority in Renaissance Science* (Chicago, IL: University of Chicago Press, 2021), chap. 6.

12 Andreas Berthold, *Terrae sigillatae nuper in Germania repertae* (Frankfurt am Main, 1583); Andreas Berthold, *The Wonderfull and Strange Effect and Vertues of a New Terra Sigillata Lately Found out in Germanie* (London, 1587).

13 Berthold, *Terrae sigillatae*, B4r–C2v; Berthold, *Wonderfull and Strange Effect*, 24–28.

14 I am quoting the English translation here. The Latin version reads similarly: "facerunt periculum … eiusmodi Terram sigillatam duplici probarunt examine." Berthold, *Terrae sigillatae*, B4v; Berthold, *Wonderfull and Strange Effect*, 27.

15 Berthold, *Wonderfull and Strange Effect*, 27.

16 Ibid., 33.

17 Ibid., 35.

18 Cod. Pal. germ. 177, fols 38r–39r, at 38r. "dennoch EFG ettliche jnn der Natur verborgene geheimbnussen, so Jch zum theil in der Thatt und proba erfaren, an mich gnedigst gesonnen, dieselbe zuoffenbaren…"

19 Charles B. Schmitt, "Experience and Experiment: A Comparison of Zabarella's View with Galileo's in De Motu," *Studies in the Renaissance* 16 (1969): 80–138; Peter Dear, *Discipline & Experience: The Mathematical Way in the Scientific Revolution* (Chicago, IL: University of Chicago Press, 1995); Dear, Peter, "The Meanings of Experience," in *Early Modern Science*, ed. Katharine Park and Lorraine Daston, vol. 3, The Cambridge

History of Science (Cambridge: Cambridge University Press, 2006), 106–31; Peter Dear, "Narratives, Anecdotes, and Experiments: Turning Experience into Science in the Seventeenth Century," in *The Literary Structure of Scientific Argument*, ed. Peter Dear (Philadelphia: University of Pennsylvania Press, 1991), 135–63; Steven Shapin and Simon Schaffer, *Leviathan and the Air-Pump: Hobbes, Boyle, and the Experimental Life* (Princeton, NJ: Princeton University Press, 1985); Steven Shapin, *The Scientific Revolution* (Chicago, IL: University of Chicago Press, 1996).

20 For an introduction to Galenic theory, see Nancy G. Siraisi, *Medieval and Early Renaissance Medicine: An Introduction to Knowledge and Practice* (Chicago, IL: University of Chicago Press, 1990); Erin Sullivan and Andrew Wear, "Materiality, Nature and the Body," in *The Routledge Handbook of Material Culture in Early Modern Europe*, ed. Catherine Richardson, Tara Hamling, and David Gaimster (London: Routledge, 2016), 141–57, https://doi.org/10.4324/9781315613161.ch9.

21 Andreas Vesalius, *The Fabric of the Human Body: An Annotated Translation of the 1543 and 1555 Editions of "De Humani Corporis Fabrica Libri Septem,"* ed. and trans. Daniel H. Garrison and Malcolm H. Hast (Basel: Karger, 2014); Roberto lo Presti, "Anatomy as Epistemology: The Body of Man and the Body of Medicine in Vesalius and His Ancient Sources (Celsus, Galen)," *Renaissance and Reformation/Renaissance et Réforme* 33, no. 3 (2010): 27–60.

22 On Paracelsus, see especially Charles Webster, *Paracelsus: Medicine, Magic and Mission at the End of Time* (New Haven, CT: Yale University Press, 2008); Bruce T. Moran, *Paracelsus: An Alchemical Life* (London: Reaktion Books, 2019). On the interest in Paracelsian remedies rather than theories, see Michael Stolberg, *Learned Physicians and Everyday Medical Practice in the Renaissance* (Berlin and Boston, MA: De Gruyter Oldenbourg, 2021), 363–77.

23 The Italian physician Pietro Andrea Mattioli (1501–1577) specifically used poison trials on condemned criminals to reify Avicenna's writings on toxicity. Rankin, *The Poison Trials*, chap 3. On the different motives of medical experimentation, see Elaine Leong and Alisha Rankin, "Testing Drugs and Trying Cures: Experiment and Medicine in Medieval and Early Modern Europe," *Bulletin of the History of Medicine* 91 (2017): 157–82.

24 Michael McVaugh, "Determining a Drug's Properties: Medieval Experimental Protocols," *Bulletin of the History of Medicine* 91, no. 2 (July 25, 2017): 183–209, https://doi.org/10.1353/bhm.2017.0024; Paula Findlen, *Possessing Nature: Museums, Collecting, and Scientific Culture in Early Modern Italy* (Berkeley: University of California Press, 1994); Paula Findlen, "Controlling the Experiment: Rhetoric, Court Patronage, and the Experimental Method of Francesco Redi," *History of Science* 31 (1993): 35–64; Harold J. Cook, "Victories for Empiricism, Failures for Theory: Medicine and Science in the Seventeenth Century," in *The Body as Object and Instrument of Knowledge*, ed. Charles T. Wolfe and Ofer Gal (Dordrecht: Springer, 2010), 9–32; Harold J. Cook, *The Decline of the Old Medical Regime in Stuart London* (Ithaca, NY: Cornell University Press, 1986); Harold J. Cook, "Global Economies and Local Knowledge in the East Indies: Jacobus Bontius Learns the Facts of Nature," in *Colonial Botany: Science, Commerce, and Politics in the Early Modern World*, ed. Londa L. Schiebinger and Claudia Swan (Philadelphia: University of Pennsylvania Press, 2005), 100–18.

25 Evan R. Ragland, "Making Trials in Sixteenth-Century European Academic Medicine," *Isis* 108 (2017): 503–28.

26 The 2017 special issue of the *Bulletin of the History of Medicine* on "Testing Drugs and Trying Cures in Premodern Europe," which I co-edited with Elaine Leong, demonstrates the widespread interest in contrived drug tests in medieval and early modern Europe. See Leong and Rankin, "Testing Drugs and Trying Cures."

27 Although the language around experimental controls did not develop until the nineteenth century, some kinds of control have been used since antiquity, as Jutta Schickore has noted. Twentieth-century philosopher of science Edwin G. Boring laid out three specific

types of control: a check or verification, a restraint to maintain constant conditions, and a manipulation of an independent variable in a specific manner. Jutta Schickore, *About Method: Experimenters, Snake Venom, and the History of Writing Scientifically* (Chicago, IL: University of Chicago Press, 2017), 151–52; Edwin G. Boring, "The Nature and History of Experimental Control," *The American Journal of Psychology* 67, no. 4 (1954): 573–89, https://doi.org/10.2307/1418483.

28 Cod. Pal. germ. 177, fol. 16r.

29 In the case of Galileo, Peter Dear has argued that written narratives helped codify experimental practice. Dear, "Narratives, Anecdotes, and Experiments."

30 Rankin, *The Poison Trials*, chaps 2–4.

31 Anita Guerrini, *The Courtiers' Anatomists: Animals and Humans in Louis XIV's Paris* (Chicago, IL: University of Chicago Press, 2015); Evan R. Ragland, "Experimental Clinical Medicine and Drug Action in Mid-Seventeenth-Century Leiden," *Bulletin of the History of Medicine* 91, no. 2 (July 25, 2017): 331–61, https://doi.org/10.1353/bhm.2017.0029.

32 Alisha Rankin, *Panaceia's Daughters: Noblewomen as Healers in Early Modern Germany* (Chicago, IL: University of Chicago Press, 2013), chap. 1.

Bibliography

Manuscript Sources

Recipe Collection of Elisabeth of Saxony, Countess Palatinate. University of Heidelberg Library, Codex Palatinum germanicum 177.

Printed Sources

Berthold, Andreas. *Terrae sigillatae nuper in Germania repertae*. Frankfurt am Main, 1583.

———. *The Wonderfull and Strange Effect and Vertues of a New Terra Sigillata Lately Found out in Germanie*. London, 1587.

Boring, Edwin G. "The Nature and History of Experimental Control." *The American Journal of Psychology* 67, no. 4 (1954): 573–89. https://doi.org/10.2307/1418483.

Cook, Harold J. *The Decline of the Old Medical Regime in Stuart London*. Ithaca, NY: Cornell University Press, 1986.

———. "Global Economies and Local Knowledge in the East Indies: Jacobus Bontius Learns the Facts of Nature." In *Colonial Botany: Science, Commerce, and Politics in the Early Modern World*, edited by Londa L. Schiebinger and Claudia Swan, 100–18. Philadelphia: University of Pennsylvania Press, 2005.

———. "Victories for Empiricism, Failures for Theory: Medicine and Science in the Seventeenth Century." In *The Body as Object and Instrument of Knowledge*, edited by Charles T. Wolfe and Ofer Gal, 9–32. Dordrecht: Springer, 2010.

Coryat, Thomas. *Coryats Crudities Hastily Gobled vp in Five Moneths Trauells in France, Sauoy, Italy, ... Some Parts of High Germany, and the Netherlands*. London: Printed by William Stansby for the author, 1611. https://search.proquest.com/docview/2240870301.

Dannenfeldt, Karl H. "The Introduction of a New Sixteenth-Century Drug, Terra Silesiaca." *Medical History* 28 (1984): 174–88.

Dear, Peter. *Discipline & Experience: The Mathematical Way in the Scientific Revolution*. Chicago, IL: University of Chicago Press, 1995.

———. "The Meanings of Experience." In *Early Modern Science*, edited by Park, Katharine and Daston, Lorraine, 3, 106–31. The Cambridge History of Science. Cambridge: Cambridge University Press, 2006.

———. "Narratives, Anecdotes, and Experiments: Turning Experience into Science in the Seventeenth Century." In *The Literary Structure of Scientific Argument*, edited by Peter Dear, 135–63. Philadelphia: University of Pennsylvania Press, 1991.

Findlen, Paula. "Controlling the Experiment: Rhetoric, Court Patronage, and the Experimental Method of Francesco Redi." *History of Science* 31 (1993): 35–64.

———. *Possessing Nature: Museums, Collecting, and Scientific Culture in Early Modern Italy*. Berkeley: University of California Press, 1994.

Guerrini, Anita. *The Courtiers' Anatomists: Animals and Humans in Louis XIV's Paris*. Chicago, IL: University of Chicago Press, 2015.

Leong, Elaine, and Alisha Rankin. "Testing Drugs and Trying Cures: Experiment and Medicine in Medieval and Early Modern Europe." *Bulletin of the History of Medicine* 91 (2017): 157–82.

McVaugh, Michael. "Determining a Drug's Properties: Medieval Experimental Protocols." *Bulletin of the History of Medicine* 91, no. 2 (July 25, 2017): 183–209. https://doi.org/10.1353/bhm.2017.0024.

Miller, Matthias, and Karin Zimmermann, eds. *Die medizinischen Handschriften unter den Codices Palatini germanici 182–303*, 2005. http://www.ub.uni-heidelberg.de/archiv/5709.

Moran, Bruce T. *Paracelsus: An Alchemical Life*. London: Reaktion Books, 2019.

———. "Wilhelm IV of Hesse-Kassel: Informal Communication and the Aristocratic Context of Discovery." In *Scientific Discovery: Case Studies*, edited by Thomas Nickles, 67–96. Dordrecht: D. Riedel, 1983.

Park, Katharine. "Country Medicine in the City Marketplace: Snakehandlers as Itinerant Healers." *Renaissance Studies* 15 (2001): 104–20.

Presti, Roberto lo. "Anatomy as Epistemology: The Body of Man and the Body of Medicine in Vesalius and His Ancient Sources (Celsus, Galen)." *Renaissance and Reformation/Renaissance et Réforme* 33, no. 3 (2010): 27–60.

Probst, Veit. "Digitization at the Heidelberg University Library: The Digital Bibliotheca Palatina Project." *Digital Philology* 6, no. 2 (2017): 213–33. https://doi.org/10.1353/dph.2017.0011.

Ragland, Evan R. "Experimental Clinical Medicine and Drug Action in Mid-Seventeenth-Century Leiden." *Bulletin of the History of Medicine* 91, no. 2 (July 25, 2017): 331–61. https://doi.org/10.1353/bhm.2017.0029.

———. "Making Trials in Sixteenth-Century European Academic Medicine." *Isis* 108 (2017): 503–28.

Rankin, Alisha. *Panaceia's Daughters: Noblewomen as Healers in Early Modern Germany*. Chicago, IL: University of Chicago Press, 2013.

———. *The Poison Trials: Wonder Drugs, Experiment, and the Battle for Authority in Renaissance Science*. Chicago, IL: University of Chicago Press, 2021.

Schickore, Jutta. *About Method: Experimenters, Snake Venom, and the History of Writing Scientifically*. Chicago, IL: University of Chicago Press, 2017.

Schmitt, Charles B. "Experience and Experiment: A Comparison of Zabarella's View with Galileo's in De Motu." *Studies in the Renaissance* 16 (1969): 80–138.

Shapin, Steven. *The Scientific Revolution*. Chicago, IL: University of Chicago Press, 1996.

Shapin, Steven, and Simon Schaffer. *Leviathan and the Air-Pump: Hobbes, Boyle, and the Experimental Life*. Princeton, NJ: Princeton University Press, 1985.

Siraisi, Nancy G. *Medieval and Early Renaissance Medicine: An Introduction to Knowledge and Practice*. Chicago, IL: University of Chicago Press, 1990.

Stolberg, Michael. *Learned Physicians and Everyday Medical Practice in the Renaissance*. Berlin and Boston, MA: De Gruyter, 2021.

Stoudt, Debra L. "The Medical Manuscripts of the Bibliotheca Palatina." In *Manuscript Sources of Medieval Medicine: A Book of Essays*, edited by Margaret Rose Schleissner, 159–81. New York: Garland, 1995.

Sullivan, Erin, and Andrew Wear. "Materiality, Nature and the Body." In *The Routledge Handbook of Material Culture in Early Modern Europe*, edited by Catherine Richardson, Tara Hamling, and David Gaimster, 141–57. London: Routledge, 2016. https://doi.org/10.4324/9781315613161.ch9.

Vesalius, Andreas. *The Fabric of the Human Body: An Annotated Translation of the 1543 and 1555 Editions of "De Humani Corporis Fabrica Libri Septem."* Edited and translated by Daniel H. Garrison and Malcolm H. Hast. Basel: Karger, 2014.

Webster, Charles. *Paracelsus: Medicine, Magic and Mission at the End of Time*. New Haven, CT: Yale University Press, 2008.

8 An Imperial Doctor's Guide to Bone Setting, 1742

Yi-Li Wu

In the fourth year of his reign, the Qianlong Emperor (r. 1735–1795) of the Qing dynasty (1644–1912) of China ordered his Imperial Medical Academy (*tai yi yuan*) to compile a comprehensive medical treatise that would set a standard of correct practice for the empire. The result was the *Imperially Compiled Golden Mirror of the Orthodox Lineage of Medicine* (*Yuzuan yizong jinjian*), printed in 1742. An imposing work comprising 90 *juan* (Chinese-style book chapters) it covered numerous subspecialties of medicine (see Table 8.1). While the *Golden Mirror* had no formal institutional power beyond the government medical bureaucracy, printed copies circulated throughout the realm, and it was a well-known medical reference. Because of its imperial provenance and influence, historians regularly use the *Golden Mirror* as a source for investigating eighteenth-century Chinese medicine generally and Qing court medicine specifically.[1] The last four *juan bear* the collective title "Rectifying Bones: Essential Knowledge about Received Learning and Techniques" (*Zhenggu xinfa yaozhi*). When I decided to research the history of medicine for injuries in China, "Rectifying Bones" was an obvious source to include.

I became interested in injuries because I wanted to understand more fully how people of the past conceptualized the human body. The conventional wisdom about Chinese medicine describes it as being concerned with the body's dynamic functions, but indifferent to bodily structure. This formulation, however, is a product of early twentieth-century modernization movements in China, when critics used Euro-American biomedical teachings to disparage Chinese medicine as unscientific. In response, as Sean Hsiang-lin Lei shows, leading Chinese doctors reconfigured older teachings to argue that Chinese medicine was not describing the anatomical body of flesh, but rather the dynamic transformations of bodily *qi*, which could not be disproven by science (*qi* was a central concept in Chinese philosophy and cosmology, simultaneously encompassing all matter and vitality).[2] Prior to the twentieth century, however, the fleshy, material body was very much present in medical discussions of illness and healing. Over the past decade, I and other scholars have been explicitly seeking to recover these historical perspectives.[3] Since injuries and wounds involve damage to the body's physical form, the history of medicine for injuries is a particularly useful vehicle for investigating how doctors thought about the structural and material aspects of the body.

DOI: 10.4324/9781003094876-11

Table 8.1 Content of the *Golden Mirror*

Juan no.	*Topic/title*
1–17	Zhang Ji, *Treatise on Cold Damage* (*shanghan* [epidemic febrile disorders])
18–25	Zhang Ji, *Essential Prescriptions from the Golden Cabinet*
26–33	The medical methods of famous doctors
34	The four diagnostic methods
35	The cosmic circulatory phases of qi
36	Cold Damage
39–43	Uncategorized internal diseases (*zabing*)
44–49	Women's diseases (*fuke*)
50–55	Children's diseases (*youke*)
56–59	Pox and rashes (*douzhen*)
60	Planting pox (*zhongdou* [smallpox variolation])
61–76	External diseases (*waike* [diseases of skin and flesh])
77–78	Eye diseases (*yanke*)
79–86	Acupuncture and moxibustion (*cijiu*)
87–90	Rectifying bones (*zhenggu*)

The *Golden Mirror*'s compilers explained that the phrase "rectifying bones" comprised "injuries caused by falls and blows."[4] These included bone fractures and dislocations as well as sprains, wrenches, and contusions. To treat these,

"Rectifying Bones" described a panoply of methods: manual manipulations and orthopedic implements to correct the body's form, and medicinal washes, plasters, ointments, pills, and decoctions to dissipate lumps and bruises, alleviate pain, prevent complications, and generate new bone and flesh. Throughout, the body's functions and its material structures were envisioned as two aspects of a whole – physical damage impaired vital functions, and restoring vital functions was essential for healing physical damage.

A distinctive feature of "Rectifying Bones" as compared to earlier texts on bone setting was that it deliberately created a standardized and comprehensive bone-setting curriculum. Its first *juan*, titled "Methods of External Treatment," described techniques of manual manipulation, explained how to fashion and use orthopedic implements, and discussed passages on injury treatment from the ancient classics. The next two *juan* divided the body into a number of sectors, describing the bony parts in each, their typical injuries, and the manual and drug-based therapies for treating these. The final *juan*, titled "Methods of Internal Treatment," discussed orally administered remedies to manage internal bleeding, pain, and many other complications.

"Rectifying Bones" thus provides a wealth of information about eighteenth-century views of the body. However, it also poses a historical puzzle – whose knowledge does it represent, why was this knowledge written down, and how was it meant to be used? We ask these questions of all texts, but the fact that "Rectifying Bones" is a work on bone setting adds an additional layer of complexity. To become an effective bone setter, one must train one's hands to feel and manipulate the bodies of living people in pain. What role, then, would a written text play in creating or disseminating bone-setting knowledge?

We can glean some answers by reading "Rectifying Bones" through the lens of eighteenth-century medical politics at court. As I discuss below, "Rectifying Bones" was the product of a predominately ethnic Chinese Imperial Medical Academy caring for a Manchu ruling house that also relied on the prowess of Mongol bone setters.[5] It was in this setting that the imperial doctors aimed to systematize and improve bone-setting knowledge. For a work that claimed to set new standards of comprehensiveness, however, the descriptions of specific manual techniques in "Rectifying Bones" vary widely in their level of detail. My reading is that "Rectifying Bones" embodies a tension between the compilers' desire to create a text-based intellectual foundation for bone setting, and their tacit recognition that the core skills would still be conveyed through hands-on training. There was thus a limit to what needed to be recorded in writing.

To show how I arrived at these conclusions, I will begin with a brief survey of Chinese medical literature and introduce the historical context in which "Rectifying Bones" was compiled. I then analyze selected passages and images from the text to illustrate its foci and silences and what we can read into them. This method of reading back and forth between a text and its historical context is a standard methodology in medical history. Here, we will use "Rectifying Bones" as our case study.

Historical Chinese Medical Writings

Bibliographic catalogs of Chinese medical texts held by Chinese libraries list thousands of titles of pre-1900 works that vary widely as to format, content, genre, and audience (see "for further reading" at the end of this chapter). The *Golden Mirror* is representative of the comprehensive treatises that aimed to cover all known ailments and diseases, and it included discussions of doctrine as well as lists of medicinal remedies. Other important textual genres include works focused on a specific disease or specialty, medical case collections, studies of drugs and medicinal formulas, and handbooks meant for household use. Some were produced by (or attributed to) people who made their living as healers, while others were compiled by amateurs with an interest in medicine or experience in treating themselves and family members. Many extant texts are manuscripts. But beginning in the seventh century, the development and spread of woodblock printing – a practical and relatively inexpensive technology – resulted in the proliferation of medical texts printed by government offices, booksellers, and well-to-do-families and individuals.

The first step in analyzing a Chinese medical text is to ascertain when it was produced, by whom, and for what purpose and readership. When such information is not recorded, we can try to extrapolate it by comparing the text's language, physical format, or content with comparable works about which we know more.[6] Printed works will often include a title page that identifies an author, year of printing, and the printing house. Many texts also contain one or more dated prefaces written by the author and his patrons, disciples, or descendants that explain the history of the text and the provenance of its contents. Some texts (including the *Golden Mirror*) also contain a "guide to the reader" (*fan li*) that explains the content and format of the text.

These paratextual elements, however informative, must also be read critically. For example, booksellers sometimes attributed texts to famous doctors to make them more marketable. More generally, the boundaries of what constituted a "book" or "authorship" in China were historically fluid. People re-edited or reorganized existing works, combined information from different medical texts, or appended new information to older texts. When people reprinted texts, they often recycled the title pages, prefaces, and author attributions, even if they altered the content. Preface writers also repeated certain rhetorical tropes. They lamented the shortcomings of other texts, which are described as biased, incomplete, or unsystematic, and they praised their text for improving on past ones. Similarly, they criticized contemporary doctors for being mediocre and self-serving while praising the text's author as perspicacious and benevolent. Such statements show how people made value judgments about medical knowledge and practitioners, but they are only a starting point for understanding the historical significance of any given text.

The history of the *Golden Mirror* is much easier to ascertain because the text opened with the Qianlong Emperor's 1739 edict to the Imperial Medical Academy commissioning the text, as well as communications from officials reporting on its progress and completion. It also included a list of 80 people who officially worked on the project, from the Emperor's brother and the Imperial Grand Secretary down to the personnel in the Imperial Printing Office. Weaving through these official records is a multi-stranded story of medicine and power. Understanding this background can help illuminate the textual choices in "Rectifying Bones."

The Compilation and Background of the *Golden Mirror*

The Qing imperial family belonged to an ethnic group from Northeast Asia known as the Manchus, whose ancestors once ruled over much of what is now Northern China as the Jin dynasty (1115–1234). The challenges that the Manchus faced as an ethnic minority ruling over a vast Chinese population are directly relevant to the history of the *Golden Mirror*. Marta Hanson describes the Qianlong Emperor as having "an obsession with defining orthodoxy (*zheng*) in all realms of Chinese knowledge as a tool of Manchu control over both Chinese culture and the Chinese."[7] The *Golden Mirror* was one of the scholarly projects that he commissioned to enhance his political legitimacy. Confucian philosophy taught that a sovereign's right to rule depended on his ability to nurture the well-being of his people. A long-recognized way to demonstrate imperial benevolence was to improve medical knowledge by compiling and publishing learned medical books.

The Qing Imperial Medical Academy was responsible for training and overseeing a corps of physicians who primarily cared for the imperial family.[8] It was dominated by ethnically Chinese doctors from the wealthy southeast, who used the *Golden Mirror* project to promote their own vision of scholarly medicine. Medicine was considered a technical trade, but literate physicians had long strived to elevate medicine into a branch of scholarly learning, rooted in natural philosophy, cosmology, and classical study.[9] Outside the governmental medical service, there were no set medical curricula or regulations governing who could practice medicine. Elite doctors thus asserted their intellectual and moral superiority by emulating the norms of Confucian scholars.

The title of the *Golden Mirror* embodied these scholarly aspirations. Hanson points out that the "mirror" metaphor was familiar in the study of history (a core field of Confucian learning), for the moral man used history as a mirror to inspect the virtues or flaws of the present day. The term *zong*, meaning "the orthodox ancestral lineage," borrowed the rhetoric of Confucian philosophical lineages. To speak of a medical *zong* meant that doctors, like scholars, were heirs to an ancient intellectual lineage.[10] Leading eighteenth-century Chinese physicians argued that this intellectual ancestor was the late 2nd to early 3rd c. doctor Zhang Ji, and they embraced new scholarly forms of philological inquiry to recover the original meaning of Zhang's texts. These dynamics converged in the person of the imperial physician Wu Qian, a noted Zhang Ji scholar and the co-chief editor of the *Golden Mirror* who ultimately determined most of its content. The influence of Wu Qian and like-minded colleagues is clear in the fact that the first 25 *juan* of the *Golden Mirror* reproduce Zhang Ji's writings, with philologically informed commentary.

The status of bone setting in the Qianlong era is also pertinent to "Rectifying Bones." Previous dynasties had included departments of bone setting in their medical bureaus, but it appears that the Qing placed an especially high value on this skill. Manchu rulers valorized mounted archery as the epitome of their culture, and bone setting was essential for soldiers and others who lived and worked on horseback. Sare Aricanli shows that by the early eighteenth century, an official corps of bone setters known as "Mongol doctors" had been established as part of the Ministry of Imperial Stables, Herds, and Carriages (*shang si yuan*), which was part of the Imperial Household Department. This was a formalization of earlier initiatives to recruit bone setters from among the Mongol units in the Qing armed forces. These Ministry bone setters treated both horses and men, and their institutional stature increased over the Qianlong era. During the early nineteenth century, the bone-setting division of the Imperial Medical Academy was closed, and its duties transferred to the Mongol doctors.[11] But "Rectifying Bones" was compiled when there were still two official groups of bone setters working for the government, and we can assume they were aware of each other. Aricanli notes that not all the equine bone setters were necessarily Mongol, and that there were analogous Manchu healers known as *coban*. However, the appellation "Mongol doctor" evoked a form of medical expertise rooted in the culture of militaristic and nomadic societies where equestrian injuries were commonplace. It was in this institutional environment that the doctors of the Imperial Medical Academy set out a scholarly curriculum for bone setting that aimed to set standards for the empire.

Some have suggested that the bone-setting knowledge in "Rectifying Bones" reflected the skills of Mongol bone setters or Manchu *coban*.[12] Further research will be required to evaluate this claim. For the moment, however, we can see that the compilers used scholarly Chinese norms to frame their bone-setting information. While asserting that skillful hands were the foundation of bone setting, they also argued that the skill of the hands was dependent on the knowledge of the mind. A healer who possessed the knowledge laid out in "Rectifying Bones" would be able to treat any injury he faced, "a far cry from those who handle matters with a rote application of apparatus and tools."[13] In the next section, I analyze how this model curriculum was textually constructed, as well as the limits of this textual approach.

Reading "Rectifying Bones"

In their "Guide to the Reader," the compilers of the *Golden Mirror* stated that "Rectifying Bones" would improve on previous works by including information on *shou fa*, literally "hand methods," or manual techniques.[14] Given that earlier texts had also described manual manipulations for treating fractured or dislocated bones, what did the compilers have in mind? What we find is that "Rectifying Bones" created a standardized, technical vocabulary of manual manipulations. Knowing the right terms to use now became part of learning the techniques.

The very first entry of the text was a discussion of manual methods, and it opened with a definition of the term "hand methods" itself: "*Shou fa* refers to using the two hands to arrange injured sinews and bones, thereby making them return to their original state."[15] Although the words "hand" and "method" were common words, "Rectifying Bones" presents *shou fa* as a technical term with a specific therapeutic connotation. This also semantically emphasized the more formalistic meanings of the term *fa*, which could mean "law" or other systematized way of doing things. The discussion that followed this definition emphasized that "hand methods" did not simply refer to manual techniques, but rather to the proper and perspicacious use of the techniques. The effective bone setter needed to have both "a clear mind and ingenious hands" (*xin ming shou qiao*) including a thorough understanding of the body's structure and all the possible forms that injury could take. Only then could he accurately assess the patient's condition and tailor his techniques to the particularities of the situation.

This rhetorical pattern of assigning special technical meanings to common words continued in the discussion of the eight manual methods that would serve as the foundation of the healer's practice: "feeling" (*mo*), "joining" (*jie*), "straightening out" (*duan*), "lifting up" (*ti*), "pressing" (*an*), "rubbing" (*mo*), "pushing" (*tui*), and "grasping" (*na*). "Feeling," for example, was defined as a diagnostic procedure in which the skilled bone setter would assess the nature of the injury entirely by touch:

> The "feeling" method: "Feeling" means to use the hand to meticulously feel the injured place, [to determine] whether the bone is broken in two, or broken in pieces; whether the bone is askew or aligned; whether the bone is soft or hard; whether the sinew is tight, soft, askew, straight, broken in two, dislodged, thick, turned over, cold, or hot; as well as if there is depletion or repletion in the exterior and interior; and whether the injury is new or of long standing.[16]

The remaining seven methods referred to therapeutic manipulations that would be used after the injury was diagnosed. In some cases, such as "straightening out," a single term denoted a set of related techniques.

> "Straightening out" means one uses one or both hands to hold fast the place that should be straightened, and then, after judging whether the case is serious or light, straightens it out by moving it from a lower to a higher position, or manipulates it from the exterior towards the interior, or rectifies it in a straight or slanted direction.[17]

This section on the eight methods concluded by reiterating that their effectiveness depended on the healer's level of insight, namely his ability to understand the nature of the injury and what method to use in a given case.

A Repertoire of Tools

Following its discussion of manual manipulations, "Rectifying Bones" described a set of orthopedic tools, or implements (*qi*), numbered one through ten. These implements were used to help realign the injured part or to protect and stabilize it during healing. The use of numbered sets was a common mnemonic device in China, but here the numbers also had the rhetorical effect of delineating a standard repertoire of bone-setting implements. The compilers also provided visual diagrams of the more complex implements that allowed the reader to understand their form and usage with much greater ease. Figure 8.1, for example, depicts the "reach ropes" (implement 4) and "stacked bricks" (implement 5). The text explained that this was used to elongate and straighten the torso of someone who was hunched over as the result of an injury to the belly, chest, or ribs.[18] The patient held onto the overhead ropes while each foot rested on a stack of three bricks. The healer would stand behind the patient and grasp his lower back. Then the bricks would be removed, one layer at a time, increasing the vertical stretch to straighten the patient's body. Figures 8.2 and 8.3 depict the form of the "bamboo screen" (implement 8) and "fir fence" (implement 9) and how to use them to stabilize fractures of the limbs. The text describes the former as a section of a bamboo window screen, and the latter as comprising slats of fir wood connected to each other with string.[19] After the broken bone was aligned, the limb would be wrapped first with cloth, next with the bamboo screen, and finally with the fir fence. The other implements in this section of "Rectifying Bones" were used to treat injuries to the head, back, kneecap, and shoulder. While we can find descriptions of some of these orthopedic implements in earlier texts, "Rectifying Bones" was novel in providing a systematic illustrated catalog of these devices.

A Catalog of Bones

In its second and third *juan*, "Rectifying Bones" created an explicit framework for organizing information about the patient's body. It divided the body into three main sectors (*bu*) called "head and face," "chest and back," and "the four limbs," with further subdivisions in each section. Each subdivision was introduced with an image depicting that portion of the body as shown on a living person, with

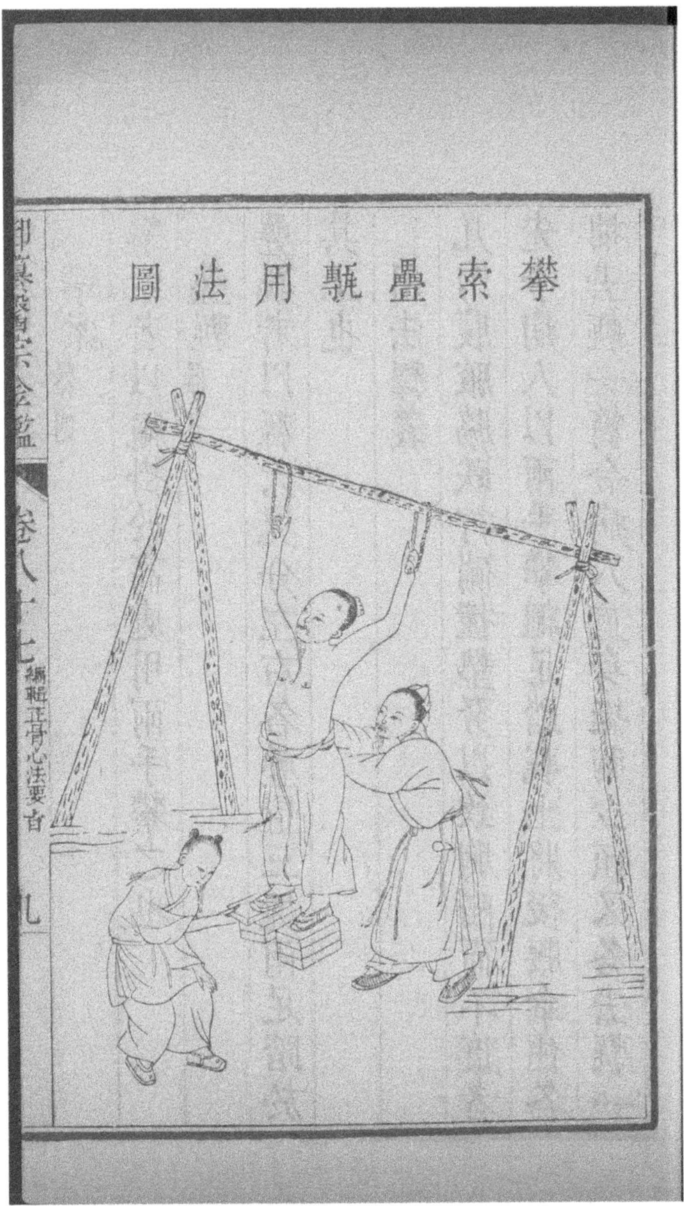

Figure 8.1 Illustration of the "reach ropes and stacked bricks" from the *Golden Mirror*. This was used to elongate and straighten the torso of someone who was hunched over from an injury to the belly, chest, or ribs. As the patient held onto the ropes, someone would remove the bricks under his feet, one layer at a time, until his body was straight. A brace consisting of a "bamboo screen" (a window shade made of strips of bamboo interwoven with string) would then be wrapped around the person's chest and bound securely with several sashes of cloth. Courtesy of the Chinese Collection, Harvard-Yenching Library, Harvard University. Accessed via the Harvard Library Digital Collections.

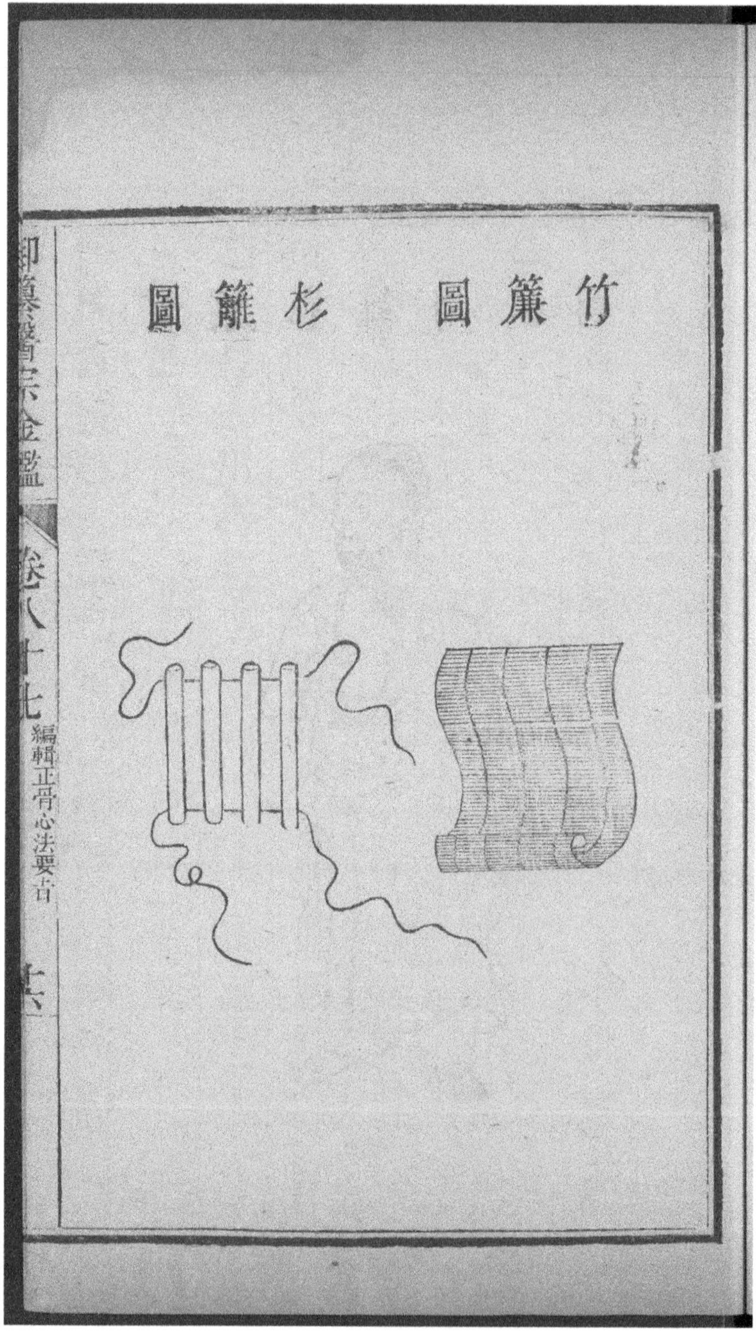

Figure 8.2 Illustration of the "bamboo screen" and the "fir fence" from *Golden Mirror*. These were used to stabilize fractured bones of the arms and legs. Courtesy of the Chinese Collection, Harvard-Yenching Library, Harvard University. Accessed via the Harvard Library Digital Collections.

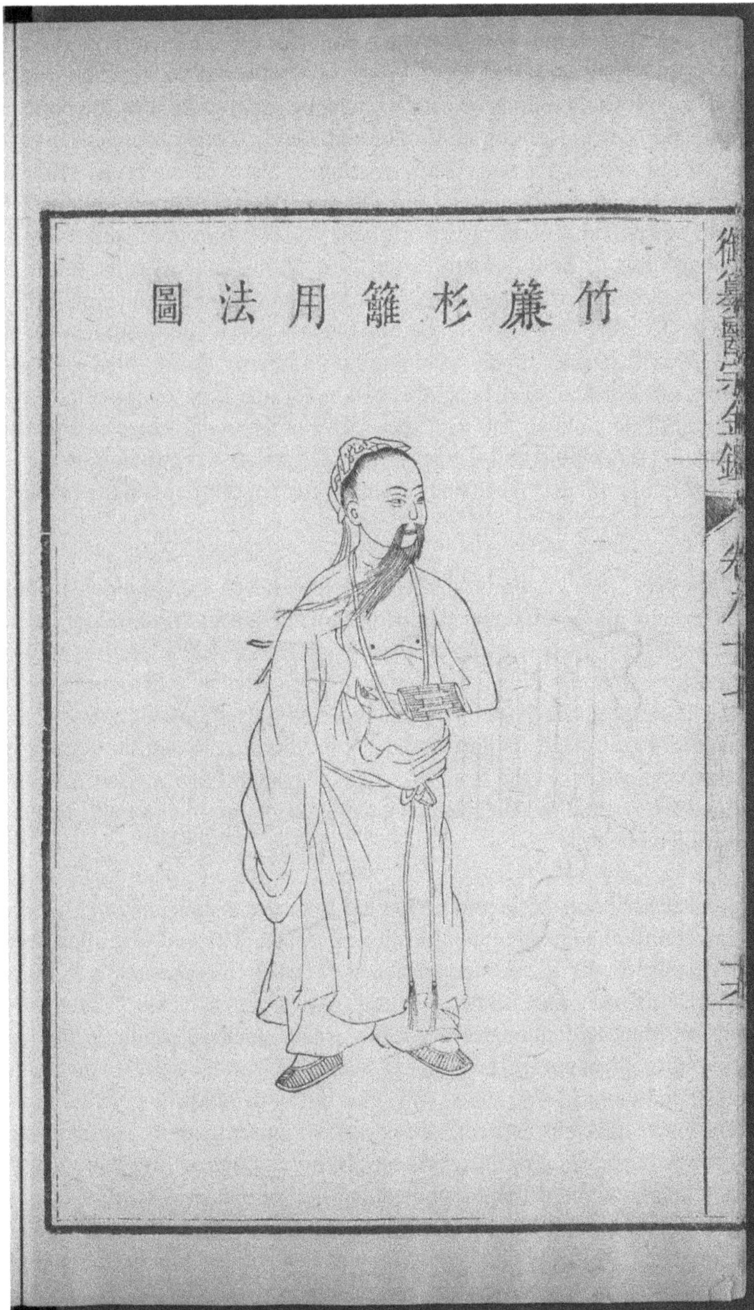

Figure 8.3 Illustration of how to use the "bamboo screen" and "fir fence" from the *Golden Mirror*. The injured limb would be wrapped in cloth, then with the bamboo screen, and lastly with the fir fence. Additional bindings would then be used to hold the fir strips in place. Courtesy of the Chinese Collection, Harvard-Yenching Library, Harvard University. Accessed via the Harvard Library Digital Collections.

labels placed on the surface of the skin to indicate the positions of the relevant bones. For example, Figure 8.4 depicts the bones of the face, while Figure 8.5 depicts the bones of the arm. Each such image was followed by a textual catalog of bone names, with explanations of what each name referred to, how the bone might be injured, and how these injuries should be treated. While some earlier writings on bone setting had also arranged information by parts of the body, "Rectifying Bones" is notable for the intentional and self-conscious way in which it used body sectors and subdivisions as an organizing schema for information about injuries.

But what kinds of body structures do these "bone" names refer to? In some cases, they correspond to anatomically discrete pieces of bone. For example, "Rectifying Bones" defines the *nao* as "the bone that is below the shoulder and above the elbow" – easily equated with the biomedical humerus. Other "bones," however, are bony protrusions that merit special attention because they are especially vulnerable to injury. This includes the *yu* ("shoulder") bone, which corresponds to what present-day doctors would call the acromion, defined as a protrusion on the upper part of the shoulder blade. "Rectifying Bones," conversely, defined the blade as the lower extension of the *yu*:

> The *yu* bone: The *yu* bone is the bone at the end of the shoulder, namely the ridge bone along the upper part of the socket end of the shoulder *jia*. Its socket contains the upper end of the *nao* bone. The place where it is located is called the "shoulder division," namely the seam where the shoulder blade and the *nao* meet each other. The popular name is "swallowing mouth," and one name is "the head of the shoulder." Its lower part, which is close to the backbone and takes the form of a flat slice resembling a wing, is called the shoulder *jia*, and is also called the shoulder *bo*, and its popular name is "shovel blade bone."[20]

This textual description is far more detailed than the visual image (Figure 8.5), which shows only the approximate location of the *yu*. The text also illustrates the compilers' desire to clarify and standardize bone terms: they present *yu* as the name of record for this body part, to be preferred over "popular names." Such work of assessing, defining, and standardizing terms was a standard scholarly device, including in philological study. It was also a feature of learned treatises on medicinal substances and acupuncture points, two other areas of medical practice in which there were many different and competing terms in circulation.[21] The existence of multiple terms for bones was unsurprising given that bone setting knowledge was historically taught within different medical families or master-disciple lineages. By selecting a standard term and recording it in a didactic text, "Rectifying Bones" aimed to impose uniformity and consistency over ideas and practices arising from diverse people distributed across time and place.

Interestingly, however, this standardized vocabulary itself also had diverse origins. The term *yu* was an ancient term for the shoulder, and it was one of the terms that medical literature had historically used to describe the shoulder, particularly when describing the position of acupuncture points. By contrast, terms like

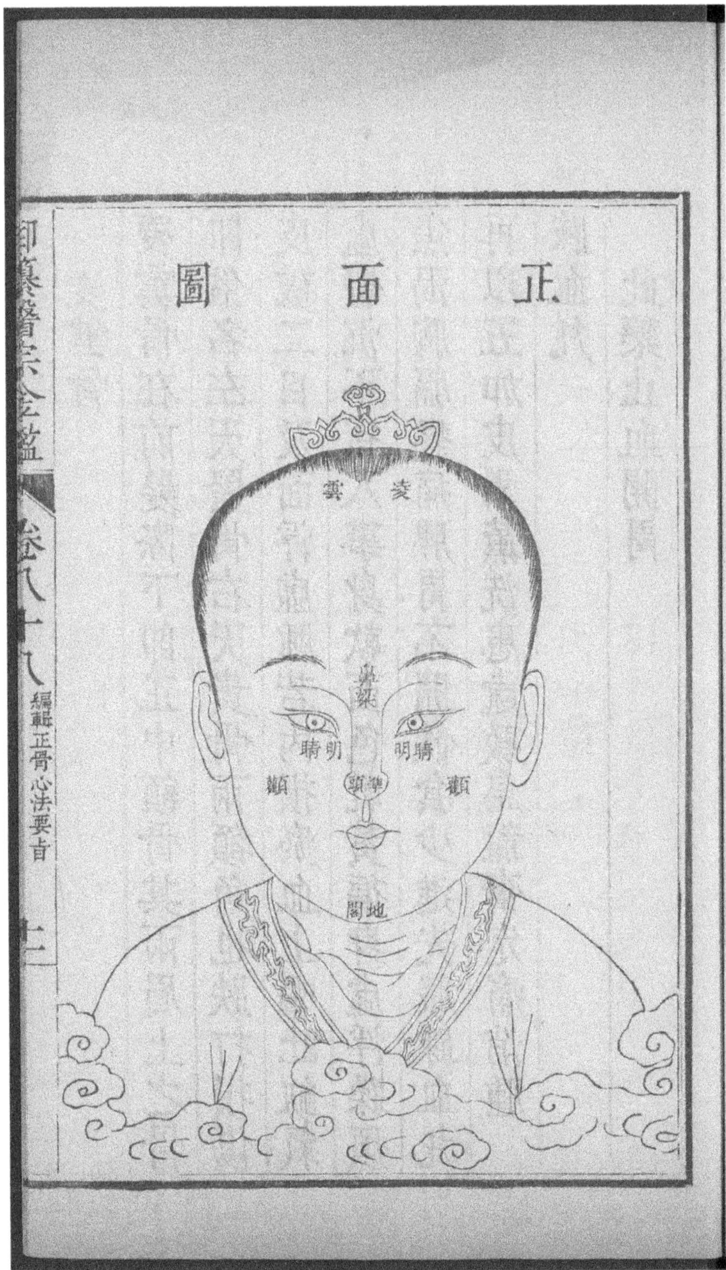

Figure 8.4 Illustration of the bones of the front of the head and the face from the *Golden Mirror*. The vertical line of labels from the top of the forehead to the chin reads "ascending to the clouds" (forehead bone), "nose beam," "the exact end" (tip of the nose) and "earthly pavilion" (chin). The other labels read "cheek" and "eye brightness." Courtesy of the Chinese Collection, Harvard-Yenching Library, Harvard University. Accessed via the Harvard Library Digital Collections.

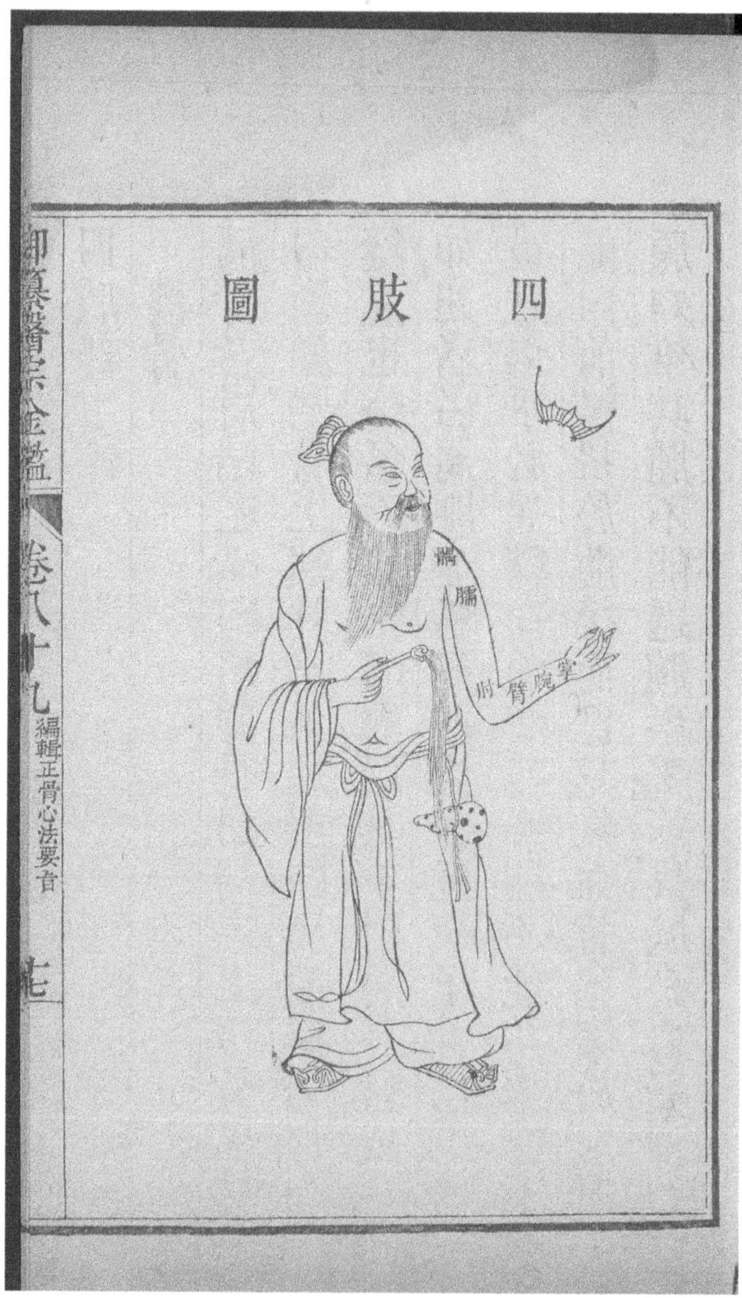

Figure 8.5 Illustration of the position of bones in the arm from the *Golden Mirror*. Starting from the shoulder and moving downward, the labels read *yu* (acromion), *nuo* (humerus), *zhou* (elbow), *bi* (ulna), *wan* (wrist), and *zhang* (palm). Courtesy of the Chinese Collection, Harvard-Yenching Library, Harvard University. Accessed via the Harvard Library Digital Collections.

"earthly pavilion" for the chin (Figure 8.4) appear to be borrowed from physiognomy (*xiang shu*), the divinatory art of reading someone's fate from the physical form of their bodily features, notably their face.[22] A close examination of the terms in "Rectifying Bones" thus reveals that its knowledge of the body was shaped by information derived from multiple bodily practices.

Reading Textual Silences

The inconsistencies and omissions in a medical text can also help us formulate hypotheses about the way that it would have been employed. In "Rectifying Bones," there are evident discrepancies between the bone sector images and the body parts described in the accompanying text. For example, the image of the front of the face does not include a label for the "central blood hall" (*zhong xue tang*, an "empty space" under the nasal cartilage) which has its own entry in the text.[23] As mentioned above, the textual descriptions also contain more details than the images. In Figure 8.5, the bones of the lower arm are designated simply with the label *bi*, located vaguely to the left of the label for "wrist" (which is at the midpoint of the forearm) and the label for "palm" (placed on the figure's wrist). By contrast, the accompanying text specifies that the term *bi* refers to the larger bone in a pair of forearm bones, namely "the one that lies beneath, which is long and large in shape, and connected to the point of the elbow" (corresponding to the ulna).[24] On top this *bi* sits a shorter and thinner bone, which is the "auxiliary bone" (*fu gu*), whose popular name is the "wrapping around bone" (*chan gu*, corresponding to the radius). In severe injuries, the text says, both bones will be broken.

The relationship between image and text in the *juan* on body sectors is thus quite different from that in the section on orthopedic implements. The orthopedic images served to convey technical details beyond what could be described in words, namely what the implements looked like and how to apply them to the body. By contrast, the body sector images served primarily as a way of categorizing and organizing knowledge. In essence, they were visual tables of contents that set the stage for learning by showing the relative position of the major bones (but not all of them).[25] The text would then carry the weight of describing the individual body parts.

But while the written word was an essential tool for recording standardized knowledge, "Rectifying Bones" also contains lacunae that point to the limits of book learning. Its descriptions of specific therapeutic manipulations are notably inconsistent in how much detail they provide, especially when compared to the consistent attention given to bone terminology. One of the fuller descriptions is this manipulation for reducing a shoulder dislocation:

> If the *nao* bone [humerus] protrudes out, it is proper to take the bone that is protruding out and push it backwards to make it enter the joining seam. Moreover, take the *nao* sinew and adjust it by rotating it towards the interior.[26]

Precise details on how one would actually do this pushing and twisting, however, are not provided. Similarly, the instructions for treating fractures of the "great pile bone" (femur) provide few details about the manipulative techniques and primarily serve to explain the general treatment strategy: "Use the two hands to press and rub any bone fragments and push and pull [them] back into position. Then press the injured spot with the tips of the fingers [to ensure] there are no bones still awry."[27] And although the entry for the "lower leg bones" describes the possibility of a compound fracture, its description of how to manipulate a broken lower leg bone is frankly perfunctory, stating simply: "Use manual techniques to press the sinews and rectify the bones and make them go back into position."[28] The tone of these descriptions conveys an assumption that the practitioner has already learned (or will learn) the specific methods for pressing, rubbing, and repositioning bones through hands-on training under the guidance of an expert teacher. In sum, while "Rectifying Bones" aimed to train the practitioner's intellect, the tactile expertise needed to manipulate bodies was beyond the text's ability to convey.

Conclusion

Although the Academy's bone setters were eventually eclipsed by the "Mongol doctors," "Rectifying Bones" itself was successful in stimulating the study of bone knowledge and injury care. Notably, during the late eighteenth and early nineteenth centuries, two doctors from southeastern China described "Rectifying Bones" as the inspiration and foundation for their own treatises on injury medicine. Both works are extant today (see Hu Tingguang and Qian Xiuchang in the bibliography). "Rectifying Bones" also influenced bone-setting treatises in Tokugawa Japan (1644–1868). Qing-era authors of forensic treatises, which discussed how to evaluate signs of trauma on skeletal remains, also referred to the *Golden Mirror*'s description of bones.[29]

After the founding of the People's Republic of China in 1949, Chinese policymakers sought to systematize and modernize historical medical practices so that they could be used in conjunction with biomedicine. This fostered the development of what is commonly referred to as "traditional Chinese medicine" (TCM). During the 1980s, the government also began initiatives to spur the growth of "TCM Osteology and Traumatology" (*Zhongyi gu shang ke*), based both on historical writings and on oral traditions of bone setting and injury healing handed down through families or master-disciple lineages. TCM researchers and practitioners have written about the *Golden Mirror* and other works, plumbing them for methods that can be adapted to present-day needs.

Meanwhile I, as a historian, examine these texts to understand the social and cultural factors that shaped the way that people in the Chinese past thought about injury and debility. The compilers of "Rectifying Bones" invested great energy into organizing and detailing knowledge about bones and their injuries, and histories of Chinese medicine will be enriched by a fuller consideration of how they and other doctors viewed the body's material and structural forms. Likewise, a study of how Qing bonesetters were trained to use their hands can diversify our understanding of how past healers selected and employed different intellectual frameworks and therapeutic techniques. By teasing apart the intricacies of "Rectifying Bones," I hope to stimulate further interest in these aspects of Chinese medical history.

For Further Reading

While the largest collections of pre-twentieth-century Chinese medical texts are held by libraries and museums in the People's Republic of China, these materials can be found in many other institutions worldwide. This includes works on bone setting and other forms of injury medicine. Beginning in the twentieth century, furthermore, scholars and publishers also reproduced many of these historical materials for wider circulation, both as facsimiles (photographic reproductions) and as reprints (re-typeset and reformatted). Scores of these historical texts, facsimiles, and reproductions have also been scanned or digitized, with many placed online in the public domain. Significant digital collections that are publicly accessible include those of the Harvard-Yenching Library of Harvard University (USA), the Princeton University East Asia Library (USA), the Waseda University Library (Japan), and the Berlin State Library (Staatsbibliotek zu Berlin, Germany), as well as the Internet Archive; undoubtedly more have appeared since I wrote this chapter.

There are voluminous Chinese-language studies of historical bone setting and injury medicine, many produced by TCM researchers (see, for example, Ding Jihua in the bibliography). By contrast, there are few such specialized studies in Western languages. Some information related to bone setting and to injury treatment can however be found in Western-language translations of medical works on other topics (see, for example, the works by Buell, Anderson, and Unschuld in the bibliography). The proliferation of such translations in recent decades owes much to the global expansion of TCM as a form of alternative medicine, as well as to burgeoning scholarly interest in the history of East Asian science, medicine, and technology. Readers should note that the nature of these translations can be quite variable. In addition to the inherent challenges of translating between Chinese and Western languages, there are numerous historical medical concepts that have no Western language equivalent. The translator's choices and goals will thus shape the style of the translations. Some translations are done by professional Sinologists and historians for an audience of those who want to understand the original historical meaning of the text as closely as possible. These translations often contain square brackets to distinguish between words that were literally there in the original and words that the translator has added for readability. Such translations are also routinely accompanied by footnotes. Other translations are written for present-day students and practitioners of Chinese medicine, and these often translate historical concepts by using a standardized terminology that was developed starting in the mid-twentieth century. Works written for present-day practitioners who want to use historical Chinese treatments for injuries include the works below by Tom Bisio and the Shaolin Monastery monk De Qian. Each of these works has its own utility; one simply needs to read them with an awareness of what the authors are hoping to achieve and what audiences they are hoping to serve.

Notes

1 When Prince Aisin-Gioro Hongli ascended the throne, he designated his reign as the era of "qianlong" (Heavenly Eminence). He is thus conventionally referred to as the Qianlong Emperor. In this chapter, the page citations for the *Golden Mirror* will reference the *Siku quanshu* edition, which is the most readily available Qing-era edition. For the history of the *Golden Mirror* see Marta Hanson, "The *Golden Mirror* in the Imperial Court of the Qianlong Emperor," *Early Science and Medicine* 8, no. 2 (2003): 111–47. Other studies that draw on the *Golden Mirror* include Che-chia Chang, "The Qing Imperial Academy of Medicine: Its Institutions and the Physicians Shaped by Them," *East Asian Science, Technology, and Medicine* 41, no. 1 (2015): 63–92; Chia-feng Chang, "Disease and Its Impact on Politics, Diplomacy, and the Military," *Journal of the History of Medicine and the Allied Sciences* 57, no. 2 (2002): 177–97; Ari Larissa Heinrich, *The Afterlife of Images: Translating the Pathological Body between China and the West* (Durham: Duke University Press, 2008); and Yi-Li Wu, "The Gendered Medical Iconography of *the Golden Mirror*," *Asian Medicine: Tradition and Modernity* 4, no. 2 (2009): 452–91.

2 Sean Hsiang-lin Lei, *Neither Donkey Nor Horse: Medicine in the Struggle over China's Modernity* (Chicago, IL: University of Chicago Press, 2014).

3 See, for example, Yi-Li Wu, "Between the Living and the Dead: Trauma Medicine and Forensic Medicine in the Mid-Qing," *Frontiers of History in China* 10, no. 1 (2015): 38–73 and Volker Scheid, "Transmitting Chinese Medicine: Changing Perceptions of Body, Pathology, and Treatment in Late Imperial China," *Asian Medicine* 8, no. 2 (2013): 299–360.

4 *Golden Mirror*, 90:1a.

5 See Hanson, "Golden Mirror;" Chang, "Qing Imperial Academy;" Chang, "Disease and Its Impact;" Sare Aricanli, "*Diversifying the Center: Authority and Representation within the Context of Multiplicity in Eighteenth Century Qing Imperial Medicine*" (Ph.D. diss., Princeton University, 2016); and Aricanli, "Reconsidering the Boundaries: Multicultural and Multilingual Perspectives on the Care and Management of the Emperors' Horses in the Qing," in *Animals through Chinese History: Earliest Times to 1911*, ed. Roel Sterckx, Martina Siebert and Dagmar Schäfer (Cambridge University Press, 2018), 199–216.

6 This method is central to Paul U. Unschuld and Jinsheng Zheng, *Chinese Traditional Healing: The Berlin Collections of Manuscript Volumes from the 16th through the Early 20th Century* (Leiden: Brill, 2012).

7 Hanson, "Golden Mirror," 112. This background section is adapted from Hanson's analysis.

8 Chang, "The Qing Imperial Academy."

9 For the scholar-physician ideal, see Asaf Goldschmidt, *The Evolution of Chinese Medicine: Song Dynasty, 960–1200* (Abingdon: Routledge, 2009); TJ Hinrichs, "The Song and Jin Periods," in *Chinese Medicine and Healing: An Illustrated History*, ed. TJ Hinrichs and Linda Barnes (Cambridge, MA: Harvard University Press, 2013), 97–128; and Yuan-ling Chao, "The Ideal Physician in Late Imperial China: The Question of *Sanshi*," *East Asian Science, Technology, and Medicine*, no. 17 (2000): 66–93.

10 Marta Hanson, "From under the Elbow to Pointing to the Palm: Chinese Metaphors for Learning Medicine by the Book (Fourth–Fourteenth Centuries)," *BJHS Themes* 5 (2020): 75–92 and Hanson, "Golden Mirror."

11 Aricanli, "Diversifying the Center," Chapter 4; and Aricanli, "Reconsidering the Boundaries." For Qing medical divisions see also Li Jingwei and Lin Zhaogeng eds., *Zhongguo Yixue Tong Shi--Gudai Juan* (Beijing: Renmin weisheng chubanshe, 2000).

12 Aricanli describes these claims in "Diversifying the Center," 141–43.

13 *Golden Mirror*, 87:2a.

14 *Golden Mirror*, prefatory *juan*, *fan li*, 5a.

15 *Golden Mirror*, 87:1a.

16 *Golden Mirror*, 87:3a.
17 *Golden Mirror*, 87:3b.
18 *Golden Mirror*, 87:9b.
19 *Golden Mirror*, 87:17a.
20 *Golden Mirror*, 89:19b.
21 For a discussion of terminological standardization in materia medica, see Carla Nappi, *The Monkey and the Inkpot: Natural History and Its Transformations in Early Modern China* (Cambridge, MA: Harvard University Press, 2009) and He Bian, *Know Your Remedies: Pharmacy & Culture in Early Modern China* (Princeton, NJ: Princeton University Press, 2020); for acupuncture see Goldschmidt, *Evolution of Chinese Medicine.*
22 Xing Wang, *Physiognomy in Ming China: Fortune and the Body* (Leiden: Brill, 2020), 154–72.
23 *Golden Mirror*, 88:21a.
24 *Golden Mirror*, 89:25a.
25 Many thanks to Marta Hanson for suggesting that I think about these images as visual tables of contents.
26 *Golden Mirror*, 89:20b.
27 *Golden Mirror*, 89:33a.
28 *Golden Mirror*, 89:35a.
29 For forensics, see Wu, "Between the Living and the Dead," and Catherine Despeux, "The Body Revealed: The Contribution of Forensic Medicine to Knowledge and Representations of the Skeleton in China," in *Graphics and Text in the Production of Technical Knowledge in China: The Warp and the Weft*, ed. Francesca Bray, Vera Dorofeeva-Lichtmann and Georges Métailié (Leiden: Brill, 2007), 635–84. For Japan, see Aricanli, "Diversifying the Center," 179–80.

Bibliography

Primary Sources

Hu Tingguang 胡廷光. *Shangke huizuan shang* 傷科彙纂. Preface dated 1815. Manuscript in the collection of the Beijing University Library. Facsimile reprint published in *Xu xiu Siku quanshu*, Shanghai: Shanghai guji chubanshe, 1995-2002. Digital copy available on the Internet Archive, www.archive.org.

Qian Xiuchang 錢秀昌. *Shangke bu yao* 傷科補要. Yinxi zhiyuan tang woodblock edition, 1818. Facsimile reprint published in *Xu xiu Siku quanshu*, Shanghai: Shanghai guji chubanshe, 1995–2002. Digital copy available on the Internet Archive, www.archive.org.

Wu Qian 吳謙, ed., *Yuzuan yizong jinjian* 御纂醫宗金鑑. Beijing: Wuying dian woodblock edition. In the collection of the Harvard Yenching Library, Harvard University. Digital copy available via the Harvard Library Digital Collections, https://library.harvard.edu/digital-collections.

Wu Qian 吳謙, ed., *Yuzuan yizong jinjian* 御纂醫宗金鑑. *Siku quanshu* manuscript edition, 1782. Facsimile reprint of the Wenyuange copy published Taipei: Taiwan shangwu yinshuguan, 1986. Digital copy available on the Internet Archive, www.archive.org.

Secondary Sources and Translations

Aricanli, Sare. "Diversifying the Center: Authority and Representation within the Context of Multiplicity in Eighteenth Century Qing Imperial Medicine." Ph.D. diss., Princeton University, 2016.

Aricanli, Sare. "Reconsidering the Boundaries: Multicultural and Multilingual Perspectives on the Care and Management of the Emperors' Horses in the Qing." In *Animals through*

Chinese History: Earliest Times to 1911, edited by Roel Sterckx, Martina Siebert and Dagmar Schäfer, 199–216. Cambridge: Cambridge University Press, 2018.

Bian, He. *Know Your Remedies: Pharmacy & Culture in Early Modern China*. Princeton, NJ: Princeton University Press, 2020.

Bisio, Tom. *A Tooth from the Tiger's Mouth: How to Treat Your Injuries with Powerful Healing Secrets of the Great Chinese Warrior*. New York: Atria Books, 2004.

Buell, Paul D., and Eugene N. Anderson. *Arabic Medicine in China*. Leiden: Brill, 2021.

Chang, Che-chia. "The Qing Imperial Academy of Medicine: Its Institutions and the Physicians Shaped by Them." *East Asian Science, Technology, and Medicine* 41, no. 1 (2015): 63–92. https://doi.org/10.1163/26669323-04101003.

Chang, Chia-feng. "Disease and Its Impact on Politics, Diplomacy, and the Military." *Journal of the History of Medicine and the Allied Sciences* 57, no. 2 (2002): 177–97.

Chao, Yuan-ling. "The Ideal Physician in Late Imperial China: The Question of *Sanshi*." *East Asian Science, Technology, and Medicine* 17 (2000): 66–93.

De Qian, Monk. *Secret Shaolin Formulas for the Treatment of External Injury*, translated by Ting-Liang Zhang and Bob Flaws. Portland, OR: Blue Poppy Press, 1995.

Despeux, Catherine. "The Body Revealed: The Contribution of Forensic Medicine to Knowledge and Representations of the Skeleton in China." In *Graphics and Text in the Production of Technical Knowledge in China: The Warp and the Weft*, edited by Francesca Bray, Vera Dorofeeva-Lichtmann and Georges Métailié, 635–84. Leiden: Brill, 2007.

Ding Jihua, ed. *Shangke jicheng*. 2 vols. Beijing: Renmin weisheng chubanshe, 1999.

Goldschmidt, Asaf. *The Evolution of Chinese Medicine: Song Dynasty, 960–1200.* Abingdon: Routledge, 2009.

Hanson, Marta. "The 'Golden Mirror' in the Imperial Court of the Qianlong Emperor." *Early Science and Medicine* 8, no. 2 (2003): 111–47.

Hanson, Marta. "From under the Elbow to Pointing to the Palm: Chinese Metaphors for Learning Medicine by the Book (Fourth–Fourteenth Centuries)." *BJHS Themes* 5 (2020): 75–92.

Heinrich, Ari Larissa. *The Afterlife of Images: Translating the Pathological Body between China and the West.* Durham: Duke University Press, 2008.

Hinrichs, TJ. "The Song and Jin Periods." In *Chinese Medicine and Healing: An Illustrated History*, edited by TJ Hinrichs and Linda Barnes, 97–128. Cambridge, MA: Harvard University Press, 2013.

Hu, Xiaofeng. "A Brief Introduction to Illustration in the Literature of Surgery and Traumatology in Chinese Medicine." In *Imagining Chinese Medicine*, edited by Vivienne Lo and Penelope Barrett, 183–94. Leiden: Brill, 2018.

Lei, Sean Hsiang-lin. *Neither Donkey nor Horse: Medicine in the Struggle over China's Modernity*. Chicago, IL: University of Chicago Press, 2014.

Leung, Angela Ki Che. "Medical Instruction and Popularization in Ming-Qing China." *Late Imperial China* 24, no. 1 (2003): 130–52.

Li, Jianmin. "Anatomy and Surgery." In *Routledge Handbook of Chinese Medicine*, edited by Vivienne Lo, Michael Stanley-Baker, and Dolly Yang, 206–16. London: Routledge, 2022.

Li Jingwei and Lin Zhaogeng, eds. *Zhongguo Yixue Tong Shi--Gudai Juan*. Beijing: Renmin weisheng chubanshe, 2000.

Li Shizhen (1518–93) and Paul U. Unschuld, translator. *Ben Cao Gang Mu* (The Classified Materia Medica). Multi-volume series. Oakland: University of California Press, 2021–2022.

Nappi, Carla. *The Monkey and the Inkpot: Natural History and Its Transformations in Early Modern China.* Cambridge, MA: Harvard University Press, 2009.

Scheid, Volker. "Transmitting Chinese Medicine: Changing Perceptions of Body, Pathology, and Treatment in Late Imperial China." *Asian Medicine* 8, no. 2 (2013): 299–360.

Unschuld, Paul U., and Jinsheng Zheng. *Chinese Traditional Healing: The Berlin Collections of Manuscript Volumes from the 16th through the Early 20th Century.* Leiden: Brill, 2012.

Wang, Xing. *Physiognomy in Ming China: Fortune and the Body*. Leiden: Brill 2020.

Wu, Yi-Li. "The Gendered Medical Iconography of *the Golden Mirror*." *Asian Medicine: Tradition and Modernity* 4, no. 2 (2009): 452–91.

Wu, Yi-Li. *Reproducing Women: Medicine, Metaphor, and Childbirth in Late Imperial China*. Berkeley: University of California Press, 2010.

Wu, Yi-Li. "Between the Living and the Dead: Trauma Medicine and Forensic Medicine in the Mid-Qing." *Frontiers of History in China* 10, no. 1 (2015): 38–73.

Wu, Yi-Li. "A Trauma Doctor's Practice in Nineteenth-Century China: The Medical Cases of Hu Tingguang." *Social History of Medicine* 30, no. 2 (2017): 299–322.

Zhang, Zhibin and Paul U. Unschuld. *Dictionary of the Ben Cao Gang Mu, Volume 1: Chinese Historical Illness Terminology*. Oakland: University of California Press, 2014.

9 Physicians' Treatises

The Ottoman Case

Miri Shefer-Mossensohn

In the early modern period, writing was a major element in the education and career of a physician. This fundamental characteristic of the early modern medical system is reflected in the sheer number of medical tracts produced at this time, and the even greater number of manuscripts in numerous languages, either the *lingua franca* of their time (Latin in Europe and Arabic and Ottoman Turkish in the Middle East) or vernaculars. This extensive writing, in turn, helped to further perpetuate the cultural value attached to medical writing. For historians of medicine, the corpus of medical tracts reveals the accepted and debated medical knowledge of the era and what the medical establishment regarded as its main challenges.

This chapter highlights one particular type of medical text: physicians writing in the Ottoman world of the sixteenth to eighteenth centuries. The medical systems in both Europe and the Islamicate worlds in the early modern period included a tradition of extensive medical writing by physicians. Many characteristics of learned Ottoman medical writing were shared with those of other contemporary medical systems in Christian Europe and Islamicate Asia. The interconnectedness of these systems stemmed from a shared tradition and led to many similarities. Greek medicine, either directly or mediated by medieval Arab-Muslim medicine, was the basis for learned urban medicine in all these medical systems until the modern period. The circulation of manuscripts, trade in *materia medica*, and travel of physicians among various medical communities perpetuated similarities well into the seventeenth and eighteenth centuries.

Ottoman Physicians: Overview

The group referred to as "Ottoman physicians" was in fact a very diverse mix of professional healers. They had different skills and varied education and training. They also based their practices on a variety of medical theories. In some cases, they did not claim any doctrinal basis for their practices.

One key medical tradition in which Ottoman doctors operated in was Ottoman humoralism. Humoralism, based on Galenic medicine from antiquity, was a physical and philosophical theory that all matter in the world, including the human body,

DOI: 10.4324/9781003094876-12

was made of four elements: earth, water, air, and fire. By the Ottoman period, Muslim physicians writing in Arabic, Persian, and Turkish made many adaptations, translations, and additions to this theory. In Ottoman society, as well as in other early or premodern societies (Christian, Jewish, and Muslim), humoralism was one claim to the niche of "scholarly medicine." In Europe, this category was related to university education, while in the Ottoman context, "scholarly medicine" was a medical tradition that privileged knowledge derived from texts and not specifically related to the institution of the university, which did not exist in the empire. Ottoman humoralism enjoyed supremacy in urban communities, in the sultanic palaces, and among the wider Ottoman elite.

There were other medical options, however, vernacular and non-learned popular medicine, sanctioned by a wide consensus from below based on varied local customs and environmental possibilities, as well as religious medicine ("Prophetic medicine," *al-Ṭibb al-Nabawī* or *Tib al-Nabbī* in Arabic and *Tibb-i Nebevī* in Ottoman Turkish), originating from, and therefore sanctioned by, the sayings of the Prophet Muhammad. Whereas popular medicine was transmitted orally and emphasized techniques and visible results, Prophetic medicine, like humoral medicine, was grounded in written traditions.[1] A related, yet distinct, Ottoman medico-religious tradition was one that relied on mysticism (Islamic Sufism and Jewish *kabbalah*). It had a written tradition of recommended cures that was part of the literature on the miraculous powers of living and dead holy figures.[2]

Ottoman physicians in the early modern period mixed and combined medical traditions. The medical reality, both on theoretical and clinical levels, was one of considerable overlaps, even ambiguities, that defied clear and easy categorization in terms of medical traditions and so-called popular/learned hierarchies. Both healers and patients did not consider the various traditions to be mutually exclusive. To some healers and patients, etiologies (that is, theories about how illness originated), were meaningful. But the bulk of the evidence suggests that most healers and patients did not concern themselves with such categorization in day-to-day medical routines. Terms like "physician" and "healer" juxtapose different professionals within the healing realm who may or may not have considered themselves as belonging to the same social and professional group.

However, we can better delineate the vague boundaries of the large group of "Ottoman physicians" by looking at writing and *who* was writing medical texts in the early modern Ottoman world. Not all Ottoman physicians wrote medical texts – far from it. Those who did write represent a particular group that is small and well defined. This is a group of practitioners who were educated to varying degrees, in either medicine or religious subjects, and on different methods (whether self-taught, school educated, family trained, or apprenticed). To them, writing was intellectually and professionally meaningful. Although they do not represent the whole group of Ottoman medical practitioners, their texts comprised a significant aspect of elite urban culture in the Ottoman world and a substantial component of the Ottoman medical realm.

Ottoman Physicians' Writings

Medical writing today takes many forms, such as review articles, case reports, editorials, letters to the editor, book reviews, book chapters, edited books, authored books, research protocols, applications for grant support, and reports of clinical research studies.[3] In the early modern period, there was a more restricted number of formats available for learned medical writing. The two main formats in the Ottoman context are prescriptions on the one hand and treatises on the other, either comprehensive encyclopedias or specialized tracts on particular medical issues.

An important starting point when approaching physicians' writing is to consider the literary models that authors followed. Contemporaries viewed medical writing primarily as a literary and social activity.[4] Therefore, understanding the literary framework at play and how it formed over time is necessary to reconstructing how authors adapted medical content into the genre.

Medical literary models that existed in the Ottoman Empire evolved over hundreds of years in the Islamicate Middle East. This tradition asserted its legitimacy by drawing on the scientific treatises of the sages of antiquity, the patronage of a Muslim urban elite, and the dominant role it played in the intellectual and literary discourses of famous medical figures. The Ottomans inherited these genres, incorporating their own adaptations as they did so. Like the works that preceded them, these works were organized internally in a manner suitable for their use, whether as a quick reference for the doctor or pharmacist, for learned and thorough discussion, or for a lexical interest (i.e., an interest in medical vocabulary). Some medical tracts formed part of a larger medical encyclopedia.

A second way to analyze these texts is to compare them, which helps to expose authors' intended purposes. Comparisons of the works of physicians who wrote more than one surviving treatise reveal that they employed different types of texts for different purposes. Dā'ūd al-Anṭākī (d. 1599) is most famous for his large medical compendia, the *Tadhkirat ʿuli al-albāb wa jāmiʿ lil-ʿajab al-ʿujāb* (*Memorandum of those who possess reason and the collection of great wonders*). However, he wrote many more treatises, some of them specific, like a description of illnesses belonging primarily to the "third life" (ages over 40), a treatise on the importance of astrology in medical interventions, and more.[5]

Physicians, being educated scholars, also engaged in other fields of writing, and medical content was sometimes incorporated into them. This was the case, for instance, with Refael Mordekhai Malki (c. 1640–1702), an Iberian Jew from a family of forced converts who studied medicine in an Italian university and worked as a physician and rabbi in Jerusalem for over two decades. Malki wrote a treatise devoted to medicine, which probably was lost and did not reach us. However, in the 1690s, Malki dedicated himself to composing a vast *Torah* commentary (a lengthy manuscript of some 766 folios), encompassing all the branches of knowledge that Malki knew: astronomy, geography, history, *kabbalah*, and medicine (including pharmacology and anatomy).[6]

The wide range of languages that physicians used in their medical writing mirrors the diversity of writing models available at the time, many of which were based on traditions from earlier Islamicate periods. The Ottoman Empire was a linguistic tower of Babylon. Spreading over large bodies of land and water from Arabia to Hungary, from Algeria to Iraq, at its greatest extent, Ottoman realities had to be multilingual. Ottoman urban centers were characterized by linguistic cacophony.[7]

This multiplicity of languages is a central characteristic of the medical scene and a key consideration when analyzing this type of material. In an ideal world, historians would be able to read and understand all relevant languages. A more attainable goal, however, is to consider the authoring physician's particular linguistic choices within a specific polyglot context of place and time. Malki, for instance, wrote his treatise in Hebrew from his seat in Jerusalem, a prevalently Arabic-speaking region. Malki's choice was an obvious one given that his medical writing was part of a religious discussion of the most basic and sacred Jewish text, intended for Jewish audience.

Another Ottoman Jewish physician-author, Tobias HaCohen (1652–1729), made a similar decision to publish his comprehensive medical compendia in Hebrew. He was a scion to a family of European rabbis who emigrated to Ottoman Palestine and then returned to Europe. Family troubles and Jewish turmoil in Europe, and then his own studies, took him from the Lorraine region northeast of France to Poland, then to Germany and Italy where he studied medicine at Padua. He obtained his medical degree in the summer of 1683 and took on a position in the Ottoman court. Tobias served four Ottoman sultans in the Ottoman Turkish speaking imperial capital cities of Edirne and Istanbul. Later in life, he lived and practiced in Jerusalem. However, Tobias intended his compendium *Maʿase Tuviyya* (*The Work of Tobias*) for a Jewish audience. In the Author Introduction, he explains that he is writing his treatise to make the cutting-edge medicine of his time accessible to Hebrew-reading physicians.[8] Paying attention to language choice allows us to better understand the author's intended audience.

Analyzing the multiple traditions and languages of Ottoman medical writing further enables us to give tangible form to subtle Ottoman contexts. One such context is the multi-religious, multi-ethnic, and multilingual environment that was the Ottoman Empire. This reality expressed itself in medical writing by way of incorporating multiple writing traditions and conferring legitimacy on the writing of learned medical treatises in multiple languages.

A second context is the Ottomanization of existing traditions in medicine, as in other social and cultural arenas. Ottoman Turkish gradually rose to prominence as a language of medical writing, at least in elite circles.[9] Thus, sixteenth-century Dā'ūd al-Anṭākī who operated from Antakya in the Eastern Mediterranean, which is today Turkey's southernmost province not far from the border with Syria, as well as in Damascus and Cairo, all Arabic-speaking environments, wrote his many medical treatises (over 30) in Arabic.[10] In contrast, Emir Çelebi (d. 1638) from Anatolia, studied and worked for many years at a Cairo hospital before being recruited by the Ottoman court and becoming the personal physician to Sultan Murad IV (r. 1623–1640) and imperial head physician. Emir Çelebi wrote his 1625 medical encyclopedia *Enmüzec-ül-tibb* (*Summary of Medicine*) in Ottoman Turkish.[11]

Turkish, which had been a minor and provincial language for medical writing during the fourteenth and fifteenth centuries, assumed an imperial and learned usage in the sixteenth century. At that point, Ottoman physicians began composing manuals in Ottoman Turkish, not just in Arabic, the language of learned medical writing in previous periods.

Nevertheless, Ottoman Turkish never entirely replaced the other languages used for medical writing, including both major Islamic languages like Arabic and Persian, and regional vernacular ones like Hebrew and Greek. For instance, Ṣāliḥ b. Naṣrallah Ibn Sallūm, a late seventeenth-century physician from Aleppo who rose to the same imperial position in Istanbul that had been held by Çelebi and companion of the sultan Mehmet IV (r. 1648–1687), wrote his famous tract on therapy and hygiene, *Ghāyat al-itqān fī tadbīr badan al-insān* (*The Greatest Thoroughness in Treatment of the Human Body*) in Arabic. Shortly after publication, it was translated into Ottoman Turkish by leading Ottoman physicians and the book enjoyed considerable popularity.

A third Ottoman context is the evolution of the urban elite's sense of their own imperial importance during the sixteenth and seventeenth centuries. Medical writing in Ottoman-Turkish arose and expanded because it was the language of the Ottoman imperial elite. It was estimated that medicine became such a central focus for Ottoman Turkish readers that about 70–80 percent of medical works written under the Ottomans were composed originally in Ottoman Turkish, in addition to the many translations into Ottoman Turkish.[12]

The growing trend of writing medical treatises in Ottoman Turkish reflects a practical necessity. Whoever wanted to engage with the imperial elite, perhaps to solicit patronage, had to approach its members in the common language in which they were literate, namely Ottoman Turkish. This included, for instance, the female members of the Ottoman elite, as well as professional bureaucrats and merchants in and around the court.[13] More broadly, the decision to write in Ottoman Turkish attests to a cultural and political choice on the part of the authors who wished to gain access to the imperial circles.

Ottoman Physicians' Writings and Clinical Realities

What can we, as historians, glean from these texts about the clinical realities of Ottoman medicine? Ottoman medical written traditions emphasized primarily a preventive system by stressing the importance of balance (*mizāj* in Arabic) to ward off illness. The balance in question operated on two levels. At the micro-level within the body, balance referred to the even distribution of the four humors, the physiological building blocks of the body: blood (air), phlegm (water), black bile (earth), and yellow bile (fire). At the macro-level, balance was understood as lifestyle on the whole and its suitability to one's humoral realities. This included everything from choosing a climate and topography to live in to deciding on a profession (in the case of men), to organizing hours of rest and activity during the day, to consuming a suitable diet, and much more. Within the humoral context, as it was inherited from antiquity, balancing regimen in this way was known as the *sex res non-naturales*, or the six non-naturals, and includes light and air, food and drink, work and rest, sleep and waking, excretions and secretions (including bathing and sexual intercourse), and finally the state of the soul.

Texts of Prophetic medicine also embraced the humoral concept of balance. By the Ottoman period, the logic of their organization resembled that of medical texts, and their authors were attentive to medical theories, diseases, and cures and not just aspects of belief, morals, and overall good Islamic conduct. Nevertheless, the treatises in Prophetic medicine added a further, spiritual dimension in which illness and medical treatment were addressed in terms of their relation to sin, reward, and ideal piety.[14] Such works were very popular and circulated among the audiences who also read the Galenic humoral treatises. They were included in the same personal libraries, both humble ones and those that were part of an elite patronage.

A good example of a Prophetic medical text relevant to the Ottoman period is the treatise that belonged to none other than Jalāl al-Dīn al-Suyūṭī (d. 1505), the Egyptian scholar and one of the most famous figures in premodern Islamic history. Al-Suyuṭi enjoyed a great reputation as a scholar and an aura of godliness surrounded him even during his lifetime. A versatile author known usually for his religious scholarly work (mostly hadith, the sayings of the Prophet, and Qur'anic studies), he was active also in the field of medicine. His treatise *Al-manhaj al-sawī wal-manhal al-rawī fī al-ṭibb al-nabawī* (*The Proper Road and the Thirst-quenching Spring of Prophetic Medicine*) is a discussion of medicine as formed by, and legitimized by, the sayings of the Prophet Muhammad. Written in Cairo, two copies of *Al-manhaj al-sawī* were kept at the libraries of Topkapı, the Ottoman imperial palace in Istanbul.[15] Numerous other copies are scattered in libraries throughout Turkey, including provincial libraries like Samsun, today a Black Sea port on the north coast of Turkey.[16]

Prophetic medicine was an intellectual phenomenon and discourse, but there is no evidence that it was a practical tradition.[17] Humoral medicine, which likewise cultivated a sophisticated textual tradition, was nonetheless a significant applied practice. Perhaps humoral medicine was even the leading clinical reality. There is abundant evidence of Ottoman humoral practitioners, humoral practice in Ottoman hospitals, and Ottoman humoral pharmacopeia.[18] By placing dozens of medical recipes from the imperial Ottoman palace together with lists of the purchases for the imperial kitchen or hospital larders, historians can begin to glimpse the possible medical influences that shaped gastronomic decisions and a humoral clinical reality overall.[19] That said, we do not necessarily know whether prescriptions were actually prepared or, if they were, whether they were used or whether the patient followed the dosage and usage instructions. We also do not always know which prescription was purchased for the kitchen and ultimately used for food rather than for medication.

The relationship between physicians' writing and clinical reality – both the intended correlation and the actual connection – is complicated and elusive. There is a gap between the learned and written tradition and the clinical one, sometimes in the practice of the same physician. In fact, like its Islamic predecessors, Ottoman medical writing did not include a scientific and literary tradition of discussing medical clinical experience.[20] Moreover, many tracts were written by authors who had a medical education but did not practice medicine. In other words, they did not make a living through medicine.[21] These authors did not necessarily intend their medical treatises to have an applied element. Furthermore, practicing physicians wrote their tracts for multiple reasons; we cannot assume that they intended to influence practice or embed their practices into medical writing.

The best example of this complex and difficult-to-define relationship between medical text and practice is writing on anatomy (the study of the structure of human and animal organisms and their parts) and surgery (invasive procedures on human and animal tissues and organs). These medical disciplines especially require the type of knowledge that stems from hands-on experience and have a particularly applicable significance. Both were an integral part of Ottoman medical knowledge.

There is a very small number of Ottoman anatomical and surgical works, much like their scarcity in other Islamicate medical systems. A rare Ottoman example is seventeenth-century Şemsüddin İtaki's *Taşriḥ-i abdān ve tarjumān-i kabāla-yi falāsufān* (*The Anatomy of the Body Parts and Expounding the Role of the Philosophers*). İtaki described in words and illustrations the simple organs that are of the same structure (blood, bone, and muscle) and the complex ones, like the systems of respiration and digestion. İtaki based this book on a number of medical texts: Ibn Sina's eleventh-century *Qanūn*, Ibn al-Nafīs's thirteenth-century summary and criticism of Ibn Sina, and Ibn Ilyās's fourteenth-century *Tashrih-i mansuri*. In addition to these fundamental texts in Islamicate medicine, İtaki was influenced by Andreas Vesalius (1514–1564) and his *De Humani Corporis Fabrica* (*The Structure of the Human Body*), incorporating some of Vesalius' three-dimensional images of body parts and anatomical systems.[22] No other similar Ottoman anatomy book is known to us.

The fifteenth-century treatise, *Cerrāhiyyetü'l-Ḥāniyye* (*The Imperial Surgical Operation*) is likewise a scarce type of Ottoman medical writing. The author is a physician from Amasya in central Anatolia by the name of Şerefeddin Sabuncuoğlu, who dedicated his tract to the reigning Sultan Mehmed II (r. 1451–1481). Sabuncuoğlu focuses on surgery and explains procedures and uses of surgical devices. He was one of the first in Anatolia to write a scientific treatise in Turkish and thus is part of the larger cultural change of Ottomanization. He prepared an Ottoman edition of an early eleventh-century chapter on surgery written by the Iberian al-Zahrawī in his self-contained medical manual for medicine. This is probably the earliest work on surgery in Arabic, and certainly the earliest one that contains illustrations of surgical and dental instruments. Sabuncuoğlu, however, went further than mere translation by also adding explanations and information on procedures, techniques, and devices, including new illustrations since he prided himself on the devices that he invented and produced.[23] This treatise is unique and there are no similar works, with or without illustrations.

The paucity of medical works on anatomy and surgery is a consequence of a theoretical hierarchy of treatments promoted by humoralism, which started with dietetics and then descended to medications and finally surgery as the last option a physician should consider. Salaries for medical personnel in Ottoman hospitals, which were reflective of professional hierarchies, reveal that surgeons were paid considerably less than physicians.

The marginality of surgery was also the result of objective problems facing surgery in the early modern Middle East: in many cases, major surgical procedures were fatal because the practices of sanitization and pasteurization had not yet begun. Interventions were also painful and difficult to endure, as this was long before the age of painkillers and anesthesia. Surgical texts included complex invasive procedures, for instance, intricate eye procedures, but for the most part surgical procedures were not invasive. There is some evidence of autopsies, but generally the clinical reality was minor surgeries of the type that do not penetrate deeply into the tissues of the body, such as bleeding, cutting, manipulating bones, and topical treatments. Even if surgeons possessed sufficient knowledge and techniques for major interventions, where would they gain experience? While cutting into a body was common and accepted as an option and there was no strict ban on doing it, such risky, painful procedures were not embraced wholeheartedly.[24]

This is yet another facet of the uncertain relationship between medical text and practice. The essays that doctors wrote about anatomy and surgery shared a descriptive and theoretical component that was only very partially based on clinical experience. Anatomy was a textual description of the systems in the body and their functions rather than depictions of actual systems and functions. Likewise, surgery was not wholly the art of actual dissections; it was about knowledge and not necessarily medical results.

Even when a physician declared that a treatise was based on experience, it should be assumed that, at least in part, this was a literary claim intended to promote his professional status, proclaim the extent of his training, and give his essay an additional layer of medical efficacy and truthfulness. Historians must approach these texts as authors' attempts to position themselves within the elite echelons of urban medical communities by claiming professional and intellectual authority – not necessarily as records of practice, although this cannot be ruled out.

Şerefeddin Sabuncuoğlu, for instance, titled his manual on drugs and their preparation, *Mücerrebname* (*The book of Tried Medications*). He wrote the work in 1468, the last of three medical treatises. Following common phrasing found in many medical treatises, he explains that he answered a plea from colleagues that he put on paper his 14-year medical experience working in a hospital. Indeed, this short manual straddles both medical theory and clinical reality. On the one hand, Sabuncuoğlu refers frequently to his techniques in preparing drugs and discusses efficacy based on experiments that he performed on himself and on animals. The title and the numerous references to trials and observations attest to this as a source of pride for him. On the other hand, the contents of the tract, with regard to the types of drugs, their ingredients, and methods of preparation, repeat earlier Arab-Islamic examples of learned written pharmacopeia.[25]

In sum, Ottoman physicians wrote about how "to think" about medicine of the time, not necessarily what was best "to do." However, during the closing decades of the seventeenth century and the opening ones of the eighteenth century, more practical medical writing rose in popularity. From the 1660s onwards, a new medical movement attributing itself to the sixteenth-century German-Swiss physician Paracelsus valorized empirical knowledge. This type of medicine was drug-based and claimed to offer cures that worked. Though they would later be proven ineffective and sometimes even fatal, these recipes enjoyed immense popularity in the major urban centers of the Ottoman Empire and eighteenth-century physicians working within this framework produced a wide range of manuscripts of this type. This is where the money was to be made in the medical market, explains historian Harun Küçük. Many physicians made do with very low wages and were interested in making a better living than theoretical and impractical medical thinking could provide. This accentuated interest in practical medicine, including writing about it, reflected a wider epistemological shift: Ottomans began to regard experience as "proof" and favored a logic based on practice instead of a formal logic based on theory.[26] Medical writing during the latter part of the eighteenth century offers traces of this medical tradition, whereas the nineteenth century would bring with it another shift, this time toward Western medicine.

The Modern Whereabouts of Ottoman Physicians' Tracts

Many manuscripts from the Ottoman period that deal with medicine have survived. These include works that either were authored in earlier periods but were copied, translated, and commented upon during the Ottoman period, or composed originally during this period. Some reach us as a single copy, but many exist in multiple copies at different levels of production, from the simplest and cheapest to the most meticulous, colorful, and expensive (illustrated manuscripts, in particular, were a status symbol). All of them together attest that there was a diverse audience and a vibrant market for such manuscripts.

The lion's share of the physicians' treatises still exist in manuscript form. Only a minority have received critical editions and commentaries or facsimile publications. Among these are mainly surgical manuals, perhaps because of the special interest in the subject and the illustrations of medical devices and anatomical drawings. Two main examples are Sabuncuoğlu's fifteenth-century treatise, *Cerrahiyyetü'l-Ḥaniyye*,[27] and Itaki's seventeenth-century *Taşriḥ-i abdān ve tarjumān-i kabāla-yi falāsufān*.[28]

Physicians' treatises are included in all the major collections of Islamic manuscripts in European and North American universities and libraries. Collections that specialize in Islamic medical manuscripts, including those from the Ottoman period, are at the National Library of Medicine in Bethesda, Maryland, and the Wellcome Library in London. Naturally, however, the largest concentration of Ottoman manuscripts in general and Ottoman medical manuscripts in particular is in Turkey. The Research Centre for Islamic History, Art and Culture in Istanbul has published bio-bibliographies in Arabic and Turkish for manuscripts on medical subjects in Turkish libraries.[29]

This foray into physicians' text is situated in a specific historical context, namely the urban centers of the early modern Ottoman world, specifically the Turkish- and Arabic-speaking Middle East. Furthermore, the chapter traces patterns specific to Ottoman medicine as a social and cultural phenomenon. Yet, the analytical methods discussed here – looking at medical texts through the lenses of scientific and literary models, addressing authors' concerns with status, paying attention to language and vocabulary, and attending to ever-changing historical contexts – are all necessary when studying physicians' treatises in other early modern Eurasian medical systems, too.

Notes

1 An introduction to the corpus of Prophetic medicine is Iremli Perho, *The Prophet's Medicine: A Creation of the Muslim Traditionalist Scholars* (Helsinki: Finnish Oriental Society, 1995).
2 Aslıhan Gürbüzel, *Taming the Messiah: The Formation of an Ottoman Political Public Sphere, 1600–1700* (Oakland: University of California Press, 2023); Yael Buchman, "Rabbi Hayyim Vital's Notebook of Practical Advice," *Cathedra: For the History of Eretz Israel & Its Yishuv* 99 (2001): 37–64.
3 Robert B. Taylor, *Medical Writing: A Guide for Clinicians, Educators, and Researchers* (Cham: Springer, 2018).
4 Lawrence I. Conrad, "Scholarship and Social Context in the Near East," in *Knowledge and the Scholarly Medical Traditions*, ed. Don Bates (Cambridge: Cambridge University Press, 1995), 81–101.
5 Raphaela Veit, "Dāʾūd al-Anṭākī," in Encyclopaedia of Islam, THREE, eds. Kate Fleet, Gudrun Krämer, Denis Matringe, John Nawas, Everett Rowson. Consulted online on November 16, 2021.
6 Minna Rozen, *Jewish Identity and Society in the Seventeenth Century: Reflections on the Life and Works of Refael Mordekhai Malki* (Tübingen: J.C.B Mohr, 1992), 1–4.
7 Leslie Peirce, "Polyglottism in the Ottoman Empire: A Reconsideration," in *Braudel Revisted: The Mediterranean World, 1600–1800*, eds. Gabriel Piterberg, Teofilo F. Ruiz, and Geoffrey Symcox (Toronto: University of Toronto Press, 2010), 76–98; Eric R. Dursteler, "Speaking in Tongues: Language and Communication in the Early Modern Mediterranean," *Past & Present* 217 (2012): 47–77.
8 Tuvia HaCohen, *Maʿase Tuvia* (Venice: Bragadina, 1708), 5–6v.
9 Cornell H. Fleischer, *Bureaucrat and Intellectual in the Ottoman Empire: The Historian Mustafa Âli* (1541–1600) (Princeton, NJ: Princeton University Press, 1986); Emine Fetvacı, *Picturing History at the Ottoman Court* (Bloomington: Indiana University Press, 2013).
10 Veit, "Dāʾūd al-Anṭākī."
11 Adnan Abdulhak Adıvar, *Osmanlı Turklerinde İlim* (Istanbul: Remzi Kitabevi, 1991), 128–29; Esin Kâhya and Aysegül D. Erdemir, *Bilimin Işığında Osmanlıdan Cumhuriyete Tıp ve Sağlık Kurumları* (Ankara: Turkiye Diyanet Vakfı Yayınları, 2000), 173–74.
12 Cevat İzgi, *Osmanlı Medreselerinde İlim* (Istanbul: İz Yayıncılık, 1997), 2:42–3.
13 M. Cağatay Ulucay, *Osmanlı Sultanlarına Aşk Mektupları* (Istanbul: Ufuk Kitapları, 2001 [Vakıt Matbaası, 1950]); Cağatay Ulucay, *Harem II* (Ankara: Türk Tarih Kurumu Basımevi, 1992), 86–7.
14 On the Islamic pious construction of illness based on the Prophetic medicine literature, although of pre-Ottoman period, see Ahmed Ragab, *Piety and Patienthood in Medieval Islam* (Abingdon: Routledge, 2018).
15 Fehmi Edhem Karatay, *Topkapı Sarayı Müzesi Kütüphanesi Arapça Kataloğu* (Istanbul: Topkapı Sarayı Müzesi, 1966), 3:859–60.

16 This is according to the online portal of the Presidency of Turkish Manuscripts Institution at the Culture and Tourism Ministry: http://www.yazmalar.gov.tr/ [accessed November 29, 2021].

17 Ahmed Ragab, "Prophetic Medicine," in *The Oxford Encyclopedia of the Islamic World: Digital Collection,* ed. John L. Esposito (Oxford: Oxford University Press, 2022).

18 On Ottoman hospitals, see Miri Shefer-Mossensohn, *Ottoman Medicine: Healing and Medical Institutions 1500–1700* (Albany: SUNY Press, 2009).

19 Topkapı Sarayı Müzesi Arşivi [Archives of Topkapi Palace, Istanbul], evrak 93/1–2, 2657/1–5, 11942/7–11, 13–16, 18, 25, 28, 30–33, 37, 41, 43–46, 48, 56, 60, 66, 67–69, 71, 73, 75, 78–82, 85, 87–90, 92, 96–98, 102–5, 112, 118, 122–25, 127–28, 131. J. Michael Rogers, "The Palace, Potions and the Public: Some Lists of Drugs in Mid-16th Century Ottoman Turkey," in *Studies in Ottoman History in Honour of Professor V. L. Menage*, eds. Colin Heywood and Colin Imber (Istanbul: Isis Press, 1994), 273–95.

20 Cristina Alvarez-Millan, "Graeco-Roman Case Histories and Their Influence on Medieval Islamic Clinical Accounts," *Social History of Medicine* 12 (1999): 19–43; Idem., "Practice versus Theory: Tenth-Century Case Histories from the Islamic Middle East," *Social History of Medicine* 13 (2000): 293–306.

21 Doris Behrens-Abouseif, "The Image of the Physician, Arab Biographies of the Post-Classical Age," *Der Islam* 66 (1989): 331–43.

22 Şemsüddin İtaki, *Teşrih-ī Ebdan* (Islamabad: al-Majlis al-Waṭanī, AH 1410 [1990]); idem. *Şemseddîn-i İtâkî'nin Resimli Anatomi Kitabı*, ed. Esin Kahya (Ankara: Atatürk Kültür Merkezi Yayını, 1996); Idem. *The Treatise on Anatomy of the Human Body and Interpretation of Philosophers* (Islamabad: National Hijra Council, AH 1410/ AD 1990); Esin Kâhya, "One of the Samples of the Influences of Avicenna on the Ottoman Medicine, Shams al-Din Itaqi," *Belleten* 64, 4 (2000): 63–8; Gül Russell, "'The Owl and the Pussycat': The Process of Cultural Transmission in Anatomical Illustration," in *Transfer of Modern Science and Technology to the Muslim World*, ed. Ekmeleddin İhsanoğlu (Istanbul: Research Centre for Islamic History, Art and Culture, 1992), 191–95.

23 Şerefeddin Sabuncuoğlu, *Cerrahiyyetü'l-Ḥāniyye*, 2 vols., trans. and ed. İlter Üzel (Ankara: Atatürk Kültür, Dil ve Tarih Yüksek Kurumu, 1992).

24 Emilie Savage-Smith, "Attitudes toward Dissection in Medieval Islam," *Journal of the History of Medicine and Allied Sciences* 50 (1995): 67–110; Emilie Savage-Smith, "The Practice of Surgery in Islamic Lands: Myth and Reality," *Social History of Medicine* 13 (2000): 307–21.

25 Şerefeddin Sabuncuoğlu, *Mücerreb-nāme*, eds. İlter Üzel and Kenan Süveren (Ankara: Atatürk Kültür Merkezi Yayınları, 1999).

26 Harun B. Küçük, *Science without Leisure: Practical Naturalism in Istanbul, 1660–1732* (Pittsburgh, PA: University of Pittsburgh Press, 2019), ch. "The Recipe: An Annotated Chronology of New Medicine in the Seventeenth Century," 143–66; idem. "New Medicine and the *Ḥikmet-i Ṭabīʿiyye* Problematic in Eighteenth-Century Istanbul," in *Texts in Transit in the Medieval Mediterranean*, eds. Y. Tzvi Langermann and Robert G. Morrison (University Park: Pennsylvania State University Press, 2016), 222–42; Akif Ercihan Yerlioğlu, "'May Those Who Understand What I Wrote Remember This Humble One": Paratextual Elements in Eighteenth-Century Ottoman Medical Manuscripts," *YILLIK: Annual of Istanbul Studies* 2 (2020): 35–51.

27 Sabuncuoğlu, *Cerrahiyyetü'l-Ḥāniyye*.

28 İtaki, Şemseddîn-I İtâkî'nin Resimli Anatomi Kitabı.

29 Ramazan Şeşen, *Fihris Makhṭūṭāt al-Ṭibb al-Islāmi bi al-Lughat al-cArabiyya wa al-Turkiyya wa al-Farisiyya fi Maktabat Turkiyya* (Istanbul: Research Centre for Islamic History, Art and Culture, 1984); *Osmanlı Tıbbi Bilimler Literatürü Tarihi*; 4 vols. (Istanbul: İslam Tarih, Sanat ve Kültür Araştırma Merkezi, 2008).

Bibliography

Primary Sources

Topkapı Sarayı Müzesi Arşivi, evrak 93/1–2, 2657/1–5, 11942/7–11, 13–16, 18, 25, 28, 30–3, 37, 41, 43–46, 48, 56, 60, 66, 67–9, 71, 73, 75, 78–82, 85, 87–90, 92, 96–8, 102–05, 112, 118, 122–25, 127–28, 131.

HaCohen, Tuvia. *Maᶜase Tuvia*. Venice: Bragadina, 1708.

İtaki, Şemsüddin. *Teşrih-ī Ebdan.* Islamabad: al-Majlis al-Waṭanī, AH 1410 [1990].

———. *Şemseddîn-I İtâkî'nin Resimli Anatomi Kitabı*, ed. Esin Kahya. Ankara: Atatürk Kültür Merkezi Yayını, 1996.

———. *The Treatise on Anatomy of the Human Body and Interpretation of Philosophers.* Islamabad: National Hijra Council, AH 1410/AD 1990.

Sabuncuoğlu, Şerefeddin. *Mücerreb-nāme*, edited by İlter Üzel and Kenan Süveren. Ankara: Atatürk Kültür Merkezi Yayınları, 1999.

———. *Cerrahiyyetü'l-Ḥāniyye*, 2 vols., translated and edited by İlter Üzel. Ankara: Atatürk Kültür, Dil ve Tarih Yüksek Kurumu, 1992.

Secondary Sources

Adıvar, Adnan Abdulhak. *Osmanlı Turklerinde İlim*; 5th ed. Istanbul: Remzi Kitabevi, 1991.

Alvarez-Millan, Cristina. "Graeco-Roman Case Histories and Their Influence on Medieval Islamic Clinical Accounts." *Social History of Medicine* 12 (1999): 19–43.

———. "Practice Versus Theory: Tenth-Century Case Histories from the Islamic Middle East." *Social History of Medicine* 13 (2000): 293–306.

Behrens-Abouseif, Doris. "The Image of the Physician, Arab Biographies of the Post-Classical Age." *Der Islam* 66 (1989): 331–43.

Buchman, Yael. "Rabbi Hayyim Vital's Notebook of Practical Advice." *Cathedra: For the History of Eretz Israel & Its Yishuv* 99 (2001): 37–64. [Hebrew]

Conrad, Lawrence I. "Scholarship and Social Context in the Near East." In *Knowledge and the Scholarly Medical Traditions*, edited by Don Bates, 81–101. Cambridge: Cambridge University Press, 1995.

Dursteler, Eric R. "Speaking in Tongues: Language and Communication in the Early Modern Mediterranean." *Past & Present* 217 (2012): 47–77.

Fetvacı, Emine. *Picturing History at the Ottoman Court.* Bloomington: Indiana University Press, 2013.

Fleischer, Cornell H. *Bureaucrat and Intellectual in the Ottoman Empire: The Historian Mustafa Âli* (1541–1600). Princeton, NJ: Princeton University Press, 1986.

Gürbüzel, Aslıhan. *Taming the Messiah: The Formation of an Ottoman Political Public Sphere, 1600–1700.* Oakland: University of California Press, 2023.

İzgi, Cevat. *Osmanlı Medreselerinde İlim*; 2 vols. Istanbul: İz Yayıncılık, 1997.

Kâhya, Esin. "One of the Samples of the Influences of Avicenna on the Ottoman Medicine, Shams al-Din Itaqi," *Belleten* 64, no. 4 (2000): 63–8.

Kâhya, Esin and Aysegül D. Erdemir. *Bilimin Işığında Osmanlıdan Cumhuriyete Tıp ve Sağlık Kurumları*. Ankara: Turkiye Diyanet Vakfı Yayınları, 2000.

Karatay, Fehmi Edhem. *Topkapı Sarayı Müzesi Kütüphanesi Arapça Kataloğu*; 3 vols. Istanbul: Topkapı Sarayı Müzesi, 1966.

Küçük, Harun B. "New Medicine and the *Ḥikmet-i Ṭabīʿiyye* Problematic in Eighteenth-Century Istanbul." In *Texts in Transit in the Medieval Mediterranean*, edited by Y. Tzvi Langermann and Robert G. Morrison, 222–42. University Park: Pennsylvania State University Press, 2016.

———. *Science without Leisure: Practical Naturalism in Istanbul, 1660–1732*. Pittsburgh, PA: University of Pittsburgh Press, 2019.

Peirce, Leslie. "Polyglottism in the Ottoman Empire: A Reconsideration." In *Braudel Revisted: The Mediterranean World, 1600–1800*, edited by Gabriel Piterberg, Teofilo F. Ruiz, and Geoffrey Symcox, 76–98. Toronto: University of Toronto Press, 2010.

Perho, Iremli. *The Prophet's Medicine: A Creation of the Muslim Traditionalist Scholars*. Helsinki: Finnish Oriental Society, 1995.

Ragab, Ahmed. *Piety and Patienthood in Medieval Islam*. New York: Routledge, 2018.

———. "Prophetic Medicine." In *The Oxford Encyclopedia of the Islamic World: Digital Collection*, edited by John L. Esposito. Oxford: Oxford University Press, 2022, Accessed 21November 2023, from https://www.oxfordreference.com/view/10.1093/acref/9780197669419.001.0001/acref-9780197669419-e-329.

Rogers, J. Michael. "The Palace, Potions and the Public: Some Lists of Drugs in Mid-16th Century Ottoman Turkey." In *Studies in Ottoman History in Honour of Professor V. L. Menage*, edited by Colin Heywood and Colin Imber, 273–95. Istanbul: Isis Press, 1994.

Rozen, Minna. *Jewish Identity and Society in the Seventeenth Century: Reflections on the Life and Works of Refael Mordekhai Malki*. Tübingen: J.C.B Mohr, 1992.

Russell, Gül. "'The Owl and the Pussycat': The Process of Cultural Transmission in Anatomical Illustration." In *Transfer of Modern Science and Technology to the Muslim World*, edited by Ekmeleddin İhsanoğlu, 180–212. Istanbul: Research Centre for Islamic History, Art and Culture, 1992.

Savage-Smith, Emilie. "Attitudes toward Dissection in Medieval Islam." *Journal of the History of Medicine and Allied Sciences* 50 (1995): 67–110.

———. "The Practice of Surgery in Islamic Lands: Myth and Reality." *Social History of Medicine* 13 (2000): 307–21.

Şeşen Ramazan. *Fihris Makhṭūṭāt al-Ṭibb al-Islāmi bi al-Lughat al-ᶜArabiyya wa al-Turkiyya wa al-Farisiyya fi Maktabat Turkiyya*. Istanbul: Research Centre for Islamic History, Art and Culture, 1984.

———. *Osmanlı Tıbbi Bilimler Literatürü Tarihi*; 4 vols. Istanbul: İslam Tarih, Sanat ve Kültür Araştırma Merkezi, 2008.

Shefer-Mossensohn, Miri. *Ottoman Medicine: Healing and Medical Institutions 1500–1700*. Albany: SUNY Press, 2009.

Taylor, Robert B. *Medical Writing: A Guide for Clinicians, Educators, and Researchers*. 3rd ed. Cham: Springer, 2018.

Ulucay, M. Cağatay. *Osmanlı Sultanlarına Aşk Mektupları*. Istanbul: Ufuk Kitapları, 2001 [Vakıt Matbaası, 1950].

———. *Harem II*. Ankara: Türk Tarih Kurumu Basımevi, 1992.

Veit, Raphaela. "Dāʾūd Al-Anṭākī." In *Encyclopaedia of Islam, THREE*, edited by Kate Fleet, Gudrun Krämer, Denis Matringe, John Nawas, and Devin J. Stewart. Accessed November 21, 2023. doi:http://dx.doi.org/10.1163/1573-3912_ei3_COM_23481.

Yerlioğlu, Akif Ercihan. "'May Those Who Understand What I Wrote Remember This Humble One": Paratextual Elements in Eighteenth-Century Ottoman Medical Manuscripts." *YILLIK: Annual of Istanbul Studies* 2 (2020): 35–51.

10 Missionary Remedies

Sebestian Kroupa

When suffering from jaundice, the people of Tarahumara of northern Mexico would traditionally bathe in a red decoction prepared from brazilwood and consume a few lice boiled in water.[1] The same therapy against jaundice was recommended by the Jesuit Johannes Steinhöffer (1664–1716) in his *Florilegio medicinal de todas las enfermedades* ("Medical anthology of all ailments"), published in Mexico City in 1712 (Figure 10.1).[2] Steinhöffer was trained in pharmacy in his native Czech lands and subsequently sent to assist his Jesuit brethren in the Mexican missions with his medical skills. *Florilegio* was the result of 20 years of experience in healing across the northern frontier of New Spain among a variety of ethno-linguistic communities. Steinhöffer listed common diseases found in the missions, described their causes and symptoms, and suggested therapies. He explained that he wrote the work primarily for fellow missionaries in the field without access to medical practitioners since he could not travel to all the widely scattered missions himself.[3] However, *Florilegio* earned wider circulation and greater longevity than Steinhöffer could probably have expected: it went through four editions in the first 50 years of its existence, and its influence on medical practices across the North American southwest can still be observed today.[4]

Missionary pharmacopoeias like that of Steinhöffer offer rich insights into colonial medical practices and cross-cultural transfers of medical knowledge in the early modern world.[5] Pharmacopoeias are a textual genre of medical writing that lists remedies, their virtues, and preparations, as well as social pharmacopoeias, or collective knowledge of medicinal virtues held by a community in textual, oral, and embodied forms.[6] Conceived as practical guides written in accessible vernacular language, missionary pharmacopoeias comprised simple recipes that even individuals without medical training could prepare. In his aptly titled *Remedios fáciles para diferentes enfermedades* ("Simple remedies for different ailments"), published in Manila in 1712, the Jesuit Paul Klein (1652–1717) listed "remedies that you can easily find in your towns, or not far from them, or if they come from a pharmacy, they can be brought as part of provisions."[7] The diseases and cures, both local and introduced, were typically interpreted through the lens of the Galenic humoral framework. The treatments combined substances and practices imported from Europe with those native to the region and brought from around the world by increasingly global trade links.

DOI: 10.4324/9781003094876-13

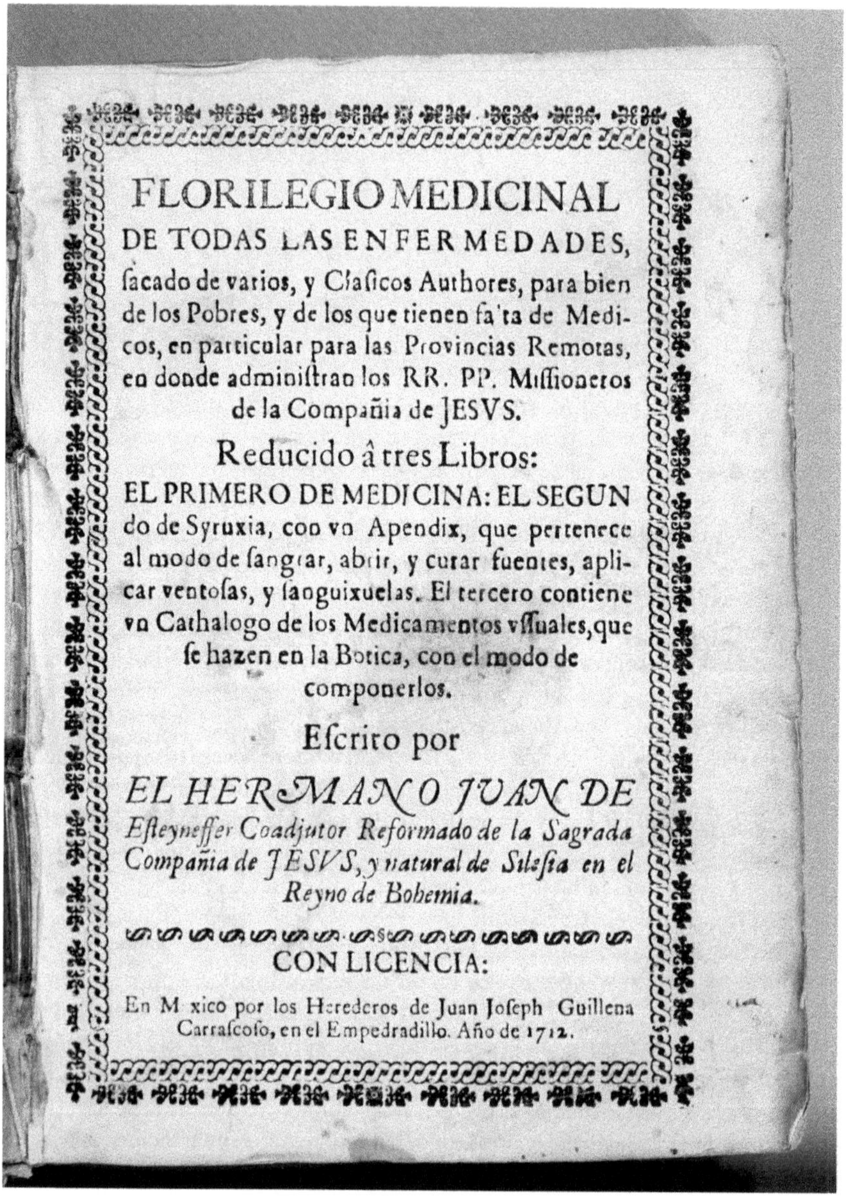

FLORILEGIO MEDICINAL
DE TODAS LAS ENFERMEDADES,
sacado de varios, y Clasicos Authores, para bien
de los Pobres, y de los que tienen falta de Medicos, en particular para las Provincias Remotas,
en donde administran los RR. PP. Missioneros
de la Compañia de JESVS.
Reducido â tres Libros:
EL PRIMERO DE MEDICINA: EL SEGUN
do de Syruxia, con vn Apendix, que pertenece
al modo de sangrar, abrir, y curar fuentes, apli-
car ventosas, y sanguixuelas. El tercero contiene
vn Cathalogo de los Medicamentos vssuales, que
se hazen en la Botica, con el modo de
componerlos.
Escrito por
EL HERMANO JUAN DE
Esteyneffer Coadjutor Reformado de la Sagrada
Compañia de JESVS, y natural de Silesia en el
Reyno de Bohemia.
CON LICENCIA:
En Mexico por los Herederos de Juan Joseph Guillena
Carrascoso, en el Empedradillo. Año de 1712.

Figure 10.1 The title page of Johannes Steinhöffer's *Florilegio medicinal* (1712).

Scholars of colonial medicine have spent recent decades examining the connections between the politics of medical care and the imperial configurations of power and control. Growing interest in the drug trade and material cultures of remedies and recipes has changed our understanding of the globalization of commerce;

the development of empirical practices and theories of the body; and the roles of agencies across cultures, gender, and social standing in the production of medical knowledge.[8] Particular attention has been devoted to bioprospecting, or the colonizers' search for new substances that could yield profit, which has been identified as a crucial driver of European imperial expansion.[9] Recent studies have increasingly focused on the local dynamics of knowledge production in a bid to deconstruct narratives built around European institutions and élite actors, and to question the hegemony of European teleologies of global modernity. Studies of Iberian colonial worlds have been at the forefront of these developments.[10] They have highlighted the limits of imperial control; the tensions between imperial, scientific, and commercial concerns; and the plurality and porosity of knowledge and practice amidst the complex cross-cultural settings, in which the worlds of Europeans and non-Europeans became entangled.[11] The helpful metaphor of "friction" has been developed by Anna Tsing to reflect the complex interactions out of which such entanglements were borne.[12]

Missionary pharmacopoeias can help us add to this growing body of scholarship. Due to their focus on medical practice and multidirectional transfers of knowledge across medical traditions and cultures, they can answer the call for writing histories of medicine that capture local, regional, and global dimensions of medicine within one frame.[13] Missionary sources can take us beyond colonial hubs to examine colonial medicine outside major cities, in missions and Indigenous reductions.[14] The works suggest that the European medical conquest involved more than just projects of bioprospecting. On the one hand, since missionaries relied extensively on Old World remedies and practices in their healing activities, the sources expose how European ideas and substances interacted with diverse pharmaceutical traditions. On the other hand, as missionaries incorporated Indigenous *materia medica* and terminologies into their repertoire, long-standing pharmaceutical traditions could be disrupted by novelty. By showing how local diseases, remedies, and practices were documented by missionaries, the works provide insights into the processes of knowledge appropriation. Collecting medical knowledge was part of a broader missionary ethnographic project, in which they documented Indigenous bodies, customs, and practices. As such, missionary pharmacopoeias fed into European discourses of Indigeneity and the constructions of the European, the "Other," and the hybrid. In the following pages, I will first discuss why religious missionaries engaged in colonial healing before analyzing the content of their works. I conclude by considering how we might read these sources for non-European agency.

Missionaries or Healers?

To analyze missionary medical accounts, we first need to situate them in their religious contexts. The clergy's ability to engage in medicine was restricted by the canon law of the Catholic Church and the precepts of individual orders. Although rules varied over time, space, and community, medical care was generally to be provided as charity rather than material gain. Ordained priests and nuns were altogether excluded from teaching and practicing medicine and surgery without special papal dispensation, mainly since such activities were considered a distraction from their higher spiritual vocation.[15] Yet religious missionaries became deeply embroiled in colonial medical care and produced vast volumes of medical writings over the early modern era. When analyzing these works, historians must be careful to acknowledge the tropes used by religious orders to justify their involvements in healing and medicine. These engagements were underpinned by a combination of religious, intellectual, and commercial considerations, all of which were closely aligned to the higher apostolic goals to spread the Gospel. As we will see, we must consider the sources as products of intersecting concerns with Christian charity, humanist natural history and medicine, and projects of colonization and evangelization.[16]

The connection between religious commitment, charitable work, and healing has been a prominent feature of Christianity since the early days of the Church.[17] The Council of Trent (1545–1563) and the ensuing Counter-Reformation reinforced these concerns and stimulated the creation of institutions and even orders dedicated to the care of the poor and sick. Both in Europe and globally, healing emerged as a central field of missionary activity, in which physical and material needs naturally overlapped with the religious message. In the Christian world, the healing of souls was inextricably linked with the healing of bodies.[18] Under the auspices of Christian charity, Catholic orders founded hospitals, shelters, and pharmacies in most Iberian colonial cities and rapidly established themselves as a major force in local medical marketplaces. Among the wide array of missionary orders, the most prominent were the Jesuits, Franciscans, Augustinians, and Dominicans. Some orders, such as the Brothers Hospitallers of St John of God, even specialized in caring for the sick. Since missionaries participated in healing in all Catholic colonies – from Chile to New France and from Angola to the Philippines – their activities offer a uniquely global and trans-national lens (Figure 10.2).

In preparing and administering medicines, religious orders commonly relied on their lay members, who also authored many of the surviving medical writings. Such individuals entered the organization by taking vows but did not seek the priesthood and could therefore devote their time to manual or technical labor in support of their ordained peers. Lay brothers and sisters were recruited as accountants, librarians – or medical practitioners. Religious orders commonly trained their own lay pharmacists through apprenticeship. Steinhöffer learned the apothecary trade during his novitiate at the Jesuit college in Brno from another lay brother, Thomas Linhardt.[19] Others entered the order with experience in the medical arts under their belt and were assigned to the role that would most benefit the organization. This was the case for Pedro de Montenegro (1663–1728), a Jesuit missionary and pharmacist among the Guaraní people of South America, who had previously worked as an infirmarian in a hospital in Madrid.[20]

Lay medical practitioners primarily served the internal needs of their congregations and provided charitable services. However, their work became an important source of income for religious orders. The difference between payment and charitable donation was inherently blurred. Although the clergy was forbidden from selling wares made by others for profit, they were allowed to vend goods that they had

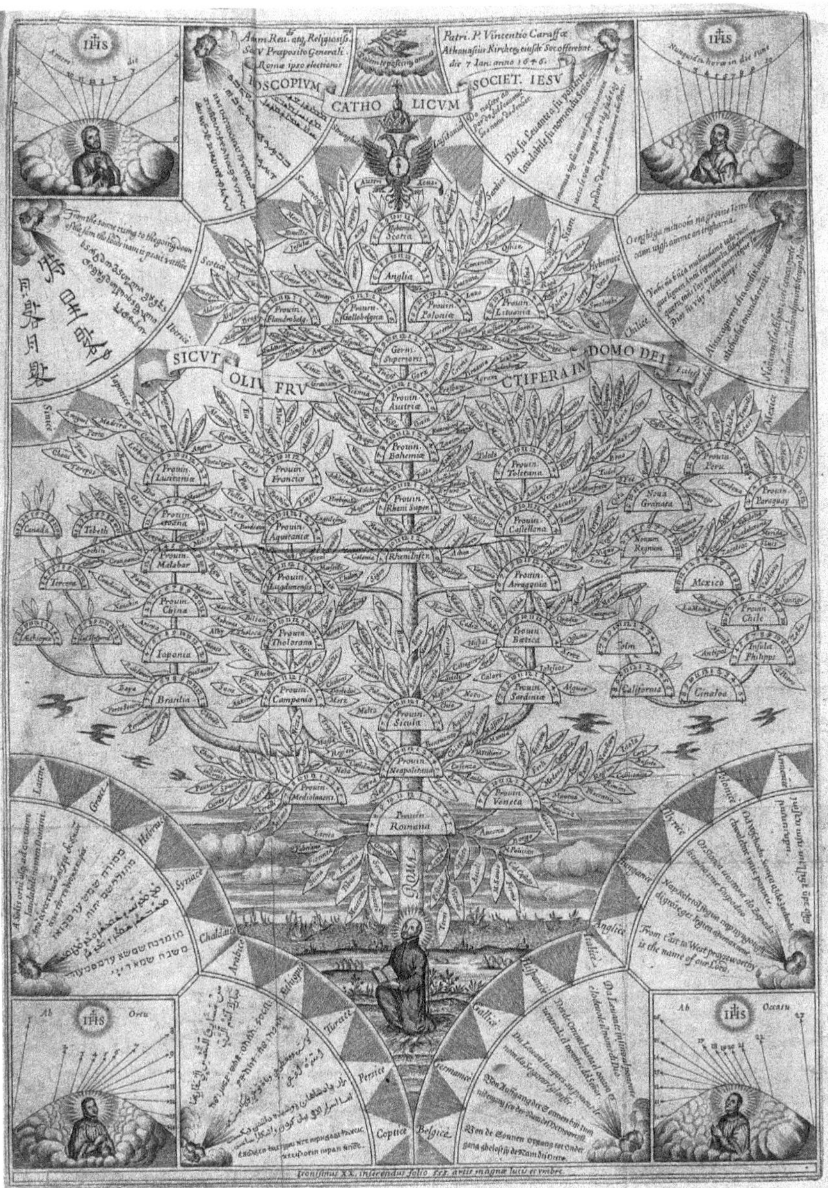

Figure 10.2 The provinces and colleges of the Society of Jesus presented as a family tree. Engraving after Athanasius Kircher, 1646. © Wellcome Library, London.

produced or grown themselves, including remedies, for their own subsistence.[21] Religious orders therefore turned to drugs as a source of revenue to fund their worldwide spiritual crusade. These activities led to tensions within the Church over the moral status of marketing medicines and to regular feuds between the clergy and licensed medical practitioners, who were displeased about unwelcome – and often unlicensed – competition.[22]

To legitimize their involvement in medicine, missionaries invoked the precepts of charity and pointed to the poor medical supply and the lack of licensed medical practitioners in colonial areas. Steinhöffer wrote that "curing and healing is part of the apostolic ministry" and subtitled his work "for the benefit of the poor and of those who lack physicians."[23] Indeed, licensed medical practitioners, if present in the colonies at all, typically served the military corps or preferred to reside in colonial hubs where they could attract wider and more affluent clienteles. Montenegro claimed to "have only seen one physician and surgeon in the 21 years" he had spent in the Americas.[24] He confessed that this dearth of medical practitioners "forced me to become an author in *materia medica*," quickly adding that he was "moved by the charity to benefit my brethren rather than the ambition to author a book."[25] In the less strictly regulated colonial spaces, even ordained clergy could engage in medical practices. In 1576, Pope Gregory XIII granted the Jesuits a special privilege that allowed priests to practice medicine, given that secular colonial physicians were unavailable.[26] This exemption enabled the ordained priest Klein to publish a pharmacopoeia based on his "expertise acquired through the study and practice of healing."[27] Missionaries therefore sought to present themselves as notable for their charitable care and as a crucial force that filled important gaps in the colonial medical infrastructure.

Considered through a more critical lens, these statements emerge as missionary tropes that served to justify colonial projects: a concern that historians must account for in their analyses. While licensed practitioners were rare, Indigenous and non-European communities possessed their own healers, whom the colonizers in Spanish territories usually termed *curanderos* and *curanderas*, or "quacks," or even *brujos* and *brujas*, "sorcerers" and "witches." This terminology highlights that for the colonizers the boundaries between medical and spiritual realms were blurred inherently. Knowledge of plants and healing was one of the sources of authority of Indigenous practitioners and spiritual leaders, whom the Catholic and imperial establishment regarded as obstacles in pursuing their projects.[28] Yet the powers of the *Protomedicato* and the *Inquisition*, the two main colonial bodies that regulated healing activities, were often limited, especially outside colonial hubs.[29] In missionary works, Indigenous healers were usually vilified or entirely absent. In *Materia medica misionera* ("Missionary materia medica," 1710), Montenegro complained that it would be "more befitting to call them quacks and butchers than surgeons and physicians." Similarly, Klein lamented the presence of "*curanderos* unskilled in medical arts" who "more often worsen the disease due to their ignorance."[30] To displace Indigenous healers and gain the locals' trust, missionaries strove to appropriate their knowledge, discredit their practices, and demonstrate the superiority of Christian rites and remedies. Steinhöffer, for example, provided a patron saint for every disease he discussed and suggested that every therapy should start with a prayer. Missionary accounts are therefore above all reflective of the competition with Indigenous healers for power and the attempts to appropriate Indigenous knowledge and erase Indigenous agency.

In the missions and colonial frontiers, which were typically distant from imperial settlements, religious orders were the main face of colonial medicine. Indigenous communities who inhabited these spaces provided a crucial source of natural and medical knowledge for the missionaries. Their agenda involved long-term residency among non-Christian communities, training in Indigenous languages, and gathering information about local inhabitants and nature, including medicinal plants and healing practices. This knowledge enabled missionaries to survive and operate in diverse regions of the world and to document and alter the ways of colonized populations. Efforts to learn about local medicinal plants and healing practices were above all motivated by a desire either to appropriate knowledge of Indigenous healers or discredit them and thus facilitate evangelization. In addition, the missionaries' interest in the natural world was underpinned by intellectual and spiritual concerns. By studying nature, missionaries contemplated and celebrated divine Creation. The collection of natural and medical knowledge was also rooted in the humanist curriculum of studying classical texts, embraced in Catholic education, among which the Roman naturalist Pliny the Elder (23/24–79 AD) held a prominent place. Rare and marvelous objects and information possessed particular appeal given the early modern passion for curiosities and the Baroque culture of spectacle – both for the missionaries and their audiences, from among which prospective members and benefactors were recruited.[31]

Indeed, the vast quantities of natural and medical knowledge accumulated by missionaries were further used by religious orders for their own benefit. With their efficient and centralized administration, the Jesuits were especially adept at deploying the information gathered to justify their monopoly of Catholic education, garner prestige as scholars, solicit favors among both European and non-European élites, and attract curious patrons.[32] The Society of Jesus established a worldwide network of pharmacies, hospitals, and plantations, which enabled it to generate immense profits. For these reasons, Jesuit medical activities have received more attention than other religious orders. Historians have increasingly acknowledged their crucial role in the nascent global drug trade, using especially the example of cinchona, or the Jesuit's bark.[33] Samir Boumediene has even argued that the Jesuits were probably the only early modern organization capable of handling every aspect of drug importation, from the extraction of materials in the colonies to their marketing in Europe.[34] In many Spanish and Portuguese colonial regions, the Jesuits came to dominate in the production and distribution of drugs. The gradual abolition of the Society between 1759 and 1773 left a gap in colonial medical infrastructure that imperial powers struggled to fill.[35]

Listing Cures, Inventing Galenic Drugs

When analyzing primary sources, we must examine the contexts of their production. Missionary accounts of remedies and medicinal plants can be found in diverse sorts of works written by a range of authors in different spaces around the world: from letters, slips, and pharmacopoeias produced by lay brothers with artisanal training to natural and civil histories written by university-educated priests.[36] In compiling their works, the authors relied on a combination of education in the medical arts and natural history, self-study, and knowledge gathered from willing informants: Indigenous and enslaved people, fellow missionaries, and European and non-European migrants. Whilst some works, like that of Steinhöffer, were published, many circulated in manuscript form across hospitals, pharmacies, missions, and other colonial spaces. Klein acknowledged drawing on "a manuscript account of home remedies that passes through the hands of many."[37] Montenegro's account survives in several manuscript versions with different additions and did not appear in print until the modern era.[38] The Jesuit manuscript of remedies titled *Coleção de várias receitas* ("Collection of various recipes"), which comprised drugs from across Portuguese possessions, has received limited attention.[39] The Real Academia de la Historia in Madrid holds numerous recipes written and received by the local Jesuit college, which await closer investigation.[40]

To gain insights into the authors' concerns and aims, we need to consider how missionaries organized their works and drew on different genres of medical writing from the period. With their practical approach and accessible style and structure, the sources mimicked the genres of European books of *materia medica*, recipes, and home remedies. The instructions were spelled out in simple vernacular language and any complex terminology was explained. The organization of these works reflected the utilitarian aims of their authors. Steinhöffer relied on schemes commonplace to medical texts: he followed the tripartite division into medicine, surgery, and pharmacy and used the arrangement of *a capite ad calcem* ("from head to heel"), which categorized ailments according to the human body part affected. To make the texts even more accessible for readers unacquainted with medical literature, Klein organized ailments alphabetically. Both authors discussed issues ranging from coughs to venomous bites and from ulcers to women's diseases, moving gradually from definitions to causes, prognoses, symptoms, and cures. They avoided complex medicines or rare ingredients but sought to include as many remedies as possible, since some might work better or be more easily available.

Montenegro organized his work by plants rather than diseases, incorporating elements from herbals and books of home remedies, cooking, and horticulture. From his arrangement of the material, we can infer Montenegro's concern with the practicalities of plant identification, harvesting, preparation, and even cultivation. For every plant, Montenegro provided both the Spanish and Indigenous names to facilitate its acquisition in local cross-cultural contexts. Each entry included an image alongside physical descriptions, virtues, and preparations, including Indigenous uses. For example, Montenegro found yerba maté, or "ibirá caá mirí" in Guaraní, "very similar to the European laurel in the smell of its leaves" (Figure 10.3). He advised that its leaves "can be used for dyes and plasters," whilst its decoction "prevents intoxication if taken before drinking" and "serves the Indigenes as the only relief in diarrhea."[41] For those less acquainted with medical terminology, diarrhea was helpfully defined in an adjoined medical vocabulary.[42] This directory of medical terms was followed by a list of plant names in Spanish, Guaraní, and Tupí, the most widely used local languages. Inclusions of Indigenous vocabularies were not uncommon: Klein also appended one with vernacular names and descriptions of local plants and diseases "that perhaps not everyone would understand."[43]

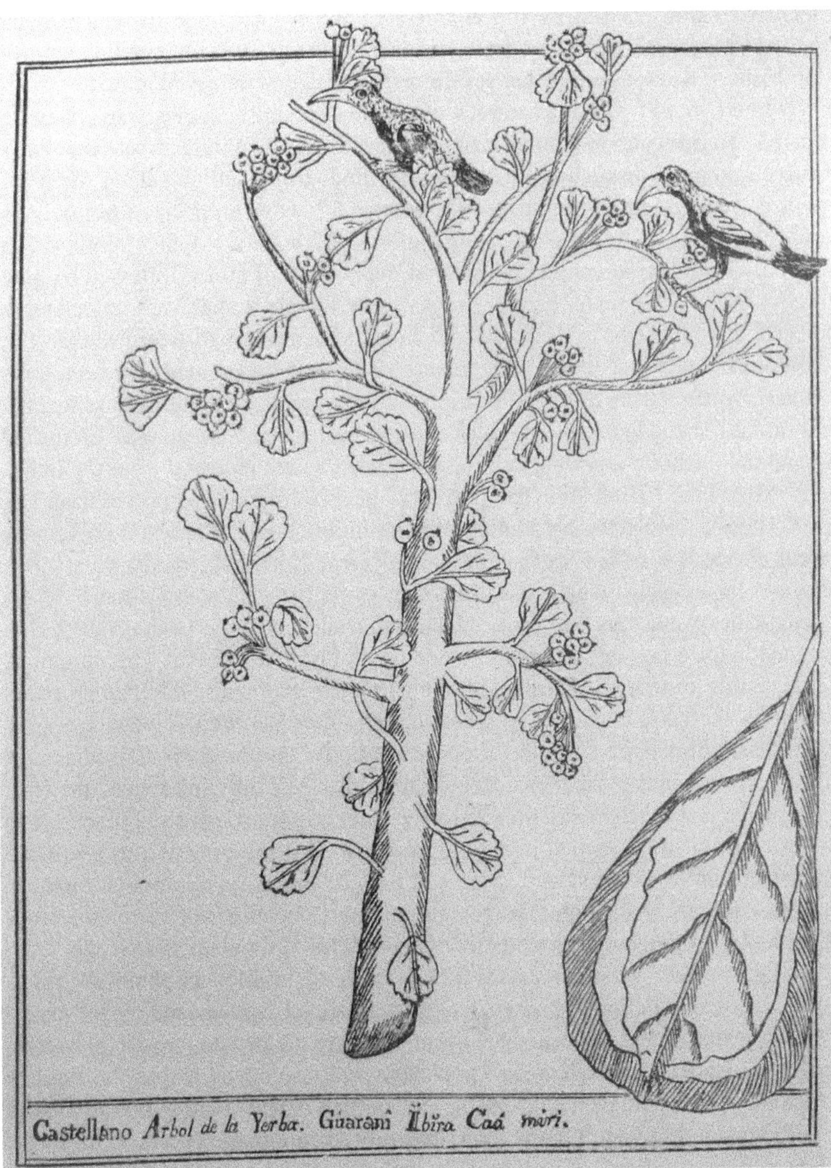

Figure 10.3 The drawing of yerba maté included in Pedro de Montenegro's *Materia medica misionera* (1710). Reproduced from Pedro de Montenegro, *Materia médica misionera*, ed. Raúl Quintana, Buenos Aires: Biblioteca Nacional, 1945, fig. 1.

Missionaries devoted attention to women's ailments and their texts therefore offer some insight into women's health, albeit through male eyes. Concerns with reproduction were paramount; for example, Montenegro warned against obstructions to menstrual flow caused by the coldness of the womb, "due to which many [women] become sterile."[44] For those reasons, Klein advised menstruating women not to bathe.[45] Klein also devoted several pages to enumerating all remedies pregnant women should avoid. Therapies offered by the missionaries were likewise gendered. To mitigate abdominal pains, for instance, Steinhöffer wrote that "it is effective (although disgusting) to squeeze the juice from stallion's dung when the patient is a man; and from a mare, if a woman."[46] Women appeared not only as targets of treatments but also as a source of *materia medica*. Mother's milk was a commonly used ingredient and considered the best of all milks, followed by goat and cow milk.[47] The texts therefore reveal how female bodies were understood, managed, and imagined in the works of Christian men who had sworn celibacy.

Missionary pharmacopoeias are characteristic of entanglements between lores of *materia medica* from different locations and traditions. Steinhöffer classified the local disease saguadodo, or "yellow vomiting in the Opata language," alongside humoral melancholic vomiting and recommended a cure prepared from the Indigenous maize-based drink atole and powdered peels of oranges, imported from Europe.[48] These exchanges were complex and multidirectional. The Jesuit lay brother Marcos Villodas (1695–1741) authored a medical handbook for the Guaraní in their own language, in which most remedies came from Indigenous lore.[49] Guaraní medicines were thus reinterpreted and reintroduced to the Guaraní through a Jesuit mediator. Knowledge transfers were not limited to missionary appropriations of Indigenous knowledge. Healers of non-European origin also adopted practices brought by the colonizers, and religious orders often recruited non-European associates and introduced them to European methods.[50] In his study on Indigenous and folk healers in the Americas, Robert Voeks has helpfully introduced the term "disturbance pharmacopoeias" to emphasize that their knowledge and practices do not derive from some ancient pristine source that predated or necessarily resisted colonialism, but were expanded in the wake of the intensifying cross-cultural encounters.[51] Recast in this light, Indigenous pharmacopoeias become dynamic products of historical interactions rather than repositories of timeless knowledge.

Taking a broader geographical outlook, we can use missionary pharmacopoeias to observe the circulation of knowledge and practice on regional and global scales. Missionary spaces and medical establishments were connected through networks, in which missionaries exchanged knowledge and specimens across the borders of regions, states, and even continents. The *mestizo* Augustinian friar stationed in Manila, Ignacio Mercado (1648–1698), described more than 200 plants in his *Libro de medicinas* ("Book of medicines"), including those native to the Philippines and introduced from Europe and the Americas.[52] Klein's recipe for theriac, the renowned ancient poison antidote and panacea, included such a worldwide assortment of substances that it would hardly be recognizable to practitioners in Europe. In addition to the principal ingredient of snake flesh, Klein listed substances native to the Philippines and imported from across Europe, Asia, and America: betel leaves and the lemongrass tanglad; Castilian saffron and rosemary; Persian bezoars, Chinese oranges, and Maluku spices; and the "Mexican tea" epazote. The mixture was to be dissolved in communion wine or, in its absence, the Mexican maize-based beverage atole.[53] By the early eighteenth century, these ingredients sourced from different corners of the world were available in Manila and circulated across Indo-Pacific worlds. Klein's recipe thus illustrates the increasing globalization of the early modern drug trade.

The missionaries typically interpreted non-European remedies and diseases through the lens of Galenic humoral medicine and the works of Graeco-Roman, Arabic, and European authors from antiquity to early modernity. Montenegro provided humoral qualities for every plant described and included a crash course in humoralism with instructions for identifying humoral qualities of different substances, primarily based on taste.[54] He identified numerous local plants with those described by medical authorities like Dioscorides (40–90 AD), Avicenna (980–1037), and Pier-Andrea Mattioli (1501–1577), who were referenced throughout and offered a source of authority. This practice with long humanist roots enabled Montenegro to recognize, for example, the plant caáisi as the almáciga of Pliny the Elder.[55] Montenegro acknowledged that some American plants were entirely new.[56] Others may have differed in form from their alleged Old World counterparts, but Montenegro asserted that they still possessed identical virtues, as proven by his experiments.[57]

Montenegro – and other missionaries around the world – therefore engaged in what Miguel de Asúa has termed the "Galenization of native herbal lore," that is "its codification in terms of Galenic theory."[58] Galenism provided missionaries a crucial tool for understanding local nature and appropriating non-European knowledge. In their efforts to Galenize foreign substances and integrate them into the humoral system, missionaries drew on the pharmaceutical tradition of *succedanea* ("substitutions") or *quid pro quo* ("this for that").[59] This established practice enabled pharmacists to use alternative substances to replace ingredients which were rare, expensive, or unavailable at the time of need. Initially, the majority of drugs from the Americas were introduced in Europe as substitutes, especially for substances native to the Far East.[60] In Europe, medical authorities regularly issued lists of accepted substitutes. Missionaries in colonial spaces, by contrast, were largely at liberty to experiment with their own *succedanea*.

Treatments in pharmacies and hospitals in Iberian colonial worlds relied predominantly on Old World drugs, supplied largely from Europe.[61] The apothecary of the Jesuit college in Córdoba, Heinrich Peschke (1672–1729), wrote in the early 1700s that "almost all medicines come from Europe, at great expense and risk."[62] In addition to the high costs, preservation remained an issue due to the long voyages. In the missions and reductions, European imports were especially hard to access. For these reasons, missionaries looked for more easily available substitutes, which could stand in for the missing Old World remedies. In his ointment against convulsions, Steinhöffer advised that one could replace fox flesh with that of the coyote.[63] The Jesuit lay brother Georg Joseph Kamel (1661–1706), stationed in Manila, adopted the lemongrass tanglad as a substitute for squinanth, a rush-like plant recommended by the ancients against obstructions of humors.[64] In the adjoined figure, Kamel strove to convey the physical similarity of tanglad to rushes (Figure 10.4). The practices of substitution call into question narratives of bioprospecting, which continue to be of prominence in the field of colonial medicine.

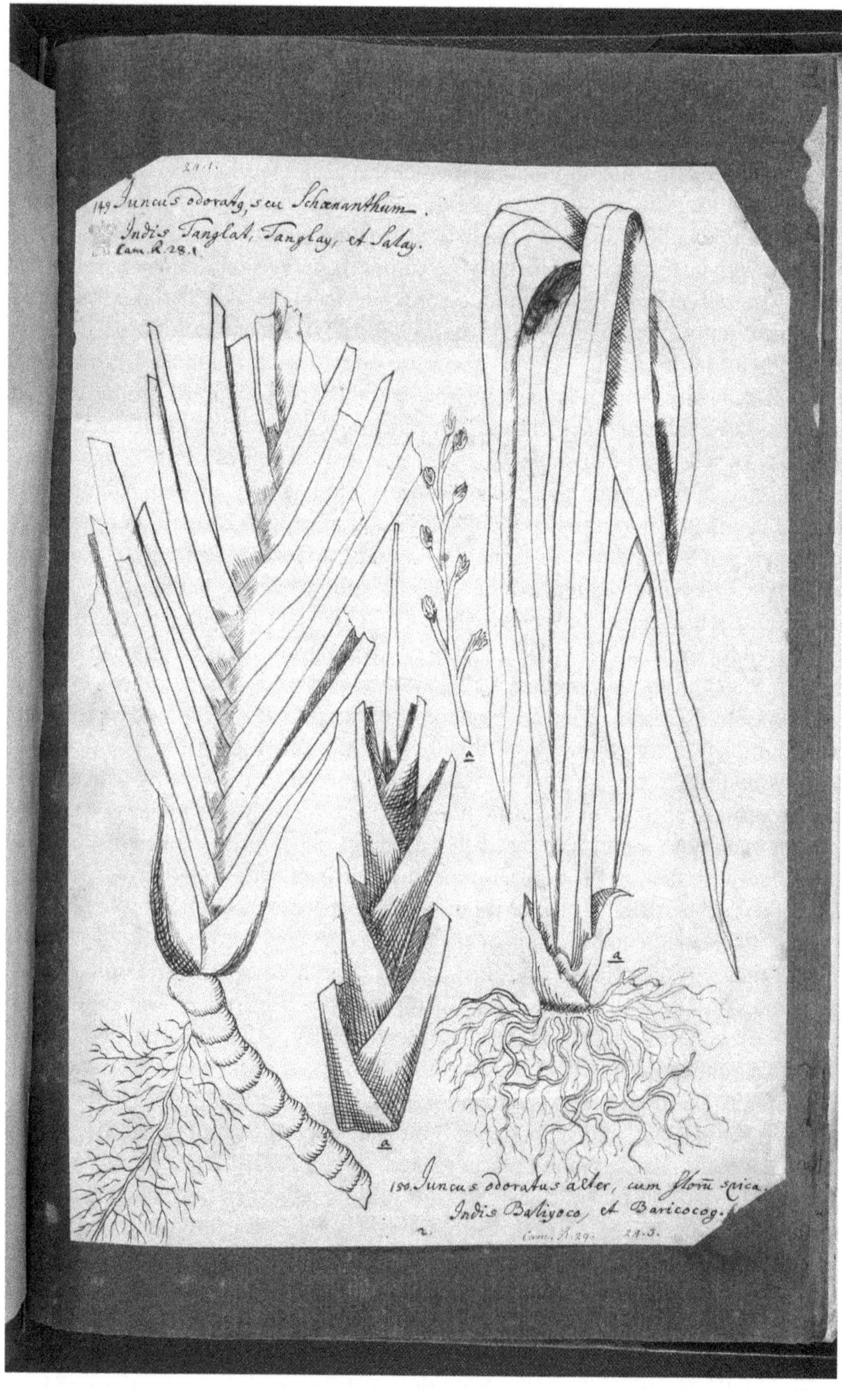

Figure 10.4 Georg Joseph Kamel's figure of tanglad (left), which he employed as a local substitute for squinanth (British Library, Sloane MS 4080, f. 130).

Missionaries often used local substances out of necessity rather than by choice. Their investigations of native *materia medica* seemed not to be motivated by the hunger to discover new profitable cures, so much as by the desire to find substitutes for those already known to them.[65]

Reading for Indigenous Voices

When interpreting missionary medical works, historians must attend to the wide variety of agencies across cultures and the social status involved in their production. Indigenous voices remained largely silenced in the sources and when they appeared, they were mediated through colonizers' eyes. Missionaries commonly sought to present themselves as simply using Indigenous plants without having received local assistance, discovering their virtues by chance, physical affinities, or divine inspiration, and testing them through experience. Knowledge derived from non-European sources was deemed inherently suspicious and its adoption raised several issues. Crucially for religious missionaries, since local communities had been pagan prior to the European arrival, the source of their knowledge could well be demonic.[66] Moreover, missionaries typically did not consider Indigenous knowledge to be the result of systematic engagement with nature, like European science. As historians have shown, Europeans ignored local theoretical constructs and pictured Indigenous information as mere know-how and raw materials used in the production of new and genuine knowledge.[67] To be recognized as valid science and medicine, non-European knowledge therefore had to be dissociated from its original contexts and grounded in medical systems acknowledged by the Europeans.

In appropriating Indigenous knowledge, missionaries drew on a combination of empirical and Christian explanations in addition to Galenization. When discussing the source of the knowledge of yerba maté, Montenegro claimed it was traditionally understood that the Guaraní had learned about the plant from St Thomas the Apostle, who was believed to have preached in the New World in apostolic times.[68] Kamel and his colleagues in the Philippines authored treatises of the Indigenous panacea igasud, in which they Galenized the plant and reinvented it as the St Ignatius bean: its powers now symbolically vested in by the holy founder of the Jesuit order.[69] They presented the drug's virtues as emerging from their own experiments rather than borrowed from local healing practices. In these trials, the missionaries used the bodies of Indigenous, migrant, and enslaved individuals as instruments. Montenegro repeatedly mentioned experimenting both on himself and the Indigenes.[70] It was this experience that enabled "the poor ignorant" Montenegro to argue with authority and even "go against the precepts of Dioscorides," a canonical medical authority.[71] Alongside references to learned authors, appeals to direct experience with Indigenous *materia medica* provided the main source of authority for the missionaries. In this way, Indigenous knowledge and spiritual beliefs were supplanted by religious and medical practices sanctioned by European authorities and thus reframed as legitimate knowledge for European audiences.

One way to gain insight into non-European worlds and cross-cultural exchanges is to examine the recurring use of local terminology in missionary writings. Some missionaries described more closely how they obtained local knowledge. One Jesuit stationed in the Philippines, Ignacio Alcina (1610–1674), maintained friendly relations with Indigenous herbalists to receive information about native plants. However, such information required verification before it could be adopted, which enabled Alcina to downplay Indigenous agency. Upon learning the virtues of the tree anonang from "an Indigenous herbalist," Alcina "did not believe him and only through its use found it to be the truth."[72] An important source of information was also provided by non-Europeans whose paid, free, or enslaved labor was extracted by religious orders. Steinhöffer acknowledged to have learned about various antidotal roots from "a herbalist physician from [the city of] México, who assists our colleges a lot."[73] Last but not least, missionary work itself offered opportunities to gain knowledge of *materia medica*, for example, through the rite of confession, as Andrés Prieto has shown.[74]

Even when their contributions were acknowledged, Indigenous informants were rarely named by the missionaries. Montenegro described how he had learned about the antidote yacaré caá from a "certain old Indigene" and foraged for the rare purgative capií catí with the assistance of three Indigenous guides.[75] Yet he mentioned only one Indigene by name: a Guaraní named Clemente, "the most skilled *curuzuyara*, or physician, I have encountered in these missions."[76] *Curuzuya* was a male infirmarian serving in the reductions, often an Indigene trained by the missionaries.[77] Although *curuzuyaras* were present in various missions, Montenegro trusted only the information provided by Clemente. In addition to his knowledge of herbs, the main attribute that qualified Clemente as a trustworthy informant was him being a "good Christian," which precluded the possibility that his knowledge had been obtained from the Devil.[78] The authority of Christianity and other European practices therefore structured colonial knowledge hierarchies and determined the difference between the skilled *curuzuyara* and the devilish *curanderos*.

To gain closer insight into Indigenous agency, we can read pharmacopoeias "against the grain" or in conversation with wider sets of sources, including visual and material culture and archaeological and anthropological evidence.[79] Montenegro's work contains 136 illustrations of plants and animals, at least some of which were produced in collaboration with Indigenous informants. The drawing of the plant aguapé came "through the relation of a trustworthy and religious person, a son of these lands."[80] Such images can be analyzed for traces of Indigenous influences and cross-cultural entanglements.[81] Pairing historical with ethnographic material offers another means of gaining insights into knowledge entanglements. In his work, Kamel classified Philippine flora into three main divisions: herbs; trees and shrubs; and climbing plants. This tripartite scheme seems to have had no parallel in European botany, which traditionally divided flora into two main groups: herbs and trees. Unlike sedentary European scholars, Kamel was confronted by plants that did not fit into the traditional dichotomy, such as lianas, which probably compelled him to add another group. This decision may have been informed by Indigenous categories of knowledge, as some Filipino folk taxonomies use schemes identical to Kamel, with vines or climbing plants as one of the main classes.[82] By expanding methodological horizons, we can therefore address some of the silences of written sources. Despite the missionaries' efforts to efface local agencies, by focusing on the processes of translation and erosion we stand to gain insights into what cross-cultural knowledge encounters entailed.

Local Remedies, Global Movements

Despite listing an abundance of remedies and therapies, missionary writings cannot necessarily show whether, by whom or how these were locally consumed. However, the longevity of many of the works discussed suggests that they were in frequent use and had a lasting impact on medical practices in colonial spaces. Montenegro's treatise circulated in the Paraguay region until the nineteenth century.[83] As the introductory anecdote suggests, the influence of Steinhöffer's work on folk medicine across the North American southwest can still be observed today. To gain insight into how the works and their therapies were employed locally, we can bring the pharmacopoeias into conversation with other sources, both historical (pharmacy registers, hospital accounts, court records) and ethnographic.

As we have seen, missionary pharmacopoeias can help us trace shifts in knowledge and practice through both space and time, from local encounters to wider circulations. Through the lens of these sources, we can observe entanglements between different medical traditions, and the power relations among various colonial actors. We can broaden our understanding of colonial healing beyond developments in major cities and narratives of bioprospecting. Missionary medical accounts offer insights into what cross-cultural encounters entailed and into the kinds of resources mobilized in the bid to – and in the name of – maintaining and restoring health. The works also unveil the complex nature of the networks that sustained circulations of knowledge, practices, and remedies across socio-cultural, national, and continental boundaries. In short, with missionary pharmacopoeias, we can examine how new forms of knowledge were produced in colonial settings and how they fed into the constructions of notions of health and disease, conceptions of the body, and colonial hierarchies of knowledge that continue to resonate to this day.

Notes

1 Margarita Artschwager Kay, *Healing with Plants in the American and Mexican West* (Tucson: University of Arizona Press, 1996), 159.

2 Johannes Steinhöffer, *Florilegio medicinal de todas las enfermedades* (México: Herederos de Juan Joseph Guillena Carrascoso, 1712), 143. Steinhöffer is better known under his Hispanicized alias Juan de Esteyneffer.

3 Steinhöffer, *Florilegio*, n.p.

4 Margarita Artschwager Kay, "The *Florilegio Medicinal*: Source of Southwest Ethnomedicine," *Ethnohistory* 24:3 (1977), 251–59.

5 For missionary remedies, see Sabine Anagnostou, "Jesuits in Spanish America: Contributions to the Exploration of the American *Materia Medica*," *Pharmacy in History* 47:1 (2005), 3–17; Andrés Prieto, *Missionary Scientists: Jesuit Science in Spanish South America, 1570–1810* (Nashville: Vanderbilt University Press, 2011), 36–89;

Miguel de Asúa, *Science in the Vanished Arcadia: Knowledge of Nature in the Jesuit Missions of Paraguay and Río de la Plata* (Leiden; Boston: Brill, 2014), 96–163; Samir Boumediene, "Jesuit Recipes, Jesuit Receipts: The Society of Jesus and the Introduction of Exotic Materia Medica into Europe," in *Cultural Worlds of the Jesuits in Colonial Latin America*, ed. Linda Newson (London: University of London Press, 2020), 227–54.

6 Pablo Gómez, *The Experiential Caribbean: Creating Knowledge and Healing in the Early Modern Atlantic* (Chapel Hill, NC: University of North Carolina Press, 2017); Matthew James Crawford and Joseph Gabriel, eds., *Drugs on the Page: Pharmacopoeias and Healing Knowledge in the Early Modern Atlantic World* (Pittsburgh, PA: University of Pittsburgh Press, 2019).

7 Paul Klein, *Remedios faciles para diferentes enfermedades* (Manila: Juan Correa, 1712), viii, "señalar remedios, que facilmente pueden hallar en sus mismos pueblos, o no lejos de ellos, o si son de botica, son de aquellos que se pueden traer de provision." Klein is better known under his Hispanicized alias Pablo Clain.

8 For example, Harold J. Cook, *Matters of Exchange: Commerce, Medicine, and Science in the Dutch Golden Age* (New Haven, CT: Yale University Press, 2007); Dániel Margócsy, *Commercial Visions: Science, Trade and Visual Culture in the Dutch Golden Age* (Chicago, IL: University of Chicago Press, 2014); Pratik Chakrabarti, *Materials and Medicine: Trade, Conquest and Therapeutics in the Eighteenth Century* (Manchester: Manchester University Press, 2015); Suman Seth, *Difference and Disease: Medicine, Race, and the Eighteenth-Century British Empire* (Cambridge: Cambridge University Press, 2018); Benjamin Breen, *The Age of Intoxication: Origins of the Global Drug Trade* (Philadelphia: University of Pennsylvania Press, 2019); He Bian, *Know Your Remedies: Pharmacy and Culture in Early Modern China* (Princeton, NJ: Princeton University Press, 2020); Paula De Vos, *Compound Remedies: Galenic Pharmacy in Colonial Mexico* (Pittsburgh, PA: University of Pittsburgh Press, 2020).

9 Especially Londa Schiebinger, *Plants and Empire: Colonial Bioprospecting in the Atlantic World* (Cambridge, MA: Harvard University Press, 2004); Antonio Barrera-Osorio, *Experiencing Nature: The Spanish American Empire and the Early Scientific Revolution* (Austin: University of Texas Press, 2006).

10 For example, Samir Boumediene, *La colonisation du savoir: Une Histoire des plantes médicinales du "Nouveau Monde" (1492–1750)* (Vaulx-en-Velin: Les Éditions des mondes à faire, 2016); Matthew James Crawford, *The Andean Wonder Drug: Cinchona Bark and Imperial Science in the Spanish Atlantic, 1630–1800* (Pittsburgh: University of Pittsburgh Press, 2016); Gómez, *The Experiential Caribbean*; De Vos, *Compound Remedies*.

11 For entanglements, see Ralph Bauer and Marcy Norton, eds., "Entangled Trajectories: Indigenous and European Histories," Special Issue of *Colonial Latin American Review* 26:1 (2017).

12 Anna Lowenhaupt Tsing, *Friction: An Ethnography of Global Connection* (Princeton, NJ: Princeton University Press, 2005).

13 Mark Jackson, ed., *A Global History of Medicine* (Oxford: Oxford University Press, 2018).

14 Reductions were urban settlements modelled on those in Spain, into which Spanish authorities relocated, often forcibly, Indigenous populations. Religious missionaries played a central role in administering reductions.

15 Especially Darrel Amundsen, "Medieval Canon Law on Medical and Surgical Practice by the Clergy," *Bulletin of the History of Medicine* 52 (1978), 22–44.

16 Ines Županov, "Conversion, Illness and Possession: Catholic Missionary Healing in Early Modern South Asia," in *Divins remèdes: Médecine et religion en Asie du Sud*, ed. Ines Županov and Caterina Guenzi (EHESS, 2008), 263–300; José Pardo-Tomás,

"Conversion Medicine: Communication and Circulation of Knowledge in the Franciscan Convent and College of Tlatelolco, 1527–1577," *Quaderni Storici* 48:1 (2013), 21–42; Gabriela Ramos, "Indian Hospitals and Government in the Colonial Andes," *Medical History* 57:2 (2013), 186–205.

17 For medicine and Christianity, see Ronald Numbers and Darrel Amundsen, eds., *Caring and Curing: Health and Medicine in the Western Religious Traditions* (Baltimore, MD: Johns Hopkins University Press, 1998); Ole Peter Grell, Andrew Cunningham, and Jon Arrizabalaga, eds., *Health Care and Poor Relief in Counter-Reformation Europe* (New York: Routledge, 1999); Maria Pia Donato et al., eds., *Médecine et religion: Compétitions, collaborations, conflits (XIIe–XXe siècles)* (Rome: École française de Rome, 2013).

18 Županov, "Conversion, Illness and Possession."

19 Archivum Romanum Societatis Jesu, Bohemia 90 II: Catalogi breves 1641–1689, 641v–42r.

20 Asúa, *Science in the Vanished Arcadia*, 113.

21 Nicholas Cushner, "Merchants and Missionaries: A Theologian's View of Clerical Involvement in the Galleon Trade," *The Hispanic American Historical Review* 47:3 (1967), 360–69; Dauril Alden, *The Making of an Enterprise: The Society of Jesus in Portugal, Its Empire, and Beyond, 1540–1750* (Stanford, CA: Stanford University Press, 1996), 529.

22 For example, Timothy D. Walker, "The Early Modern Globalization of Indian Medicine: Portuguese Dissemination of Drugs and Healing Techniques from South Asia on Four Continents, 1670–1830," *Portuguese Literary & Cultural Studies* 17/18 (2010), 83; Sharon Strocchia, "The Nun Apothecaries of Renaissance Florence: Marketing Medicines in the Convent," *Renaissance Studies* 25:5 (2011), 627–47; Asúa, *Science in the Vanished Arcadia*, 105.

23 Steinhöffer, *Florilegio*, n.p., "el curar, y el sanar, es una parte del ministerio Apostolico," "para bien de los pobres, y de los que tienen falta de Medicos."

24 Pedro de Montenegro, "Materia medica misionera (I)," in *Revista patriótica del pasado argentino*, ed. Manuel Ricardo Trelles, vol. 1 (Buenos Aires: Europea, 1888), 268, "en veintiun años que há que entré en ella, solo un medico y cirujano he visto."

25 Ibid., 266, "por hallarme en estas tierras de la América sin botica ni boticarios, me ha forzado á que con ellas hacerme autor de botica [...] me mueve mas la caridad de hacer bien á mis hermanos, que la ambicion de autor de un libro."

26 John W. O'Malley, *The First Jesuits* (Cambridge, MA: Harvard University Press, 1993), 171.

27 Klein, *Remedios faciles*, viii, "con el estudio, y practica de curar los pobres enfermos, he adquirido de esta ciencia."

28 Fernando Cervantes, *The Devil in the New World: The Impact of Diabolism in New Spain* (New Haven, CT: Yale University Press, 1994); Prieto, *Missionary Scientists*, 48–89.

29 *Protomedicato* was an official colonial board of medicine charged with training, examining, and supervising medical practitioners in the Spanish and Portuguese realms.

30 Montenegro, "Materia Medica Misionera (I)," 268–69, "mas les cuadra el nombre de matasano que el de cirujano, y el de carnicero que el de medico"; Klein, *Remedios faciles*, vii, "curanderos indios, imperitos de la ciencia medica; y que a veces por su ignorancia mas pueden servir para aumentar la enfermedad."

31 Prieto, *Missionary Scientists*, 143–220; Asúa, *Science in the Vanished Arcadia*, 25–163.

32 Steven J. Harris, "Long-Distance Corporations, Big Sciences, and the Geography of Knowledge," *Configurations* 6:2 (1998), 269–304; John W. O'Malley et al., eds., *The Jesuits: Cultures, Sciences, and the Arts 1540–1773*, 2 vols. (Toronto: University of Toronto Press, 2000, 2006); Beatriz Puente-Ballesteros, "Jesuit Medicine in the Kangxi

Court (1662–1722): Imperial Networks and Patronage," *East Asian Science, Technology, and Medicine* 34 (2011), 86–162.

33 Timothy D. Walker, "The Medicines Trade in the Portuguese Atlantic World: Acquisition and Dissemination of Healing Knowledge from Brazil (c. 1580–1800)," *Social History of Medicine* 26:3 (2013), 403–31; Boumediene, *La Colonisation*; Crawford, *The Andean Wonder Drug*.

34 Boumediene, "Jesuit Recipes," 230.

35 Luis Martín, *The Intellectual Conquest of Peru: The Jesuit College of San Pablo* (New York: Fordham University Press, 1968), 110; Timothy D. Walker, "Crown Authorities, Colonial Physicians, and the Exigencies of Empire: The Codification of Indigenous Therapeutic Knowledge in India and Brazil During the Enlightenment Era," in Crawford and Gabriel, *Drugs on the Page*, 102.

36 See esp. Boumediene, "Jesuit Recipes."

37 Klein, *Remedios faciles*, vii, "un cuaderno manuscrito, que anda en manos de muchos, de algunos remedios caseros."

38 Asúa, *Science in the Vanished Arcadia*, 319–20.

39 Archivum Romanum Societatis Jesu, Opera Nostrorum 17. For a modern edition in Portuguese, see Ana Carolina de Carvalho Viotti and Jean Marcel Carvalho França, eds., *Coleção de várias receitas e segredos particulares das principais boticas da nossa Companhia de Portugal, da Índia, de Macau e do Brasil* (São Paulo: Edições Loyola, 2019).

40 Real Academia de la Historia, 9/3426, no. 2; 9/3631; 9/3671, no. 65; 9/3823. Cited in Boumediene, "Jesuit Recipes," 236.

41 Montenegro, "Materia Medica Misionera (I)," 304–07, "En el olor de sus hojas, muy semejantes á las del laurel de Europa […] se puede usar de ella para los tintes y engobes, como para las medicinas emplásticas […]. A los indios les es único remedio para las cámaras de relajacion del estómago, que es la diarrea […]. Tomándola antes de beber, impide la embriaguez."

42 Ibid., 286.

43 Klein, *Remedios faciles*, x, "porque en esta obrilla algunas veces uso de términos de vocablos vulgares de esta tierra, que quizás no entenderán todos."

44 Pedro de Montenegro, "Materia medica misionera (II)," in *Revista patriótica del pasado argentino*, ed. Manuel Ricardo Trelles, vol. 2 (Buenos Aires: Europea, 1888), 50, "las mujeres resfriadas del vientre y matriz, que no les viene la regla, y muchas por tal causa se hacen estériles."

45 Klein, *Remedios faciles*, 152.

46 Steinhöffer, *Florilegio*, 122, "(aunque es feo) es efficaz; exprimir el jugo de la buñigas del cavallo para quando el enfermo es hombre; y de yegua, siendo muger."

47 Klein, *Remedios faciles*, 96.

48 Steinhöffer, *Florilegio*, 117, "saguadodo, que llaman en legua Opata, el Vomito Amarillo."

49 Asúa, *Science in the Vanished Arcadia*, 148–50.

50 Ibid., 138; Gómez, *The Experiential Caribbean*, 77.

51 Robert A. Voeks, "Disturbance Pharmacopoeias: Medicine and Myth from the Humid Tropics," *Annals of the Association of American Geographers* 94:4 (2004), 868–88. See also Matthew James Crawford, "An Imperial Pharmacopoeia? The *Pharmacopoeia Matritensis* and *Materia Medica* in the Eighteenth-Century Spanish Atlantic World," in Crawford and Gabriel, *Drugs on the Page*, 63–78.

52 Ignacio de Mercado, "Libro de medicinas de esta tierra," in *Novissima appendix ad Floram philippinarum Emmanuëlis Blanco*, ed. Andrea Naves and Celestino Fernandez-Villar (Manila: Plana et socios, 1880), 1–59.

53 Klein, *Remedios faciles*, 248–249.

54 Montenegro, "Materia Medica Misionera (I)," 273–83.

55 Montenegro, "Materia Medica Misionera (II)," 225.

56 Ibid., 128.
57 Montenegro, "Materia Medica Misionera (I)," 266.
58 Asúa, *Science in the Vanished Arcadia*, 134, 136. For Galenization, see also Gianamar Giovannetti-Singh, "Galenizing the New World: Joseph-François Lafitau's 'Galenization' of Canadian Ginseng, ca. 1716–1724," *Notes and Records of the Royal Society of London* 75 (2021), 59–72; Sebestian Kroupa, "Spanish Bodies and Jesuit Beans: Consuming Drugs in Late Seventeenth-Century Manila," in *Exoticizing Consumption: European Drug Cultures Around 1700*, ed. Justin Rivest and Emma Spary (forthcoming).
59 Samir Boumediene and Valentina Pugliano, "The Substitute Route: Exotic Remedies, Medical Innovation and the Market for Substitutes in the 16th Century," *Revue d'histoire moderne et contemporaine* 66:3 (2019), 24–54.
60 José Pardo-Tomás and María Luz López Terrada, *Las primeras noticias sobre plantas americanas en las relaciones de viajes y crónicas de Indias, 1493–1553* (Valencia: CSIC, 1993).
61 Linda Newson, *Making Medicines in Early Colonial Lima, Peru* (Leiden: Brill, 2017); De Vos, *Compound Remedies*; Kroupa, "Spanish Bodies."
62 Renée Gicklhorn, *Missionsapotheker: Deutsche Pharmazeuten im Lateinamerika des 17. und 18. Jahrhunderts* (Stuttgart: Wissenschaftliche Verlagsgesellschaft MBH, 1973), 34.
63 Steinhöffer, *Florilegio*, 32.
64 Kroupa, "Spanish Bodies."
65 Ibid.
66 Cervantes, *The Devil in the New World*; Prieto, *Missionary Scientists*, 48–89.
67 Kathleen Murphy, "Translating the Vernacular: Indigenous and African Knowledge in the Eighteenth-Century British Atlantic," *Atlantic Studies* 8:1 (2011), 29–48; Prieto, *Missionary Scientists*, 83; Christopher Parsons, "The Natural History of Colonial Science: Joseph-François Lafitau's Discovery of Ginseng and Its Afterlives," *The William and Mary Quarterly* 73:1 (2016), 58–59.
68 Montenegro, "Materia Medica Misionera (I)," 307.
69 Kroupa, "Spanish Bodies."
70 Montenegro, "Materia Medica Misionera (II)," 341, 355–56.
71 Montenegro, "Materia Medica Misionera (I)," 272, "este pobre ignorante quiera ir contra las reglas de un Dioscórides."
72 Ignacio Alcina, "Breve resumen de las raices, hojas o plantas medicinales mas conocidas," ed. Cantius Koback and Lucio Gutiérrez, *Philippiniana Saccra* 32:94 (1997), 98, "aunque me lo habia dicho un indio herbolario, no la creia, y con el uso conoci ser verdad."
73 Steinhöffer, *Florilegio*, 383, "de todas ellas tiene conocimiento en mexico un medico herbolario que asiste mucho nuestros collegios."
74 Prieto, *Missionary Scientists*, 53–61.
75 Montenegro, "Materia Medica Misionera (II)," 56, 82, "cierto indio Viejo."
76 Ibid., 186–87, "cierto curuzuyára, ó médico, el mas perito que en estas misiones he hallado, llamado Clemente."
77 Asúa, *Science in the Vanished Arcadia*, 138–39.
78 Montenegro, "Materia Medica Misionera (II)," 229, "buen cristiano." Discussed in Asúa, *Science in the Vanished Arcadia*, 137–38.
79 For example, Ann Laura Stoler, *Along the Archival Grain: Epistemic Anxieties and Colonial Common Sense* (Princeton, NJ: Princeton University Press, 2008); Neil Safier, "Global Knowledge on the Move: Itineraries, Amerindian Narratives, and Deep Histories of Science," *Isis* 101 (2010), 133–45; Bauer and Norton, "Entangled Trajectories."
80 Montenegro, "Materia Medica Misionera (II)," 61, "doy su estampa solo por relacion de persona fidedigna y religioso, hijo de aquella patria."

81 For example, Serge Gruzinski, *La Colonisation de l'imaginaire: Sociétés indigènes et occidentalisation dans le Mexique espagnol, XVI*[e]*–XVIII*[e] *siècle* (Paris: Gallimard, 1988); Pardo-Tomás, "Conversion Medicine."

82 Sebestian Kroupa, "Georg Joseph Kamel (1661–1706): A Jesuit Pharmacist at the Frontiers of Colonial Empires," PhD diss. (University of Cambridge, 2019), 145–49.

83 Asúa, *Science in the Vanished Arcadia*, 123.

Bibliography

Printed Primary Sources

Alcina, Ignacio. "Breve resumen de las raices, hojas o plantas medicinales mas conocidas," edited by Cantius Koback and Lucio Gutiérrez. *Philippiniana Saccra* 32:94 (1997): 96–135.

de Mercado, Ignacio. "Libro de medicinas de esta tierra." In *Novissima appendix ad Floram philippinarum Emmanuëlis Blanco*, edited by Andrea Naves and Celestino Fernandez-Villar, 1–59. Manila: Plana et socios, 1880.

de Montenegro, Pedro. "Materia medica misionera." In *Revista patriótica del pasado argentino*, edited by Manuel Ricardo Trelles, vols. 1–2. Buenos Aires: Europea, 1888.

Klein, Paul. *Remedios faciles para diferentes enfermedades*. Manila: Juan Correa, 1712.

Steinhöffer, Johannes. *Florilegio medicinal de todas las enfermedades*. México: Herederos de Juan Joseph Guillena Carrascoso, 1712.

Secondary Sources

Alden, Dauril. *The Making of an Enterprise: The Society of Jesus in Portugal, Its Empire, and Beyond, 1540–1750.* Stanford, CA: Stanford University Press, 1996.

Amundsen, Darrel. "Medieval Canon Law on Medical and Surgical Practice by the Clergy." *Bulletin of the History of Medicine* 52 (1978): 22–44.

Anagnostou, Sabine. "Jesuits in Spanish America: Contributions to the Exploration of the American *Materia Medica*." *Pharmacy in History* 47:1 (2005): 3–17.

Barrera-Osorio, Antonio. *Experiencing Nature: The Spanish American Empire and the Early Scientific Revolution.* Austin: University of Texas Press, 2006.

Bauer, Ralph and Marcy Norton, eds. "Entangled Trajectories: Indigenous and European Histories." Special Issue of *Colonial Latin American Review* 26:1 (2017).

Bian, He. *Know Your Remedies: Pharmacy and Culture in Early Modern China*. Princeton, NJ: Princeton University Press, 2020.

Boumediene, Samir. *La colonisation du savoir: Une Histoire des plantes médicinales du "Nouveau Monde" (1492–1750)*. Vaulx-en-Velin: Les Éditions des mondes à faire, 2016.

Boumediene, Samir. "Jesuit Recipes, Jesuit Receipts: The Society of Jesus and the Introduction of Exotic Materia Medica into Europe." In *Cultural Worlds of the Jesuits in Colonial Latin America*, edited by Linda Newson, 227–54. London: University of London Press, 2020.

Boumediene, Samir and Valentina Pugliano. "The Substitute Route: Exotic Remedies, Medical Innovation and the Market for Substitutes in the 16th Century." *Revue d'histoire moderne et contemporaine* 66:3 (2019): 24–54.

Breen, Benjamin. *The Age of Intoxication: Origins of the Global Drug Trade*. Philadelphia: University of Pennsylvania Press, 2019.

Cervantes, Fernando. *The Devil in the New World: The Impact of Diabolism in New Spain.* New Haven, CT: Yale University Press, 1994.

Chakrabarti, Pratik. *Materials and Medicine: Trade, Conquest and Therapeutics in the Eighteenth Century.* Manchester: Manchester University Press, 2015.

Cook, Harold J. *Matters of Exchange: Commerce, Medicine, and Science in the Dutch Golden Age.* New Haven, CT: Yale University Press, 2007.

Crawford, Matthew James. *The Andean Wonder Drug: Cinchona Bark and Imperial Science in the Spanish Atlantic, 1630–1800.* Pittsburgh, PA: University of Pittsburgh Press, 2016.

Crawford, Matthew James. "An Imperial Pharmacopoeia? The *Pharmacopoeia Matritensis* and *Materia Medica* in the Eighteenth-Century Spanish Atlantic World." In *Drugs on the Page: Pharmacopoeias and Healing Knowledge in the Early Modern Atlantic World*, edited by Matthew James Crawford and Joseph Gabriel, 63–78. Pittsburgh, PA: University of Pittsburgh Press, 2019.

Crawford, Matthew James and Joseph Gabriel, eds. *Drugs on the Page: Pharmacopoeias and Healing Knowledge in the Early Modern Atlantic World.* Pittsburgh, PA: University of Pittsburgh Press, 2019.

Cushner, Nicholas. "Merchants and Missionaries: A Theologian's View of Clerical Involvement in the Galleon Trade." *The Hispanic American Historical Review* 47:3 (1967): 360–69.

de Asúa, Miguel. *Science in the Vanished Arcadia: Knowledge of Nature in the Jesuit Missions of Paraguay and Río de la Plata.* Leiden; Boston, MA: Brill, 2014.

de Carvalho Viotti, Ana Carolina, and Jean Marcel Carvalho França, eds. *Coleção de várias receitas e segredos particulares das principais boticas da nossa Companhia de Portugal, da Índia, de Macau e do Brasil.* São Paulo: Edições Loyola, 2019.

De Vos, Paula. *Compound Remedies: Galenic Pharmacy in Colonial Mexico.* Pittsburgh, PA: University of Pittsburgh Press, 2020.

Donato, Maria Pia, Luc Berlive, Sara Cabibbo, Raimondo Michetti, and Marilyn Nicoud, eds. *Médecine et religion: Compétitions, collaborations, conflits (XIIe–XXe siècles).* Rome: École française de Rome, 2013.

Gicklhorn, Renée. *Missionsapotheker: Deutsche Pharmazeuten im Lateinamerika des 17. und 18. Jahrhunderts.* Stuttgart: Wissenschaftliche Verlagsgesellschaft MBH, 1973.

Giovannetti-Singh, Gianamar. "Galenizing the New World: Joseph-François Lafitau's 'Galenization' of Canadian Ginseng, ca. 1716–1724." *Notes and Records of the Royal Society of London* 75 (2021): 59–72.

Gómez, Pablo. *The Experiential Caribbean: Creating Knowledge and Healing in the Early Modern Atlantic.* Chapel Hill: University of North Carolina Press, 2017.

Grell, Ole Peter, Andrew Cunningham, and Jon Arrizabalaga, eds., *Health Care and Poor Relief in Counter-Reformation Europe.* New York: Routledge, 1999.

Gruzinski, Serge. *La Colonisation de l'imaginaire: Sociétés indigènes et occidentalisation dans le Mexique espagnol, XVIe–XVIIIe siècle.* Paris: Gallimard, 1988.

Harris, Steven J. "Long-Distance Corporations, Big Sciences, and the Geography of Knowledge." *Configurations* 6:2 (1998): 269–304.

Jackson, Mark, ed., *A Global History of Medicine.* Oxford: Oxford University Press, 2018.

Kay, Margarita Artschwager. "The *Florilegio Medicinal*: Source of Southwest Ethnomedicine." *Ethnohistory* 24:3 (1977): 251–259.

Kay, Margarita Artschwager. *Healing with Plants in the American and Mexican West.* Tucson: University of Arizona Press, 1996.

Kroupa, Sebestian. "Georg Joseph Kamel (1661–1706): A Jesuit Pharmacist at the Frontiers of Colonial Empires." PhD Dissertation. University of Cambridge, 2019.

Kroupa, Sebestian. "Spanish Bodies and Jesuit Beans: Consuming Drugs in Late Seventeenth-Century Manila." In *Exoticizing Consumption: European Drug Cultures Around 1700*, edited by Justin Rivest and Emma Spary (forthcoming).

Margócsy, Dániel. *Commercial Visions: Science, Trade and Visual Culture in the Dutch Golden Age*. Chicago, IL: University of Chicago Press, 2014.

Martín, Luis. *The Intellectual Conquest of Peru: The Jesuit College of San Pablo*. New York: Fordham University Press, 1968.

Murphy, Kathleen. "Translating the Vernacular: Indigenous and African Knowledge in the Eighteenth-Century British Atlantic." *Atlantic Studies* 8:1 (2011): 29–48.

Newson, Linda. *Making Medicines in Early Colonial Lima, Peru*. Leiden; Boston, MA: Brill, 2017.

Numbers, Ronald and Darrel Amundsen, eds. *Caring and Curing: Health and Medicine in the Western Religious Traditions*. Baltimore, MD: Johns Hopkins University Press, 1998.

O'Malley, John W. *The First Jesuits*. Cambridge, MA: Harvard University Press, 1993.

O'Malley, John W., Gauvin Alexander Bailey, Steven J. Harris, and T. Frank Kennedy, eds. *The Jesuits: Cultures, Sciences, and the Arts 1540–1773*, 2 vols. Toronto: University of Toronto Press, 2000, 2006.

Pardo-Tomás, José. "Conversion Medicine: Communication and Circulation of Knowledge in the Franciscan Convent and College of Tlatelolco, 1527–1577." *Quaderni Storici* 48:1 (2013): 21–42.

Pardo-Tomás, José and María Luz López Terrada. *Las primeras noticias sobre plantas americanas en las relaciones de viajes y crónicas de Indias, 1493–1553*. Valencia: CSIC, 1993.

Parsons, Christopher. "The Natural History of Colonial Science: Joseph-François Lafitau's Discovery of Ginseng and Its Afterlives." *The William and Mary Quarterly* 73:1 (2016): 37–72.

Prieto, Andrés. *Missionary Scientists: Jesuit Science in Spanish South America, 1570–1810*. Nashville: Vanderbilt University Press, 2011.

Puente-Ballesteros, Beatriz. "Jesuit Medicine in the Kangxi Court (1662–1722): Imperial Networks and Patronage." *East Asian Science, Technology, and Medicine* 34 (2011): 86–162.

Ramos, Gabriela. "Indian Hospitals and Government in the Colonial Andes." *Medical History* 57:2 (2013): 186–205.

Safier, Neil. "Global Knowledge on the Move: Itineraries, Amerindian Narratives, and Deep Histories of Science." *Isis* 101 (2010): 133–45.

Schiebinger, Londa. *Plants and Empire: Colonial Bioprospecting in the Atlantic World*. Cambridge, MA: Harvard University Press, 2004.

Seth, Suman. *Difference and Disease: Medicine, Race, and the Eighteenth-Century British Empire*. Cambridge: Cambridge University Press, 2018.

Stoler, Ann Laura. *Along the Archival Grain: Epistemic Anxieties and Colonial Common Sense*. Princeton, NJ: Princeton University Press, 2008.

Strocchia, Sharon. "The Nun Apothecaries of Renaissance Florence: Marketing Medicines in the Convent." *Renaissance Studies* 25:5 (2011): 627–47.

Tsing, Anna Lowenhaupt. *Friction: An Ethnography of Global Connection*. Princeton, NJ: Princeton University Press, 2005.

Voeks, Robert A. "Disturbance Pharmacopoeias: Medicine and Myth from the Humid Tropics." *Annals of the Association of American Geographers* 94:4 (2004): 868–88.

Walker, Timothy D. "The Early Modern Globalization of Indian Medicine: Portuguese Dissemination of Drugs and Healing Techniques from South Asia on Four Continents, 1670–1830." *Portuguese Literary & Cultural Studies* 17/18 (2010): 77–97.

Walker, Timothy D. "The Medicines Trade in the Portuguese Atlantic World: Acquisition and Dissemination of Healing Knowledge from Brazil (c. 1580–1800)." *Social History of Medicine* 26:3 (2013): 403–31.

Walker, Timothy D. "Crown Authorities, Colonial Physicians, and the Exigencies of Empire: The Codification of Indigenous Therapeutic Knowledge in India and Brazil During the Enlightenment Era." In *Drugs on the Page: Pharmacopoeias and Healing Knowledge in the Early Modern Atlantic World*, edited by Matthew James Crawford and Joseph Gabriel, 101–20. Pittsburgh, PA: University of Pittsburgh Press, 2019.

Županov, Ines. "Conversion, Illness and Possession: Catholic Missionary Healing in Early Modern South Asia." In *Divins remèdes: Médecine et religion en Asie du Sud*, edited by Ines Županov and Caterina Guenzi, 263–300. EHESS, 2008.

11 Vernacular Medical Print

Or How to Read a Recipe Book

Elaine Leong

The Family Physitian or a Collection of Choice, Approv'd and Experienc'd Remedies for the Cure of Almost all Diseases appeared on London bookshelves in 1696.[1] Authored by George Hartman, self-described as a "Phylo Chymist," the book contained "hundreds of considerable Receipts and Secrets of great Vallue, with Observations of great Cures." On its debut, the book joined a long and crowded list of similar titles all offering instructions to make drugs and cures in early modern English homes. Recipe books joined a wide array of printed medical texts in English in sixteenth- and seventeenth-century London. Available at various price points, these books covered a range of topics, such as first-aid, physic and surgery, and pharmacy and dietary advice, and these were targeted toward broad audiences from medical practitioners of all stripes and experience levels to householders. As such, vernacular printed books offer rich possibilities to study past ideas and practices of health and the body and have long been studied by historians of medicine.

Centered on Hartman's *The Family Physitian*, this essay offers an introduction to the world of vernacular medical print, recipes, and household medicine in early modern England. It opens with a brief outline of how scholars have approached the study of early modern books with an emphasis on medical print, bringing together methodologies from book history, literary studies, and cultural histories of medicine. The article then guides the reader through Hartman's book from cover to cover, illustrating how analysis of different "book parts" can extend our understanding of the past knowledge practices.[2]

The study of book production, reading, and use is a long-standing field of inquiry, and scholars have approached past "book worlds" using a number of different analytical frameworks. Historians of the Book have shone light on production methods, publication conventions, and the various actors involved in the creation and dissemination of a book object.[3] Literary scholars have focused on topics such as authorship and anonymity, processes of editing, translation, and reading.[4] Bibliographers have constructed a robust vocabulary to describe and analyze different aspects of books, including physical size and length, paper quality, watermarks, stitching, and bindings.[5] Together, these scholars have shown us how material aspects of the book can tell us much about the intentions of book producers, target audiences, and eventual book use.[6] In a period where the cost of paper constituted a large proportion of production costs, the size of the book and thus the amount of

DOI: 10.4324/9781003094876-14

paper required for its production is one indication of intended audiences, or at least the size of their purses.[7] The inclusion of images, whether as woodcuts or engravings, will also raise production costs, thus impacting the kinds of readers and users who could afford the text.[8]

Historians of medicine interested in English vernacular print have drawn heavily on this rich tradition and on the tremendous work conducted by early bibliographers to identify, describe, and catalog extant pre-1800 English printed books. Consequently, the study of English medical print largely takes the form of three connected trajectories. First, scholars such as Paul Slack and Mary Fissell have conducted robust surveys of medical print from c. 1475 to 1700.[9] By identifying emerging and fading trends in book genres and topics and offering an overview of the occupations and interests of authors and other book producers, these essays are crucial to our understanding of the contours of medical print. We now have a clear idea of what was printed, when and by whom, and which genres grew in popularity over the early modern period. For example, it is clear that recipe books such as Hartman's *The Family Physitian* gained popularity over the course of the seventeenth century and became one of the best-selling genres of vernacular medical print by the end of the century.[10] Likewise, scholars such as Fissell and Slack have shown that while long-standing genres such as regimens (or guides to healthy living) were often issued in the early sixteenth century, their popularity with readers gradually declined over the time period examined.[11]

Second, parallel to these general surveys of medical print, historians have also conducted in-depth case studies of particular genres or kinds of books, tracing continuity and change in book content, authors, and production methods in response to political, social, and cultural contexts. Exemplary works include Agnes Arber and Sarah Neville's work on herbals, Bernard Capp's study of almanacs, Lauren Kassell's detailed article on alchemical books and medical cases, and Mary Fissell's *Vernacular Bodies,* which examines midwifery manuals in sixteenth- and seventeenth-century England.[12] Inspired again by historians of the book, the third strand of research concerns book reception and reading. Here, historians, such as Peter Murray Jones, have reconstructed book collections and libraries and analyzed readers' engagement with printed texts via handwritten marginalia and reading notes in notebooks.[13] If the first two strands of study tend to prioritize book production and assess what kinds of knowledge and information was made available, this third strand emphasizes the agency of readers to recover how early modern men and women might have selected, engaged with, and used book-based knowledge in their everyday health practices.[14] Furthermore, by attending to the afterlives of print, it has also traced long-view narratives of medical ideas and concepts.[15]

Scholars analyzing vernacular medical print examine a number of different components or "book parts" to gain further understandings of past health cultures. In recent years, scholars have played increasing attention to "paratextual" materials.[16] These are conventional apparatus framing the main body of text in any book, including but not limited to titlepages, table of contents, front matter such as prefaces and letters to the reader, chapter and marginal headings, and indexes. Together, these different "book parts" can tell us a great deal about a printed work.

Titlepages and front matter often reveal information about intended audiences, authors' reasons for writing and publishing the work, and the different book producers (printers, publishers, booksellers) involved in the project. Tables of contents and chapter arrangements offer indicators of knowledge organization schemes and hint at particular knowledge hierarchies via the amount of space devoted to particular topics or the sequential listing of topics. In what follows, I will briefly take you through Hartman's *The Family Physitian* from cover to cover to illustrate the kinds of questions we might ask of a vernacular printed medical book and the sorts of insights that might be gained.

The titlepage of *The Family Physitian* is divided into four distinct sections. Like many similar offerings, Hartman gave his work a long and unwieldy title: *The Family Physitian or a Collection of Choice, Approv'd and Experience'd Remedies for the Cure of Almost all Diseases incident to Humain Bodies, whether Internal or External; useful for Families, and very serviceable to Country People.*[17] Right off the bat, then, Hartman indicates that his work is comprehensive ("almost all diseases"); intended for lay practitioners ("families" and "country people"); designed to be "useful" and "serviceable;" and contains tried and tested cures ("approv'd and experience'd"). The second section of the titlepage offers more details for curious readers, revealing that the volume contains "hundreds" of "Receipts and Secrets" of "great vallue," as well as "Observations of great Cures." Additionally, Hartman has decided to pair the collection with a tract titled the "Wine-Celler," proffering instructions to make English wines and metheglin (spiced mead), as well as additional instructions for the production of "Choicest and Safest cosmetic Remedies." Crucially, he adds, the know-how offered was "never before publish'd."

For historians, this dense titlepage is revealing of early modern health cultures. First, we note that there was evidently a market for manuals for health practices within families or in non-urban areas.[18] Second, know-how gained value via hands-on testing, personal observations, and endorsements, hence the repeated use of verbs such as "approve" or "observe," and "experience."[19] Finally, it was common to bind together how-to knowledge about the production of drugs, alcohol, and cosmetics due to the close connections between food, drink, and medicines, and the contemporary attention to the surface of the body as a way to monitor health and sickness.[20]

If the first two sections of the titlepage tell us much about contemporary attitudes to recipe knowledge and health practices, the second two sections are revealing about our actors, their authority claims, and their roles as knowers. Hartman describes himself as a "Phylo chymist" or a lover of chemistry and boasted that he had "liv'd and Travell'd with the Honourable and Renoun'd Sir KENELM DIGBY in several parts of Europe, the space of Seven Years till he died."[21] Hartman's biographical statement suggests that contemporaries and, particularly readers and buyers of such books, considered Hartman's association with an aristocrat well known for his experimentations and knowledge *and* his travels outside England to be markers of medical authority.[22] The careful note that his service with Digby was lengthy and that Digby had died hints that Hartman had access to Digby's stash of secret knowledge. The final section of the titlepage contains the imprint, which lists information about the various actors (printers, publishers, booksellers, etc.) involved in the production and sale of this book. In this case, it notes that the work was "printed by H. Hills for the Author" and offers Hartman's current address. As we will see later, this self-published book was part of a larger scheme to sell medical services and goods.[23]

Once we flip open the book, we encounter two additional pieces of paratextual materials, both penned by Hartman. First is a letter dedicating the book to William Paston, Viscount, and Earl of Yarmouth, and second is a detailed letter to the reader outlining Hartman's intentions for the work and hopes for its place in the hearts of the English reading public.[24] Dedicatory letters are commonplace in early modern books and served as a space for authors to seek or firm up their connections with wealthy and/or well-connected patrons.[25] In this dedication, Hartman connects his work with another aristocratic family renowned for their interests in medical and alchemical practices.[26] As Hartman's letter is careful to note, William's father Robert Paston was known for his skills in iatrochemistry (medical alchemy) and was the dedicatee of Hartman's earlier publications. Moreover, it seems that William had promised Hartman access to his father's famed "Manuscripts and Secrets" learned from the famous physician Sir Theodore Mayerne.[27] Thus, Hartman's short dedicatory letter not only reveals his connections and past support from another aristocratic expert but also puts in print and thus public, William Paston's promise to open his books of secrets to Hartman. In other words, these often brief letters enable historians to trace and reconstruct networks of patronage and knowledge communities.

If the dedicatory letter was a masterpiece of name-dropping, the letter to the reader is rather more of an advertisement of the authors' expertise and the utility of the work at hand.[28] Hartman begins by telling readers that *The Family Physitian* is his fourth book in print, thus reminding them of his considerable experience as a practitioner and as an author. The rest of the letter reinforces themes already introduced on the titlepage. Hartman is keen to remind readers that much of book was "never Printed," alluding to the value of the knowledge that had previously only circulated in manuscript form within select circles. This volume of the "Marrow of Collections" represented know-how tested by "an able Physitian and Chyrurgion," that is approved and backed by an expert practitioner. There is again language about the value of these "Secrets" and "Observations of Famous Cures." Very quickly though, Hartman turns to a series to disclaimers, emphasizing that these instructions were not for "any Man exactly to follow" but rather a "light and Guide" to those who have "wisdom prudently to use."[29] It was also intended to be of "good use" to others such as "well dispos'd worthy Ladies and Gentlewomen, that take delight in the Charitable Contributing to the Health as well as Sustenance of their Poor Neighbours and Domestical Servants" and also those based in the country where "Physitians and Chyrurgions are scarce, if at all to be had."[30]

Three points are significant here. First, women were encouraged to engage in medical activities within their own households, particularly if it concerned patients who were unable to pay for other kinds of medical services.[31] Second, there is recognition that while medical practitioners of all stripes were common in urban centers, they were hard to come by in rural areas. In these cases, readers were encouraged to fill in this gap in healthcare provision. In other words, while Hartman was eager to open medical knowledge to all those who could read, but he was careful to delineate that this knowledge was not to be used in place of services or advice from paid medical practitioners. As part of a community of practitioners offering various kinds of health services, Hartman was careful not to be a threat or to take business away from his colleagues.[32] By closely analyzing Hartman's letter to the reader, historians can recover not only how authors promoted themselves but also their subtler intentions for how readers should use their books.

The final piece of the front matter of this publication, the index, follows the dedication and address to readers. It is somewhat unusual to see the index at the front rather than the back of the work, but even by the late seventeenth century, printing conventions were still in flux and works could include both a table of contents and an index or just one or the other.[33] Indexes can tell us much about contemporary attitudes toward disease entities and medical knowledge schemes. The one in *The Family Physitian* is listed alphabetically, and I will explore the letter B as an example. There are 16 entries listed under the letter B, starting with "Barreness" and ending with "Balsam of St. Johnswort;" the indexer was clearly comfortable listing bodily states (to be barren) with instruction to make specific drugs. Interestingly, readers looking to learn more about "barreness" are instructed to see "conception" instead. Under the heading "C" is an entry "Conception to procure." Other entries addressed ailments visible on the surface of the body such as "Burns," "Bruises and Swellings," or "Breasts in Women Swell'd hard and painful, cur'd." Others alluded to issues inside the body, including "Beating of the Heart" or "Back weak to strengthen." Elsewhere, the indexer included disease entities such as "Apoplexie," "Dropsie," "Green Sickness," "Kings Evil," and "Yellow Jaundice." While brief and often one-word long, these entries richly reveal the various bodily signs that early modern men and women searched for and noted. It also gives historians a sense of the language and vocabulary used by our historical actors to describe sickness, which included terminology for bodily symptoms and for ailments and diseases. As many have noted, this broad and fluid view of sickness and disease was common throughout the early modern period and is reflected across different genres of medical writings (Figure 11.1).[34]

Turning to the body of the text, the "First volume of the Family Physitian," as Hartman optimistically termed it (he had high hopes for a follow-up publication which did not materialize), is a lengthy work of more than 520 pages.[35] The hundreds of medical recipes in the book covered all sorts of bodily pains, ailments, and diseases and were organized into 65 chapters. Hartman begins by listing the remedies by parts of the body or the organs addressed, starting from the head and moving down the body, and then proceeds to address ailments pertinent to the whole body, such as fevers or plague.[36] The listing of recipes from head to toe (in Latin *a capite ad calem*) was a widespread practice in medieval texts on practical medicine, and Hartman's use of this convention not only presented the information in a familiar organizational structure but also connected his work (for some readers at least) to long-standing traditions of learned medical writing. Around halfway

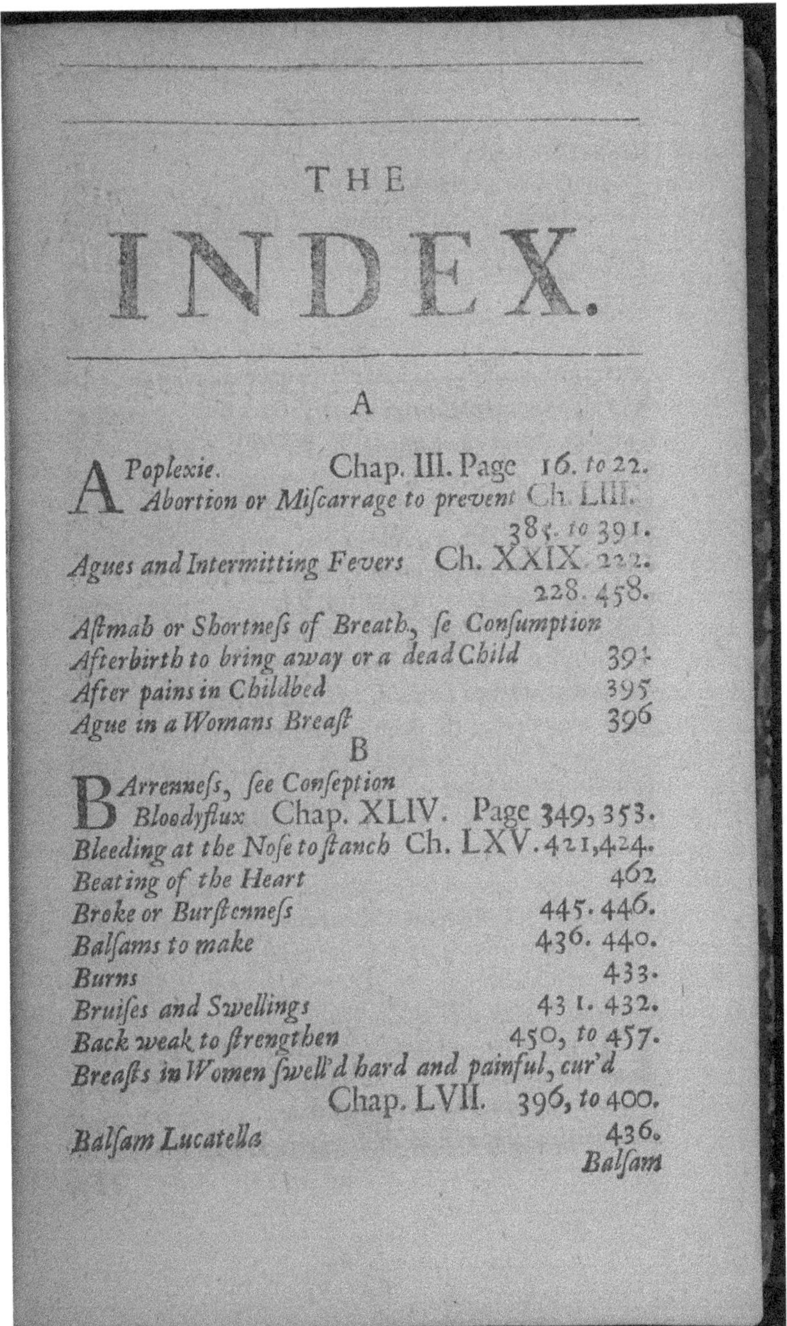

THE

INDEX.

A

APoplexie. Chap. III. Page 16. *to* 22.
Abortion or Miſcarrage to prevent Ch. LIII. 385. *to* 391.
Agues and Intermitting Fevers Ch. XXIX. 222. 228. 458.
Aſtmah or Shortneſs of Breath, ſe Conſumption
Afterbirth to bring away or a dead Child 394
After pains in Childbed 395
Ague in a Womans Breaſt 396

B

B*Arrenneſs, ſee Conception*
Bloodyflux Chap. XLIV. Page 349, 353.
Bleeding at the Noſe to ſtanch Ch. LXV. 421, 424.
Beating of the Heart 462
Broke or Burſtenneſs 445. 446.
Balſams to make 436. 440.
Burns 433.
Bruiſes and Swellings 431. 432.
Back weak to ſtrengthen 450, *to* 457.
Breaſts in Women ſwell'd hard and painful, cur'd Chap. LVII. 396, *to* 400.
Balſam Lucatella 436.
Balſam

Figure 11.1 First page of the Index, George Hartman, *The family physitian, or A collection of choice, approv'd and experienc'd remedies...* (London: Printed for Richard Wellington, 1696), Wellcome Collection EPB/B/59444.

through the chapters, Hartman switches the organizational categories from ailments to types of medicine with a strong focus on distilled waters, these included instructions to make cordial waters, strong waters, and cordial juleps.[37] This is followed by sections on medicines which purge the body and, relatedly, remedies which control vomiting, bleeding, and sweating, and a long list of remedies addressing women's health issues and children's illnesses.[38] The volume concludes with a section on miscellaneous recipes (including for veterinary medicines) and subsections titled "The True English Wine Celler," "Preserving and Pickling," and "The Cabinet of Safe Cosmetik Remedies."[39] These section headings suggest that Hartman went to considerable efforts to organize and make accessible and retrievable the vast information contained in his work.

From this brief description above, it is clear that Hartman's weighty tome contained a wealth of health-related information, and *The Family Physitian* aimed to offer comprehensive medical know-how geared to deal with all sorts of health and bodily issues arising within a household.[40] In terms of content and structure, *The Family Physician* followed in footsteps of other popular household recipe books such as *A Choice Manual of Rare and Select Secrets in Physick and Chirurgery* (London 1653) which was accredited to Elizabeth Grey, the Countess of Kent and *The Queens Closet Opened* (London 1655), connected with Henrietta Maria. Both of these texts likewise cover a wide range of ailments and offered sections on food preservation and cosmetics.[41] The bringing together of pharmaceutical knowledge with that on fermentation and preservation and beauty know-how is reflective of the close affinity between these areas within early modern mentalities. Not only did they require similar skills, techniques, and tools but, within contemporary ideas of the body, these different substances also would have worked together to balance humors and maintain health.[42]

Historians of medicine have demonstrated that the household was likely the first port of call for early modern healthcare provision, and books such as *The Family Physitian* provided much needed support for householders taking on medical roles. Supplemented by other vernacular texts such as general medical guides, surgical books or herbals and informal hands-on training and knowledge exchange with friends and family, printed recipe books such as *The Family Physitian* stood at the center of a range of home-based health activities.[43] These included all sorts of "body work" such as caring and nursing, diagnosis, observation, and tending to different kinds of ailments and medicine production.[44] While it was not unusual for husbands and wives or fathers and mothers to both take an interest and contribute to these health activities, in general, women took on the lion's share of such work.[45] Women's expertise in recipe knowledge is evident by the survival of a large number of manuscript recipe books, a number of printed works fronted by gentlewomen and by the common citation of female recipe donors in both manuscript and printed collections.[46]

Like many other printed recipe books, *The Family Physitian* is a compilation of know-how drawing from Hartman's own medical and reading practices, both of which were shaped by his service to Sir Kenelm Digby.[47] The work contains a number of recipes for which Digby was well known, including his "Wound-drink for the Kings Evil, Fistula, Corroding Ulcers, or old Soree" and cure testimonies from Digby's own practice.[48] Furthermore, Hartman offers medical and beauty know-how from a number of Royalist courtiers such as Prince Rupert and Lady Crisp, demonstrating how political and social networks framed knowledge transfer in this period.[49] Hartman also included successful cases from his own healing activities, including his observations on how a powder for "Kings Evil and other desperate scorbutick Diseases" cured an unnamed gentleman, the daughter of Sir Nathaniel Johnson and Mrs Pannel.[50] By the late seventeenth century, the inclusion of experiential knowledge such as testimonies and observations in medical texts about drugs, cures, and recipes was fairly commonplace and served as a marker for authority.[51]

The Family Physitian also existed within a network of books as Hartman's extensive reading of contemporary medical books provided him with a wealth of information. For example, the recipe for Digby's wound water was actually taken from the *Pharamcopoeia Bateana*, the dispensatory of the physician George Bate compiled by the apothecary James Shipton and published in Latin in 1688 and translated by the popular medical writer William Salmon in 1694. Here, Hartman reproduces not only the recipe but also Salmon's comments on the medicine.[52] Other contemporary authors name-checked by Hartman include the French physician and professor of practical medicine at Montpellier, Lazare Rivière, and the physicians William Harvey, Theodore Mayerne, Thomas Sydenham, and Thomas Willis.[53] This is a key characteristic of vernacular medical literature in this period, and rather than thinking of it as plagiarism, we might think of it as reading for others much like students crib notes or study guides. At a time when printed books were expensive and inaccessible for many, these "digested reads" played a key role in knowledge transfer.

Finally, while *The Family Physitian* has much in common with other popular recipe books of the day, it also has one standout feature: the inclusion of an intricate copper engraving of a distillation apparatus usually placed near the front of the book.[54] The text accompanying the image describes the apparatus as an "Engine of Still" invented by Hartman and debuted in his earlier publication *The Preserver and Restorer of Health*.[55] Made of tin, brass, or copper, the engine was designed to boil and stew meat and distill medicinal waters, depending on which of the many different components were fitted together. Heated either by charcoal or by a spirit lamp, it presented a fuel-efficient means to make many of the recipes offered in the book. Helpfully, Hartman would be very happy to direct buyers to expert artisans to have the engine made, particularly if readers visited him at his house at the "lower end of Cherry-garden street near the Jamaica-house" in Rotherhithe (Figure 11.2).[56]

Depictions of apparatus such as Hartman's engine suggest a lively trade in health-related technologies and instruments in late-seventeenth-century London. From Hartman's various descriptions of the "Engine," it was evidently a rather popular item, especially with the seafaring communities in Wapping and Rotherhithe and with fashionable gentry.[57] Like many other scientific and medical instruments of the period, consumers often obtained bespoke creations of these engines or instruments which were created to their specification in terms of size and materials by local artisans.[58] The inclusion of the engine schematics and directions on where to

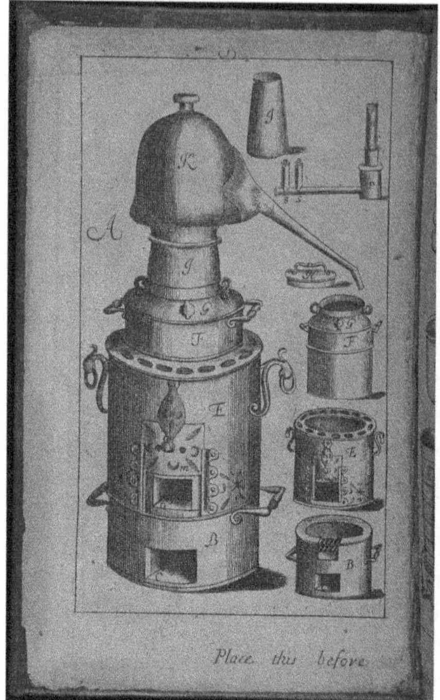

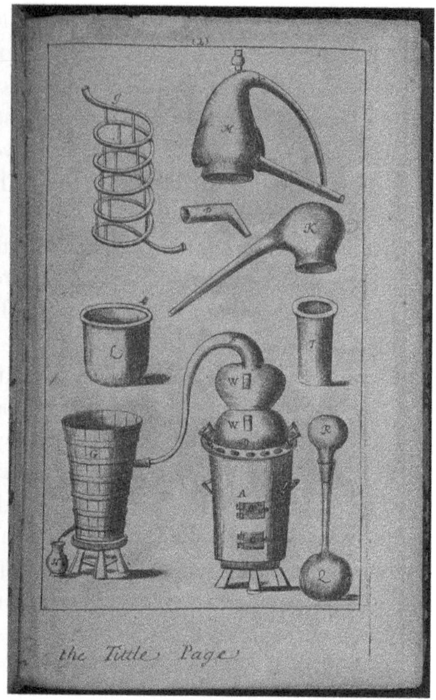

Figure 11.2 Engraving illustrating Hartman's "Engine." George Hartman, *The family physitian, or A collection of choice, approv'd and experienc'd remedies*... (London: Printed for Richard Wellington, 1696), Wellcome Collection EPB/B/59444.

obtain the apparatus in *The Family Physitian* reveals the close connections between the touting of medical knowledge and of medical goods and services.

Earlier we noted from the titlepage imprint that one edition of *The Family Physitian* was published for the author – that is, funded by Hartman – and likely sold at his listed address in Rotherhithe. In fact, Hartman offered many other medical items aside from books and engines. The final section of *The Family Physitian* is titled "Catalogue of some choice Medicines which I have by me ready prepar'd" and lists over 40 different compound medicines and their prices. Some of these, such as the "true Royal Hungarian-water," are specific famous medicines made from secret recipes passed through various hands in Royalist circles but not all of the medicines listed here are made from such guarded know-how.[59] In fact, the main text of *The Family Physitian* offers the recipes for many of these medicines, along with their virtues or use, dosage information, and endorsements from various medical practitioners. In other words, Hartman offered a drug *production* service, promising medicines made by a trustworthy expert using popular or sought-after recipes.

Hartman's more service-orientated commercial outfit existed alongside contemporary enterprises touting proprietary medicines, such as Daffy's Elixir or Anderson's Pills, highlighting market needs for different kinds of medical services.[60]

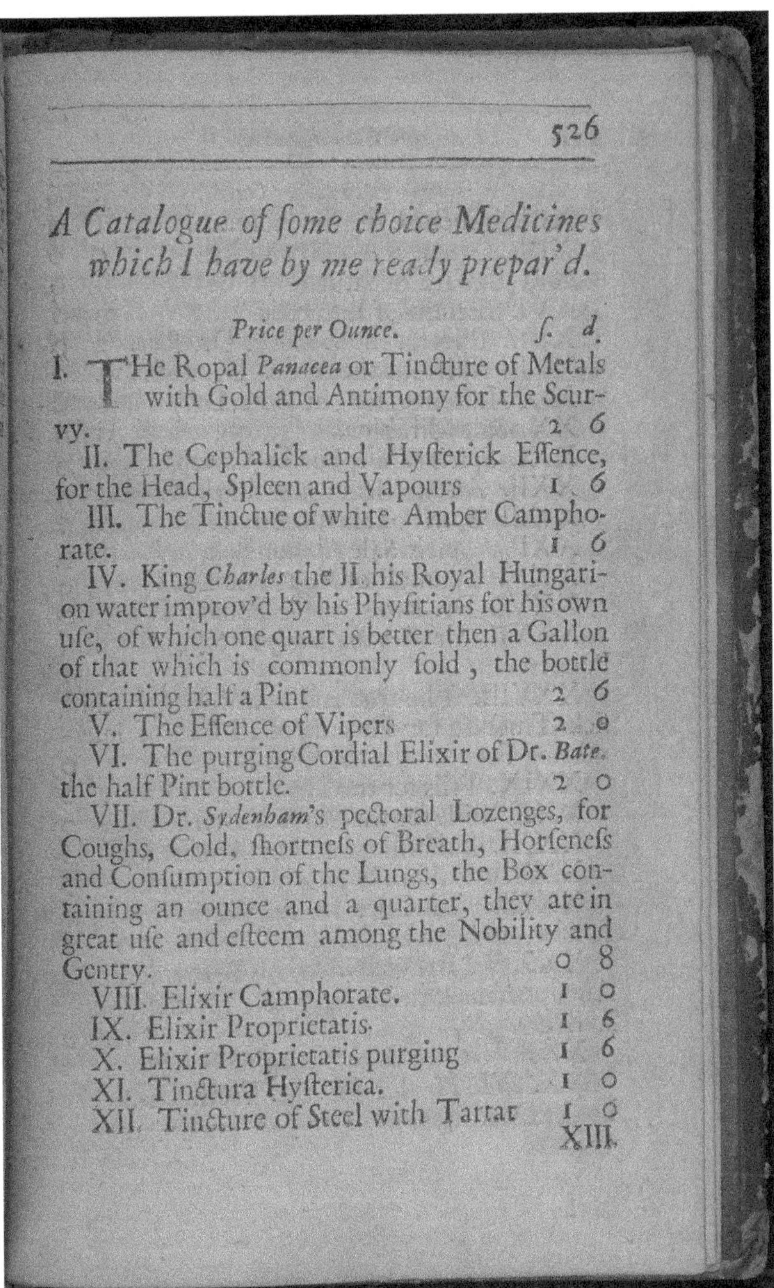

526

A Catalogue of ſome choice Medicines which I have by me ready prepar'd.

Price per Ounce. ſ. d.

I. THe Ropal *Panacea* or Tincture of Metals with Gold and Antimony for the Scurvy. 2 6

II. The Cephalick and Hyſterick Eſſence, for the Head, Spleen and Vapours 1 6

III. The Tinctue of white Amber Camphorate. 1 6

IV. King *Charles* the II his Royal Hungarion water improv'd by his Phyſitians for his own uſe, of which one quart is better then a Gallon of that which is commonly ſold, the bottle containing half a Pint 2 6

V. The Eſſence of Vipers 2 0

VI. The purging Cordial Elixir of Dr. *Bate*. the half Pint bottle. 2 0

VII. Dr. *Sydenham's* pectoral Lozenges, for Coughs, Cold, ſhortneſs of Breath, Horſeneſs and Conſumption of the Lungs, the Box containing an ounce and a quarter, they are in great uſe and eſteem among the Nobility and Gentry. 0 8

VIII. Elixir Camphorate. 1 0

IX. Elixir Proprietatis. 1 6

X. Elixir Proprietatis purging 1 6

XI. Tinctura Hyſterica. 1 0

XII. Tincture of Steel with Tartar 1 0

XIII.

Figure 11.3 First page of "A Catalog of some choice Medicines which I have by me ready prepar'd," George Hartman, *The family physitian, or A collection of choice, approv'd and experienc'd remedies...* (London: Printed for Richard Wellington, 1696), Wellcome Collection EPB/B/59444.

The overlap between Hartman's book contents and his list of medicines for sale also suggests that just because recipes are accessible via printed works, it did not mean that they were widely made by householders. Then, like now, householders might have been interested in how particular medicines were made and what they contained *and yet* still obtain them from a specialized or expert producer. A good modern analogy might be coffee table cookbooks from internationally renowned restaurants or lengthy baking tomes with instructions for making intricate celebratory cakes; in both cases, readers eagerly pore over pages for theoretical know-how but few actually make the recipes themselves, leaving that to top chefs and bakers (Figure 11.3).

Printed at the close of the seventeenth century, *The Family Physitian* entered a well-developed market in vernacular medical print offering all sorts of health-related information and advice to a wide-ranging readership. Many surviving copies of these books are heavily annotated and record how contemporary and later readers engaged with the works, underlining particularly important parts, adding supplementary information, and contesting information which with they disagreed. Thus, we know that these works were read, used, and played a crucial part in the making, transfer, and circulation of health knowledge. The example of Hartman's *Family Physitian* brings out several important points about early modern vernacular medical print. First, many of these texts presented a mix of "learned" and "popular" ideas sourced from a range of places – books by university-trained physicians and professors, personal experience and observations, and even informal conversations. As such, they suggest that for the everyday reader, the lines between "learned" and "popular" medical ideas were considerably blurred. Second, the medical book trade was bound up with all kinds of health-related businesses including the sale of new-fangled medical technologies such as Hartman's engine and drug production services. In that sense, the sale of books was an integral part of medical markets. Finally, as suggested by Hartman's title *The Family Physitian*, the early modern home was a primary site for medical activities. Recipe collections were the mainstay of book producers and sellers, reflecting lively circulation of recipe knowledge and home-based health cultures. Women, as mothers, wives, housekeepers, and drug producers, played a central role in these activities and were both producers and consumers of vernacular medical print. In this way, books as *The Family Physitian* serve as excellent introductions to the multi-faceted world of early modern healthcare and related knowledge practices.

Notes

1 Two editions of this work, with the same title and pagination, were printed in 1696. One is printed by H. Hills for the author (Wing 1003A) and the other is printed for Richard Wellington (Wing 1003). For ease, all references to the work in this article refer to the work printed for the author (Wing 1003A) and especially to the copy now in the William Andrews Clark Memorial Library and digitally available on Early English Books Online, https://www.proquest.com/books/family-physitian-collection-choice-approvd/docview/2240894383/se-2?accountid=14511. This copy is hereafter referenced as Hartman. Images of the work included in this essay are taken from the Wellcome Collection copy which is digitized and available in Public Domain. However, the Wellcome

Collection copy is the edition printed for Richard Wellington (Wing 1003). While the two editions contain slightly different prefatory materials, there are no significant differences in the reproduced pages.

2 Dennis Duncan and Adam Smyth, eds., *Book Parts* (Oxford: Oxford University Press, 2019).

3 The there is a rich literature on book history. For a recent overview see, James Raven, ed., *The Oxford Illustrated History of the Book* (Oxford: Oxford University Press, 2020). Seminal works include the following: Robert Darnton, "What Is the History of Books?," *Daedalus* 111, no. 3 (1982): 65–83; Donald Francis McKenzie, *Bibliography and the Sociology of Texts* (London: British Library, 1986); Thomas R. Adams and Nicolas Barker, "A New Model for the Study of the Book," in *A Potencie of Life: Books in Society. The Clark Lectures 1986–1987*, ed. Nicolas Barker (London: British Library, 1993), 5–43; Donald Francis McKenzie, *Making Meaning: "Printers of the Mind" and Other Essays*, ed. Peter D. McDonald and Michael Felix Suarez (Amherst: University of Massachusetts Press, 2002); Robert Darnton, "'What Is the History of Books?' Revisited," *Modern Intellectual History* 4, no. 3 (2007): 495–508. For the early modern British context, see, for example, Adrian Johns, *The Nature of the Book: Print and Knowledge in the Making* (Chicago, IL: University of Chicago Press, 1998); Joad Raymond, ed., *The Oxford History of Popular Print Culture: Cheap Print in Britain and Ireland to 1660* (Oxford: Oxford University Press, 2011).

4 See, for example, Marcy North, *The Anonymous Renaissance: Cultures of Discretion in Tudor-Stuart England* (Chicago, IL: University of Chicago Press, 2003); Sara K. Barker and Brenda M. Hosington, *Renaissance Cultural Crossroads: Translation, Print and Culture in Britain, 1473–1640* (Leiden: Brill, 2013).

5 See, for example, Philip Gaskell, *A New Introduction to Bibliography* (New Castle, DE: Oak Knoll Press, 1995) and more recently, Sarah Werner, *Studying Early Printed Books, 1450–1800: A Practical Guide* (Hoboken, NJ: Wiley, 2018).

6 See, for example, Adam Smyth, *Material Texts in Early Modern England* (Cambridge: Cambridge University Press, 2018).

7 D. F. Mckenzie, "Printing and Publishing 1557–1700: Constraints on the London Book Trades," in *The Cambridge History of the Book in Britain*, vol. 4: 1557–1695, ed. D. F. McKenzie and John Barnard, (Cambridge: Cambridge University Press, 2002), 553–67 (556).

8 Maureen Bell, "Mise-En-Page, Illustration, Expressive Form," in *The Cambridge History of the Book in Britain*, vol. 4: 1557–1695, ed. D. F. McKenzie and John Barnard (Cambridge: Cambridge University Press, 2002), 632–62; Alexandra Franklin, "Woodcuts," in *Book Parts*, 209–22; Sean Roberts, "Engravings," in *Book Parts*, 81–94.

9 Paul Slack, "Mirrors of Health and Treasures of Poor Men: The Uses of the Vernacular Medical Literature of Tudor England," in *Health, Medicine and Mortality in the Sixteenth Century*, ed. Charles Webster (Cambridge: Cambridge University Press, 1979), 237–73; Mary E. Fissell, "The Marketplace of Print," in *The Medical Marketplace and Its Colonies c. 1450-c 1850*, ed. Mark Jenner and Patrick Wallis (Basingstoke: Palgrave Macmillan, 2007), 108–32; Mary E. Fissell, "Popular Medical Writing," in *The Oxford History of Popular Print Culture: Cheap Print in Britain and Ireland to 1660*, ed. Joad Raymond (Oxford: Oxford University Press, 2011), 417–30.

10 Fissell, "The Marketplace of Print," 116.

11 Slack, "Mirrors of Health," 243 and Fissell, "The Marketplace of Print," 116.

12 Agnes Arber, *Herbals: Their Origin and Evolution: A Chapter in the History of Botany, 1470–1670* (Cambridge: Cambridge University Press, 1953); Sarah Neville, *Early Modern Herbals and the Book Trade: English Stationers and the Commodification of Botany* (Cambridge: Cambridge University Press, 2022); Bernard Capp, *Astrology and the Popular Press: English Almanacs 1500–1800* (London: Faber and Faber, 1979); Lauren Kassell, "Secrets Revealed: Alchemical Books in Early modern England," *History of*

Science 49, no. 1 (2011): 61–125; Lauren Kassell, "Casebooks in Early Modern England: Medicine, Astrology, and Written Records," *Bulletin of the History of Medicine* 88, no. 4 (2014): 595–625; Mary E. Fissell, *Vernacular Bodies: The Politics of Reproduction in Early Modern England* (Oxford: Oxford University Press, 2004).

13 Sample works include: Peter Murray Jones, "Reading Medicine in Tudor Cambridge," in *The History of Medical Education in Britain*, ed. Vivian Nutton and Roy Porter (Amsterdam: Rodopi, 1995), 153–83; Peter Murray Jones, "The Tabula Medicine: An Evolving Encyclopaedia," *English Manuscript Studies: 1100–1700* 14 (1, 2008): 60–85.

14 There is a rich literature on the history of reading. Key works on the history of reading, in general, include the following: Robert Darnton, "First Steps Toward a History of Reading," *Australian Journal of French Studies* 23, no. 1 (1986): 5–30; Lisa Jardine and Anthony Grafton, "'Studied for Action': How Gabriel Harvey Read His Livy," *Past & Present* 129, no. 1 (1990): 30–78; William H. Sherman, *Used Books. Marking Readers in Renaissance England* (Philadelphia: University of Pennsylvania Press, 2008). On medical reading, see, for example, Mary E. Fissell, "Readers, Texts, and Contexts: Vernacular Medical Works in Early Modern England," in *The Popularization of Medicine, 1650–1850*, ed. Roy Porter (London: Routledge, 1992), 72–96 and Vanessa Harding, "Reading Plague in Seventeenth-Century London," *Social History of Medicine* 32, no. 2 (2019): 267–86. On gender and medical reading, see Rebecca Laroche, *Medical Authority and Englishwomen's Herbal Texts, 1550–1650* (Aldershot: Ashgate Publishing, 2009) and Elaine Leong, "'Herbals She Peruseth': Reading Medicine in Early Modern England," *Renaissance Studies* 28, no. 4 (2014): 556–78.

15 For a long view history of Galenism, see Petros Bouras-Vallianatos and Barbara Zipser, eds., *Brill's Companion to the Reception of Galen* (Leiden: Brill, 2019). See also Elaine Leong, "Transformative Itineraries and Communities of Knowledge in Early Modern Europe: The Case of Lazare Rivière's *The Practice of Physick*," in *Civic Medicine: Physician, Polity, and Pen in Early Modern Europe*, ed. J. Andrew Mendelsohn, Annemarie Kinzelbach, and Ruth Schilling (Abingdon: Routledge, 2019), 257–79 and Lori Jones, "Itineraries and Transformations: John of Burgundy's Plague Treatise," *Bulletin of the History of Medicine* 95, no. 3 (2021): 277–314.

16 Helen Smith and Louise Wilson, eds., *Renaissance Paratexts* (Cambridge: Cambridge University Press, 2011).

17 Hartman, Titlepage.

18 See, for example, Anne Stobart, *Household Medicine in Seventeenth-Century England* (London: Bloomsbury Publishing, 2016).

19 For a recent overview on experiential knowledge in early modern medicine, see, Alisha Rankin, "Experience," in *A Cultural History of Medicine: The Renaissance*, ed. Elaine Leong and Claudia Stein (London: Bloomsbury Academic, 2021), 141–62. For a recent overview on drug testing, see Elaine Leong and Alisha Rankin, "Testing Drugs and Trying Cures: Experiment and Medicine in Medieval and Early Modern Europe," *Bulletin of the History of Medicine* 91, no. 2 (2017): 157–82.

20 For an overview see, David Gentilcore, *Food and Health in Early Modern Europe* (London: Bloomsbury Academic, 2015).

21 On the definition of "Phylochymist," see Nathan Bailey, *An universal etymological English dictionary* (London, 1721), sig. Kkkk7.

22 On books of secrets and the trope of the wandering professor of secrets, see William Eamon, *Science and the Secrets of Nature: Books of Secrets in Medieval and Early Modern Culture* (Princeton, NJ: Princeton University Press, 1994).

23 Roy Porter, *Health for Sale: Quackery in England, 1660–1850* (Manchester: Manchester University Press, 1989) and Peter Isaac, "Pills and Print," in *Medicine, Mortality and the Book Trade*, ed. Robin Myers and Michael Harris (Folkestone, Oak Knoll Press, 1998), 25–47.

24 Hartman, sigs., A2r-A3v.

25 See, for example, Helen Smith, "Acknowledgements and Dedications," in *Book Parts*, 95–108.

26 Andrew Moore, Nathan Flis, and Francesca Vanke, eds., *The Paston Treasure: Microcosm of the Known World*, (New Haven, CT: Yale University Press, 2018); Spike Bucklow, *The Anatomy of Riches: Sir Robert Paston's Treasure* (London: Reaktion Books, 2018).

27 Hartman, sig., A2v. On Mayerne, see Brian Nance, *Turquet de Mayerne as Baroque Physician: The Art of Medical Portraiture* (Amsterdam: Rodopi, 2001). The manuscript in question might be MS Osborn fb255 in the Beinecke Rare Book and Manuscript Library, Yale University, New Haven, CT.

28 On these letters as a genre of writing see, Meaghan J. Brown, "Addresses to the Reader," in *Book Parts*, 81–94.

29 Hartman, sig., A3r.

30 Hartman, sig., A3v.

31 See, for example, Linda A. Pollock and Lady Grace Mildmay, *With Faith and Physic: The Life of a Tudor Gentlewoman, Lady Grace Mildmay, 1552–1620* (New York: St. Martin's Press, 1995); Alisha Rankin, *Panaceia's Daughters: Noblewomen as Healers in Early Modern Germany* (Chicago, IL: University of Chicago Press, 2013).

32 On medical economies and markets, see, Mark Jenner and Patrick Wallis, eds., *Medicine and the Market in England and Its Colonies, c.1450–c.1850* (Basingstoke: Palgrave Macmillan, 2007).

33 See, for example, Denis Duncan, "Indexing," in Ann Blair et al., *Information: A Historical Companion* (Princeton, NJ: Princeton University Press, 2021), 491–95.

34 For a recent overview, see, Olivia Weisser, "Disease," in *A Cultural History of Medicine: The Renaissance*, ed. Elaine Leong and Claudia Stein (London: Bloomsbury Academic, 2021), 63–84.

35 Hartman, 524.

36 Hartman, 222–29 (agues and fevers) and 259–73 (plague).

37 Hartman, 274–94 (cordial waters); 294–316 (strong waters) and 317–30 (cordial juleps) and 330–43.

38 Hartman, 330–60 and 360–402 (women's health) and 402–413 (remedies specifically designated for children), 414–25 (remedies addressing measles, smallpox, nosebleeds and more).

39 Hartman, 425- ("Miscellanea"); 468–70 (remedies for ailments in horses); 471–98 ("The True English Wine Celler"); 498–510 (preserving and pickling) and 511–24 ("The Cabinet of Safe Cosmetick Remedies").

40 Alun Withey, *Physick and the Family: Health, Medicine and Care in Wales 1600–1750* (Manchester: Manchester University Press, 2011).

41 Lynette Hunter, "Women and Domestic Medicine: Lady Experimenters, 1570–1620," in *Women, Science and Medicine, 1500–1700: Mothers and Sisters of the Royal Society*, ed. Lynette Hunter and Sarah Hutton (Stroud: Sutton Publishing, 1997), 89–107; Elizabeth Spiller, "Introduction," in *Seventeenth-Century English Recipe Books: Cooking, Physic and Chirurgery in the Works of Elizabeth Talbot Grey and Aletheia Talbot Howard: Essential Works for the Study of Early Modern Women: Series III, Part Three, Volume 3* (Aldershot: Ashgate Publishing, 2008), ix–li.

42 Gentilcore, *Food and Health in Early Modern Europe*; Edith Snook, *Women, Beauty, and Power in Early Modern England: A Feminist Literary History* (Basingstoke: Palgrave Macmillan, 2011); Montserrat Cabré, "Keeping Beauty Secrets in Early Modern Iberia," in *Secrets and Knowledge in Medicine and Science, 1500–1800*, ed. Elaine Leong and Alisha Rankin (Farnham: Ashgate Publishing, 2011), 167–90.

43 See, for example, Alisha Rankin, "The Housewife's Apothecary in Early Modern Austria: Wolfgang Helmhard von Hohberg's Georgica Curiosa (1682)," *Medicina & Storia* 8, no. 15 (2008): 55–76; Elizabeth Spiller, "Printed Recipe Books in Medical, Political,

and Scientific Contexts," in *The Oxford Handbook of Literature and the English Revolution*, ed. Laura Knoppers (Oxford: Oxford University Press, 2012), 516–33; Michelle DiMeo and Sara Pennell, eds., *Reading and Writing Recipe Books, 1550–1800* (Manchester: Manchester University Press, 2013); Elaine Leong, *Recipes and Everyday Knowledge: Medicine, Science and the Household in Early Modern England* (Chicago, IL: University of Chicago Press, 2018), Chapter 5.

44 Mary E. Fissell, "Women, Health and Healing in Early Modern Europe," *Bulletin for the History of Medicine* 82 (2008): 1–17; Sharon Strocchia, "Introduction: Women and Healthcare in Early Modern Europe," *Renaissance Studies* 28, no. 4 (2014): 496–514; Debra Blumenthal, "Domestic Medicine: Slaves, Servants and Female Medical Expertise in Late Medieval Valencia," *Renaissance Studies* 28, no. 4 (2014): 515–32; Stobart, *Household Medicine*.

45 Lucinda McCray Beier, "In Sickness and in Health: A Seventeenth Century Family's Experience," in *Patients and Practitioners: Lay Perceptions of Medicine in Pre-Industrial Society*, ed. Roy Porter (Cambridge: Cambridge University Press, 1985), 101–28; Lisa Smith, "The Relative Duties of a Man: Domestic Medicine in England and France, ca. 1685–1740," *Journal of Family History* 31, no. 3 (2006): 237–56.

46 See, for example, Sara Pennell, "Perfecting Practice? Women, Manuscript Recipes and Knowledge in Early Modern England," in *Early Modern Women's Manuscript Writing: Selected Papers from the Trinity/Trent Colloquium*, ed. Jonathan Gibson and Victoria E. Burke (Aldershot: Ashgate, 2004), 237–58; Lynette Hunter, "Women and Domestic Medicine: Lady Experimenters, 1570–1620," in *Women, Science and Medicine*, 89–107; Michelle DiMeo, "Authorship and Medical Networks: Reading Attributions in Early Modern Manuscript Recipe Books," in *Reading and Writing Recipe Books*, 25–46 and references in footnote 37.

47 Michael Foster, "Digby, Sir Kenelm (1603–1665), Natural Philosopher and Courtier," in *Oxford Dictionary of National Biography*, 2004, https://doi.org/10.1093/ref:odnb/7629; Lawrence Principe, "Sir Kenelm Digby and His Alchemical Circle in 1650s Paris: Newly Discovered Manuscripts," *Ambix* 60 (2013): 3–24.

48 Hartman claims that Digby "cur'd the Daughter of Sir William Curtius at Franckfort in Germany, in the year 1[6]59 of a corroding Ulcer in her Leg." Another example of a cure testimony is the recipe titled "An experienc'd Remedy against the Falling-sickness, wherewith Sir K Digby cur'd a Ministers Son at Franckfort in Germany in the year 1659" where Hartman claimed that the patient "was perfectly cur'd to which I was an Eyewitness, helping to prepare the said Remedy with my own hands." Hartman, 214–15 and 41–2.

49 Lady Crisp is likely the wife of Sir Nicholas Crisp, a royalist who also spent time exiled in France. She is credited as the author of a purging powder. See, for example, "Prince Rupert's Receipt to prepare the said Frankfurt Pills" and other references to his role as a recipe creator and knowledge mediator, Hartman, 198 (Lady Crisp), 132, 195, 290–91 (Prince Rupert). On Nicholas Crisp, see Ashton, R. Crisp, Sir Nicholas, first baronet (c. 1599–1666), merchant and royalist. *Oxford Dictionary of National Biography*. Retrieved 7 Oct. 2021, from https://www.oxforddnb.com/view/10.1093/ref:odnb/9780198614128.001.0001/odnb-9780198614128-e-6705.

50 Hartman, 218–20.

51 Rankin, "Experience." On observations and cases as medical genres, see Gianna Pomata, "Observation Rising: Birth of an Epistemic Genre, Ca. 1500–1650," in *Histories of Scientific Observation*, ed. Lorraine Daston and Elizabeth Lunbeck (Chicago, IL: University of Chicago Press, 2011), 55-88; Kassell, "Casebooks in Early Modern England."

52 Hartman, 424. The same recipe can be found in the *Pharmacopoeia Bateana* (London, 1694), 32.

53 Hartman, see, for example, for Riviére: 6, 345, 366, 406, 463; Harvey: 102, 131, 133, 235, 330–31; Mayerne: 6, 56, 228, 385; Sydenham: 201–202, 330, 366, 371, 378,

411–13 and Willis: 27, 43, 136, 142, 188, 192, 211, 224, 358, 370, 406. This list is illustrative and not exhaustive.

54 Early modern books were often sold as unbound sheets, enabling book owners to decide on the binding materials and style, as well as other accompanying titles to bind together as a volume. In the case of *The Family Physitian*, many surviving copies, such as the Clark library copy on EEBO, have the image bound in between the letter to the reader and the "explanation of the Figures" on signature A4r.

55 George Hartman, *The Preserver and Restorer of Health* (London, 1682), sigs., A6r-7v and engraving.

56 Hartman, Sig. A5v. Samuel Pepys and his wife visited Jamaica House in April 1667 and it seems that the building was part of a pleasure garden called Cherry Garden: see, "Parishes: Bermondsey," in *A History of the County of Surrey*: Volume 4, ed. H.E. Malden (London: Victoria County History, 1912), 17–24. British History Online, accessed September 22, 2021, http://www.british-history.ac.uk/vch/surrey/vol4/pp17-24.

57 Hartman, *Preserver*, Sig. A6v.

58 See, for example, Larry Stewart, "Science, Instruments, and Guilds in Early-Modern Britain," *Early Science and Medicine* 10, no. 3 (2005): 392–410; Mario Biagioli, "From Print to Patents: Living on Instruments in Early Modern Europe," *History of Science* 44, no. 2 (2006): 139–86.

59 Hartman provides instructions to the "The Queen of Hungary's Water as they make it in France"; however, he claims that the "true Royal Hungarian water as it was prepar'd for King Charles the II' exceeds the other in "Vertue against all cold Distempers of the Head and Brain, all affects of the Nerves and Joints &c." The recipe for this version of the water was given to Hartman by an "honourable Lady, who had it of the Illustrious Prince Rupert." As Hartman is under "an obligation not to publish it," he "prepare[s] it and sell[s] it to many of the Nobility and Gentry in this Kingdom," Hartman, 289–91 and 526.

60 David Boyd Haycock and Patrick Wallis, "Quackery and Commerce in Seventeenth-Century London: The Proprietary Medicine Business of Anthony Daffy," *Medical History.* Supplement no. 25 (2005): 1–216; Porter, *Health for Sale.*

Bibliography

Primary Sources

Hartman, George. *The Family Physitian, or A Collection of Choice, Approv'd and Experienc'd Remedies, for the Cure of Almost All Diseases Incident to Humane Bodies, Whether Internal or External; Useful in Families, and Very Serviceable to Country People. Containing Some Hundreds of Considerable Receipts and Secrets of Great Vallue, with Observations of Great Cures. Together with the True English Wine-Celler, and the Right Method of Making the English-Wines, or Metheglin: With a Collection of the Choicest and Safest Cosmetick Remedies for Preserving the Beauty and Complection of Ladies, Never before Publish'd. By Geo. Hartman, Phylo Chymist, Author of the Preserver and Restorer of Health, Who Liv'd and Travell'd with the Honourable Sir Kenelm Digby in Several Parts of Europe, the Space of Seven Years till He Died.* London: printed for Richard Wellington, at the Lute in St. Pauls-Church-Yard, 1696.

———. *The True Preserver and Restorer of Health: Being a Choice Collection of Select and Experienced Remedies for All Distempers Incident to Men, Women and Children. Selected from, and Experienced by the Most Famous Physicians and Chyrurgions in Europe. Together with Excellent Directions for Cookery; as Also for Preserving, and Conserving, and Making All Sorts of Metheglin, Sider, Cherry-Vvine, &c. With the Description of an Ingenious and Useful Engin for Dressing of Meat, and for Distilling the Choicest Cordial

Waters without Wood, Coals, Candle, or Oyl. Published for the Publick Good, by G. Hartman, Chymist. London: printed by T. B[raddyll]. for the author and are to be sold at his house in Hewes-Court in Black-Friers, 1682.

Secondary Sources

Adams, Thomas R., and Nicolas Barker. "A New Model for the Study of the Book." In *A Potencie of Life: Books in Society. The Clark Lectures 1986-1987*, edited by Nicolas Barker, 5–43. London: British Library, 1993.

Arber, Agnes Robertson. *Herbals: Their Origin and Evolution: A Chapter in the History of Botany, 1470-1670*. 3rd ed. Introduction and Annotations by William T. Stearn. Cambridge: Cambridge University Press, 1953.

Ashton, R. Crisp, Sir Nicholas, first baronet (c. 1599–1666), merchant and royalist. *Oxford Dictionary of National Biography*. Accessed 7 October 2021, https://www.oxforddnb.com/view/10.1093/ref:odnb/9780198614128.001.0001/odnb-9780198614128-e-6705.

Barker, Sara K., and Brenda M. Hosington. *Renaissance Cultural Crossroads: Translation, Print and Culture in Britain, 1473-1640*. Leiden: Brill Academic Publishing, 2013.

Beier, Lucinda McCray. "In Sickness and in Health: A Seventeenth Century Family's Experience." In *Patients and Practitioners. Lay Perceptions of Medicine in Pre-Industrial Society*, edited by Roy Porter, 101–28. Cambridge: Cambridge University Press, 1985.

Bell, Maureen. "Mise-en-Page, Illustration, Expressive Form." In *The Cambridge History of the Book in Britain: Volume 4: 1557–1695*, edited by D. F. McKenzie and John Barnard, 4:632–62. Cambridge: Cambridge University Press, 2002.

Biagioli, Mario. "From Print to Patents: Living on Instruments in Early Modern Europe." *History of Science* 44, no. 2 (2006): 139–86.

Blumenthal, Debra. "Domestic Medicine: Slaves, Servants and Female Medical Expertise in Late Medieval Valencia." *Renaissance Studies* 28, no. 4 (2014): 515–32.

Bouras-Vallianatos, Petros, and Barbara Zipser, eds. *Brill's Companion to the Reception of Galen*. Leiden: Brill, 2019.

Brown, Meaghan J. "Addresses to the Reader." In *Book Parts*, edited by Dennis Duncan and Adam Smyth, 81–94. Oxford: Oxford University Press, 2019.

Bucklow, Spike. *The Anatomy of Riches: Sir Robert Paston's Treasure*. London: Reaktion Books, 2018.

Cabré, Montserrat. "Keeping Beauty Secrets in Early Modern Iberia." In *Secrets and Knowledge in Medicine and Science, 1500-1800*, edited by Elaine Leong and Alisha Rankin, 167–90. Farnham: Ashgate, 2011.

Capp, Bernard. *Astrology and the Popular Press: English Almanacs 1500-1800*. London: Faber and Faber, 1979.

Darnton, Robert. "First Steps Toward a History of Reading." *Australian Journal of French Studies* 23, no. 1 (1986): 5–30.

———. "What Is the History of Books?" *Daedalus* 111, no. 3 (1982): 65–83.

———. "'What Is the History of Books?' Revisited." *Modern Intellectual History* 4, no. 3 (2007): 495–508.

DiMeo, Michelle. "Authorship and Medical Networks: Reading Attributions in Early Modern Manuscript Recipe Books." In *Reading and Writing Recipe Books 1550-1800*, edited by Michelle DiMeo and Sara Pennell, 25–46. Manchester: Manchester University Press, 2013.

DiMeo, Michelle, and Sara Pennell, eds. *Reading and Writing Recipe Books, 1550-1800*. Manchester: Manchester University Press, 2013.

Duncan, Dennis. "Indexing." In *Information: A Historical Companion*, edited by Ann Blair, Paul Duguid, Anja-Silvia Goeing, and Anthony Grafton, 491–95. Princeton, NJ: Princeton University Press, 2021.

Duncan, Dennis, and Adam Smyth, eds. *Book Parts*. Oxford: Oxford University Press, 2019.

Eamon, William. *Science and the Secrets of Nature: Books of Secrets in Medieval and Early Modern Culture*. Princeton, NJ: Princeton University Press, 1994.

Fissell, Mary E. "Popular Medical Writing." In *The Oxford History of Popular Print Culture: Volume One: Cheap Print in Britain and Ireland to 1660*, edited by Joad Raymond, 417–30. Oxford: Oxford University Press, 2011.

———. "The Marketplace of Print." In *The Medical Marketplace and Its Colonies c. 1450-c 1850*, edited by Mark Jenner and Patrick Wallis, 108–32. Basingstoke: Palgrave Macmillan, 2007.

———. *Vernacular Bodies: The Politics of Reproduction in Early Modern England*. Oxford: Oxford University Press, 2004.

———. "Readers, Texts, and Contexts: Vernacular Medical Works in Early Modern England." In *The Popularization of Medicine, 1650-1850*, edited by Roy Porter, 72–96. London: Routledge, 1992.

———. "Women, Health and Healing in Early Modern Europe." *Bulletin for the History of Medicine* 82 (2008): 1–17.

Foster, Michael. "Digby, Sir Kenelm (1603–1665), Natural Philosopher and Courtier." In *Oxford Dictionary of National Biography*, 2004.

Franklin, Alexandra. "Woodcuts." In *Book Parts*, edited by Dennis Duncan and Adam Smyth, 209–22. Oxford: Oxford University Press, 2019.

Gaskell, Philip. *A New Introduction to Bibliography*. New Castle, DE: Oak Knoll Press, 1995.

Gentilcore, David. *Food and Health in Early Modern Europe*. London: Bloomsbury Academic, 2015.

Harding, Vanessa. "Reading Plague in Seventeenth-Century London." *Social History of Medicine* 32, no. 2 (2019): 267–86.

Haycock, David Boyd, and Patrick Wallis. "Quackery and Commerce in Seventeenth-Century London: The Proprietary Medicine Business of Anthony Daffy." *Medical History. Supplement*, no. 25 (2005): 1–216.

Hunter, Lynette. "Sisters of the Royal Society: The Circle of Katherine Jones, Lady Ranelagh." In *Women, Science and Medicine, 1500-1700: Mothers and Sisters of the Royal Society*, edited by Lynette Hunter and Sarah Hutton, 187–97. Stroud: Sutton Publishing, 1997.

———. "Women and Domestic Medicine: Lady Experimenters, 1570-1620." In *Women, Science and Medicine, 1500-1700: Mothers and Sisters of the Royal Society*, edited by Lynette Hunter and Sarah Hutton, 89–107. Stroud: Sutton Publishing, 1997.

Isaac, Peter. "Pills and Print." In *Medicine, Mortality, and the Book Trade*, edited by Robin Myers and Michael Harris, 25–47. Folkestone, Oak Knoll Press, 1998.

Jenner, Mark, and Patrick Wallis, eds. *Medicine and the Market in England and Its Colonies, c.1450-c.1850*. Basingstoke: Palgrave Macmillan, 2007.

Jardine, Lisa, and Anthony Grafton. "'Studied for Action': How Gabriel Harvey Read His Livy." *Past & Present* 129, no. 1 (1990): 30–78.

Johns, Adrian. *The Nature of the Book: Print and Knowledge in the Making*. Chicago, IL: University of Chicago Press, 1998.

Jones, Lori. "Itineraries and Transformations: John of Burgundy's Plague Treatise." *Bulletin of the History of Medicine* 95, no. 3 (2021): 277–314.

Jones, Peter Murray. "Reading Medicine in Tudor Cambridge." In *The History of Medical Education in Britain*, edited by Vivian Nutton and Roy Porter, 153–83. Amsterdam: Rodopi, 1995.

———. "The Tabula Medicine: An Evolving Encyclopaedia." *English Manuscript Studies: 1100-1700* 14 (2008): 60–85.

Kassell, Lauren. "Casebooks in Early Modern England: Medicine, Astrology, and Written Records." *Bulletin of the History of Medicine* 88, no. 4 (2014): 595–625.

———. "Secrets Revealed: Alchemical Books in Early Modern England." *History of Science* 49, no. 1 (2011): 61–125.

Laroche, Rebecca. *Medical Authority and Englishwomen's Herbal Texts, 1550-1650*. Aldershot: Ashgate, 2009.

Leong, Elaine. "'Herbals She Peruseth': Reading Medicine in Early Modern England." *Renaissance Studies* 28, no. 4 (2014): 556–78.

———. *Recipes and Everyday Knowledge: Medicine, Science, and the Household in Early Modern England*. Chicago, IL: University of Chicago Press, 2018.

———. "Transformative Itineraries and Communities of Knowledge in Early Modern Europe: The Case of Lazare Rivière's *The Practice of Physick*." In *Civic Medicine: Physician, Polity, and Pen in Early Modern Europe*, edited by J. Andrew Mendelsohn, Annemarie Kinzelbach, and Ruth Schilling, 257–79. New York: Routledge, 2019.

Leong, Elaine, and Alisha Rankin. "Testing Drugs and Trying Cures: Experiment and Medicine in Medieval and Early Modern Europe." *Bulletin of the History of Medicine* 91, no. 2 (2017): 157–82.

McKenzie, D. F. *Bibliography and the Sociology of Texts: The Panizzi Lectures*. London: The British Library, 1986.

———. *Making Meaning: "Printers of the Mind" and Other Essays*. Edited by Peter D. McDonald and Michael Felix Suarez. Amherst: University of Massachusetts Press, 2002.

———. "Printing and Publishing 1557–1700: Constraints on the London Book Trades." In *The Cambridge History of the Book in Britain: Volume 4: 1557–1695*, edited by D. F. McKenzie and John Barnard, 553–67. Cambridge: Cambridge University Press, 2002.

Moore, Andrew, Nathan Flis, and Francesca Vanke, eds. *The Paston Treasure: Microcosm of the Known World*. New Haven, CT: Yale University Press, 2018.

Nance, Brian. *Turquet de Mayerne as Baroque Physician: The Art of Medical Portraiture*. Amsterdam: Rodopi, 2001.

North, Marcy. *The Anonymous Renaissance: Cultures of Discretion in Tudor-Stuart England*. Chicago, IL: University of Chicago Press, 2003.

"Parishes: Bermondsey." In *A History of the County of Surrey*, 17–24. Volume 4. Edited by H E Malden. London: Victoria County History, 1912. British History Online. Accessed 22 September 2021, http://www.british-history.ac.uk/vch/surrey/vol4/pp17-24.

Pennell, Sara. "Perfecting Practice? Women, Manuscript Recipes and Knowledge in Early Modern England." In *Early Modern Women's Manuscript Writing. Selected Papers from the Trinity/Trent Colloquium*, edited by Jonathan Gibson and Victoria E. Burke, 237–58. Aldershot: Ashgate, 2004.

Pollock, Linda A., and Lady Grace Mildmay. *With Faith and Physic: The Life of a Tudor Gentlewoman, Lady Grace Mildmay, 1552-1620*. New York: St. Martin's Press, 1995.

Pomata, Gianna. "Observation Rising: Birth of an Epistemic Genre, 1500–1650." In *Histories of Scientific Observation*, edited by Lorraine Daston and Elizabeth Lunbeck, 55–88. Chicago, IL: University of Chicago Press, 2011.

Porter, Roy. *Health for Sale: Quackery in England, 1660-1850*. Manchester: Manchester University Press, 1989.

Principe, Lawrence. "Sir Kenelm Digby and His Alchemical Circle in 1650s Paris: Newly Discovered Manuscripts." *Ambix* 60 (2013): 3–24.

Rankin, Alisha. "Experience." In *A Cultural History of Medicine: The Renaissance*, edited by Elaine Leong and Claudia Stein, 141–62. London: Bloomsbury Academic, 2021.

———. *Panaceia's Daughters: Noblewomen as Healers in Early Modern Germany*. Chicago, IL: University of Chicago Press, 2013.

———. "The Housewife's Apothecary in Early Modern Austria: Wolfgang Helmhard von Hohberg's Georgica Curiosa (1682)." *Medicina & Storia* 8, no. 15 (2008): 55–76.

Raymond, Joad, ed. *The Oxford History of Popular Print Culture: Cheap Print in Britain and Ireland to 1660*. Oxford: Oxford University Press, 2011.

Raven, James, ed. *The Oxford Illustrated History of the Book*. Oxford: Oxford University Press, 2020.

Roberts, Sean. "Engravings." In *Book Parts*, edited by Dennis Duncan and Adam Smyth, 81–94. Oxford: Oxford University Press, 2019.

Sherman, William H. *Used Books: Marking Readers in Renaissance England*. Philadelphia: University of Pennsylvania Press, 2008.

Slack, Paul. "Mirrors of Health and Treasures of Poor Men: The Uses of the Vernacular Medical Literature of Tudor England." In *Health, Medicine, and Mortality in the Sixteenth Century*, edited by Charles Webster, 237–73. Cambridge: Cambridge University Press, 1979.

Smith, Helen. "Acknowledgements and Dedications." In *Book Parts*, edited by Dennis Duncan and Adam Smyth, 95–108. Oxford: Oxford University Press, 2019.

Smith, Helen, and Louise Wilson, eds. *Renaissance Paratexts*. Cambridge: Cambridge University Press, 2011.

Smith, Lisa. "The Relative Duties of a Man: Domestic Medicine in England and France, ca. 1685–1740." *Journal of Family History* 31, no. 3 (2006): 237–56.

Smyth, Adam. *Material Texts in Early Modern England*. Cambridge: Cambridge University Press, 2018.

Snook, Edith. *Women, Beauty, and Power in Early Modern England: A Feminist Literary History*. Basingstoke: Palgrave Macmillan, 2011.

Spiller, Elizabeth. "Introduction." In *Seventeenth-Century English Recipe Books: Cooking, Physic and Chirurgery in the Works of Elizabeth Talbot Grey and Aletheia Talbot Howard: Essential Works for the Study of Early Modern Women: Series III, Part Three, Volume 3*, ix–li. Aldershot: Ashgate, 2008.

———. "Printed Recipe Books in Medical, Political, and Scientific Contexts." In *The Oxford Handbook of Literature and the English Revolution*, edited by Laura Knoppers, 516–33. Oxford: Oxford University Press, 2012.

Stewart, Larry. "Science, Instruments, and Guilds in Early-Modern Britain." *Early Science and Medicine* 10, no. 3 (2005): 392–410. http://www.jstor.org/stable/4130335.

Stobart, Anne. *Household Medicine in Seventeenth-Century England*. London: Bloomsbury Publishing, 2016.

Strocchia, Sharon. "Introduction: Women and Healthcare in Early Modern Europe." *Renaissance Studies* 28, no. 4 (2014): 496–514.

Weisser, Olivia. "Disease." In *A Cultural History of Medicine: The Renaissance*, edited by Elaine Leong and Claudia Stein, 63–84. London: Bloomsbury Academic, 2021.

Werner, Sarah. *Studying Early Printed Books, 1450-1800: A Practical Guide*. Hoboken: Wiley, 2018.

Withey, Alun. *Physick and the Family: Health, Medicine, and Care in Wales 1600-1750*. Manchester: Manchester University Press, 2011.

Part III

The Everyday

12 Life Writing

Olivia Weisser

Thomas Thistlewood moved from rural England to a Jamaican sugar plantation at the age of 29. He worked there as an overseer for years, later purchasing his own plantation. Throughout his time in Jamaica, he was a brutal manager and enslaver. He was horrifically abusive toward captive men and repeatedly forced enslaved women to have sex with him. There is much to say about this cruel man, but I began reading his diary in search of one small piece of it: near ever-present venereal disease. Shortly after moving to his new tropical home in 1751, Thistlewood developed sores and swellings in his groin, burning while urinating, painful involuntary erections, small fleshy caruncles on his penis, and continual discharges that he referred to as "runnings."[1] He offers a rare first-hand narrative of a stigmatizing disease that few individuals in the era admitted to having in writing. I consulted the diary in search of what I might glean from this unusually candid commentary on venereal disease.

A diary like this one is a valuable historical source, most obviously because it offers a first-person narrative. But also, the impressive size and detail of Thistlewood's archive – his diary spans 10,000 pages, and he also left behind 35 weather journals, among numerous other items – provide insights into one man's life and illness that would be challenging to access otherwise. I learned, for example, the books on medicine that he owned and likely consulted, the recipes he recorded (and presumably used), and subtle changes in how he viewed and wrote about his own ailment over the years. In 1755, he hinted at a familiarity with venereal disease when he noted a "sort of tickling in the urethra" that he associated with imminent improvement. A year later, he found a caruncle "in the old Place," a turn of phrase that suggests a recurring and well-known condition. And after struggling to describe a sensation in his sore thighs – it was like a muscle ache "just as after hard leaping" – he resorted to the more reliable memory of experiences past: "this I have observed beffore."[2] What began as a litany of complaints in the early volumes of the diary developed into references to familiar sensations and expectations just a few years later. The sheer length and detail of Thistlewood's diary expose a subtle, growing awareness of the disease and how to treat it.

While some diaries offer a trove of fruitful information, others are more like haystacks with a handful of precious needles buried deep inside. William Byrd's diary spanning 1717–1721 is filled with notes about propositioning prostitutes in

DOI: 10.4324/9781003094876-16

London's "bagnios." Much like Thistlewood, Byrd suffered from recurring symptoms of venereal disease and did not seem to harbor much, if any, guilt about continuing to "roger" women at bathhouses while obviously infected with a sexually transmitted disease. Yet as a source of information about the pox, Byrd's diary is starkly different than Thistlewood's. Byrd provides scant information about his illness other than its appearance and disappearance: "My running was very bad. My physic worked by once."[3] The entries that mention health are terse and repetitive, with little reflection on how the disease felt or what it meant. What do we do with a source like this one? This chapter offers some strategies for analyzing life writing – an umbrella term for first-hand accounts of lived experiences – that range from detailed diaries like Thistlewood's to terse and seemingly impenetrable writing like Byrd's.

For all its value, Thistlewood's archive is not an easy one to use. His handwriting is messy and the diary is massive, spanning 38 years. I came to this source from a particularly advantageous position, however. Not only is the entire archive digitized and available online through Yale University's Beinecke Rare Book and Manuscript Library but also an exceedingly generous historian, Claire Gherini, shared transcriptions of several volumes of the diary with me. Added to this gift, a final piece of luck: Thistlewood coded the days he felt sick with the symbol #. Those marks could serve as a guide through the mire, an imperfect map of moments of illness. Skimming an existing transcription of the diary for the symbol # would make quick work of an otherwise daunting task, effectively capturing episodes of venereal disease that I wanted to study. While tempting, this approach is problematic. I surely would miss entries that were not coded. But most importantly, I would not develop a full sense of the author nor his writing. Such an approach would invite a surface-level report, unmoored from the man and the context in which he wrote. It would result in a superficial account of an otherwise rich and complex source.

There is immense value to embracing other approaches to analyzing life writing, ones that may be more time-consuming but that invite deeper interpretation. This chapter offers a few possible strategies, including how to ask questions, attend to genre conventions and authors' predilections, and locate and explain patterns. Such methods require reading and thinking about sources in their totality, beyond discrete episodes of interest. Analyzing an entire source (or substantial portions of it, in the case of Thistlewood) may not always be possible on account of limited access, time, or even our own ingrained ways of reading. Some scholars have suggested that fragmentary reading is the new normal, a result of technologies like databases and digitization.[4] Yet attempting to read sources in their totality, if possible, can bear rich fruit. It can lead to fuller, more textured, and more compelling findings. And it can turn the elements of life writing that are most challenging – in the instance of Thistlewood, scope and detail – into virtues. (So, too, examining original manuscripts that contain marginalia, scribbles, or changes in ink can be instructive, although accessing manuscripts is not always feasible.) Life writing that covers several years and documents the dailiness of life allows historians to chart medical matters over long time spans and to situate debility within everyday events and beliefs. We might learn, for instance, how an illness disrupted routines, fractured relationships, or intersected with other, seemingly unrelated events. One enormous value of life writing is that it places medical events in non-medical contexts. We can view illness within a constellation of a life, a personality, a community, and a writing practice. In telling us what it meant to be sick, life writing exposes so much more, including what it meant to be well.

Perhaps a most obvious, initial step to approaching any historical source is to consider its content: What is it that you want to know? Classic histories of early modern medicine centered on life writing have tended to focus on the patient's point of view, while more recent scholarship has showcased a broad range of medical themes, including reproductive health, disability, occupational hazards, reading practices, conceptions of emotions, approaches to death, household medicine, and relationships with practitioners, among others.[5]

As I began reading Thistlewood's diary, I was looking for information about how he treated his recurring venereal symptoms at home. Very few people documented such self-treatment because few admitted to having venereal disease at all. Finding this information in a first-person account seemed unlikely, but I saw hints of it early on in Thistlewood's diary. In 1751, he paid a physician to supply a wide range of anti-venereal therapies, including mercury pills, cooling powders and salts, an electuary, and balsam drops. Added to these prescribed treatments, he chose to bathe his penis twice daily in warm "new milk" and rubbed protuberances with a silver probe. These small examples compelled me to keep reading in search of others. Sure enough, as the years passed, he experimented with variations of these home therapies. He altered his bath to rum and warm water and, for a while, rum and soap. And he swapped out the silver probe for a lead one and made alterations to his diet by avoiding lime juice, punch, and spirits that might "hinder my mending."[6] Over the years, he became ever confident about his own self-care. By 1757, he regularly consumed *balsam caprivi* drops, a mixture of herbs dissolved in turpentine prescribed by the plantation's doctor. But he was doing so on his own terms. After taking the remedy one November day, he noted: "am afraid it is too soon." And when the doctor sent over eight papers of cinchona bark to treat a fever, Thistlewood chose "to recover without." Although he sought out help from several medical authorities in the first few years after moving to Jamaica, about six years later, Thistlewood was barely consulting anyone at all.[7] Finding this information took time – it spans many years and involved reading entries that did not mention medicine at all – and demonstrates the challenges and rewards of using life writing to answer specific content-driven questions.

But summing up Thistlewood's self-treatments is not the work of analysis. One way to shift from surface-level reporting to deeper interpretation is to ask analytical questions: who, what, where, when, and why. Any question is fair game, but "how" and "why" questions tend to be more rewarding than "what" or "when" questions because they require complex, thoughtful answers. Reading a diary and asking, "what were the symptoms of gout" would result in a fairly definitive list. But reading that same diary and asking, "how did gout affect reputation," requires interpretation of the text to answer. Where is the author writing and how is location a factor in his or her construction of medical issues? Who is the author and how might their gender, spiritual beliefs, age, marital status, economic background, race, and so on determine the ways they wrote about ill health, pain, reproductive health, clinical relationships, emotional health, and so on? I wrote a book that analyzed how gender norms and assumptions shaped patients' perceptions of illness.[8] One of my findings was that numerous women in early modern England seemed to mirror the illnesses of their loved ones, a kind of mimetic suffering that, I argue, was informed by gendered ways of thinking, writing, and conceptualizing bodies. Asking an analytical question ("how did gender shape ways of writing about illness?") allowed me to find this pattern in the sources (so many women seemed to fall sick from grief and fear, and their sicknesses mirrored the conditions of family members they were grieving) and connect that pattern to gendered ways of writing, working, and emoting. I had to read primary sources in their entirety to do that work, which allowed me to situate women's accounts of illness within their particular ways of writing and thinking more generally.

My own work on gender, as well as the other analytical questions posed above, presumes that there is a "self" behind life writing – an identity that can be removed and analyzed apart from the content left behind. Analyzing that self and how or why it created the writing it did requires asking questions that may not be medical per se but are still relevant to work on the history of medicine. You might ask, for example, how authors construct a sense of themselves in writing, a long-enduring interest of literary scholars and historians alike.[9] Questions about authors' biographical backgrounds and self-constructions also can lead to new, related questions that open up larger, possibly exciting realms of analysis. Let's say you are interested in social status and medicine. A starting question might be: How did an author's status affect their experiences of health and illness? Or, to frame this in a way that gets at the self: How did an author's status affect the ways they conceptualized and documented experiences of health and illness? Sometimes it is easier to pose a question in a comparative way: How did a middling-status bookseller write about health differently than a wealthy land owner? This starting point can open up related questions that invite explorations of additional ways that social status might have informed constructions of illness and/or the self in early modern life writing. Did less well-off patients express different bodily concerns than wealthy ones? Did the bookseller forge particular kinds of relationships with his healers? Or have different priorities than his wealthier counterpart? How might occupations or daily work inform how people made sense of various aspects of health? What about how they treated or described specific conditions like pain? When a shopkeeper named Roger Lowe fell ill from a "cramp" in his back, for example, he measured his recovery by his ability to open his shop.[10] What was the barometer of debility for a well-to-do individual?

Questions about genre, authorial intent, and audience also can be particularly useful strategies for analyzing life writing and the self. What kind of source is this? Why was it written? How did genre shape the ways the author documented health issues? Why is an author focusing on this or that particular theme? These types of questions are useful, foremost, because there were many and often overlapping genres of life writing in this period, each with their own conventions and norms. The term "diary" is tempting to use when writing about sources like Thistlewood's, but it can be misleading. Much of the life writing from the early modern period does not fit the genre of a diary as we think of it (i.e., private, introspective record keeping). Rather than confidential, most of the diaries in the period were written for public or semi-public consumption. Some authors were explicit about their audiences: they wrote to future generations or to posterity. Others circulated their writing among friends and family.[11] In addition to being far from private, much of the early modern writing resembling diaries was composed retrospectively. What seems like a daily diary at first sight might, in reality, be edited, re-written, or compiled long after documented events took place. One author recorded information on scraps of paper that he later copied into his "great diurnell," sometimes adding new information along the way. And by studying editing marks and handwriting, scholars have determined that some diarists likely wrote entries in batches long after the fact.[12] Many published editions of early modern diaries and autobiographies are actually the complex productions of nineteenth-century editors, patched together from several manuscript sources to create a chronological narrative. Multiple accounts of the same event can reveal contradictory information and diverging tones, challenging any notion of a single, lived truth captured in life writing.[13]

Diaries and autobiographies are just two of a vast range of genres of life writing in the period. There also were spiritual accounts, travel logs, memoranda, calendars, reading notes, weather journals, memoirs, and more. Some surviving sources are hybrids of more than one of these categories. A man named Thomas Tyldesley kept a diary that doubled as an account book, for example, which he used to record business transactions alongside descriptions of his debilitating bowel disorders. Another diarist kept a massive seven-volume journal that functioned as both diary and commonplace book, a popular form of writing that entailed recording and reflecting on passages and quotations sort of like a literary scrapbook.[14] Perhaps more difficult to parse are the types of life writing that take non-narrative forms, such as annotations in the margins of almanacs and recipe books. Scholars studying marginal notes have re-conceptualized these kinds of texts as key forms of life writing in the early modern period. They were, after all, places where individuals recorded their lives and constructed a sense of themselves in writing.[15]

Determining genre is not always straightforward. Sometimes authors offer hints in their titles or in the text itself. A spiritual diary might be titled, "A Spiritual Diary," which leaves little guesswork. One seventeenth-century diary begins with a helpful explainer: "A Diary of the Actions & accidents of my Life: tending partly to observe & memorize the Providences therein manifested; & partly to investigate the Measure of Time in Astronomical Directions, and to determine the Astrall Causes."[16] This diarist outlines his two (perhaps surprisingly) compatible goals of documenting daily events for signs of divine providence and for evidence that the positions of celestial bodies can predict terrestrial events. If genre is not so easily discernable, another tack is to consider authorial intent. Was the author recording travels for posterity? Documenting military feats? Tabulating debts? Tracking spiritual progress?

Asking questions about genre and authorial intent are useful analytical strategies because they shaped content. Explaining the relationship between form and content requires unpacking the production of a source and explaining what it reveals or obscures about medicine. Memoirs and autobiographies tend to chart extraordinary or memorable life events. As a result, they are likely to include different kinds of information (brushes with death, miraculous recoveries) than diaries that focus on the minutiae of daily life. Autobiographies are also likely to contain less detail than diaries, as authors often wrote them retrospectively. Most terse of all are "memorandum books." An entry from one such book reads: "I had a feavour at York, which lasted 10 days."[17] The length of this illness is noteworthy, but the author provides little else about the incident other than its location. Such brevity perhaps explains why this text is archived as a memorandum book rather than an autobiography, but such genre distinctions can be blurry.

A spiritual journal, on the other hand, is likely to include copious details within a religious frame. Mary Rich was a deeply pious gentlewoman whose first-person accounts offer an illustrative example of how a particular genre of life writing can determine content. Exposing and explaining those connections, as I attempt to do here, is one approach to analysis. Rich compiled her diary, foremost, as a daily religious exercise: writing offered her a tool for tabulating her daily devotional routines, as well as a way to reflect on her life and assign it divine meaning. This dual use of writing as a form of spiritual account keeping and self-reflection was quite common among the godly in the period and there were well-understood conventions that dictated it. Most of Rich's entries begin with a careful account of her devotional duties, which included meditation and prayer:

> in the morneing as sone as I waked I blest God, then I reatired in to the willderness to meditate, but finding upon my selfe auery disturbeing fitt of the spleene I was by it much unfitted for the duty.

She used this wording so often that she resorted to abbreviations by the fourth volume of the diary: "in the m as sone as I w I B G I spent not so much time as useall at my deuotiones haueing a distemper then upon me."[18] Analysis can be the work of linking a particular formulation – in this instance, recurring accounts of devotional duties – to the written conventions of a source.

So, too, is making connections between Rich's genre of writing and her constructions of health. She continually refers to her own illnesses as "afflictions," a term that was commonly used in religious writing to describe the divine significance of life's trials, medical or otherwise. As an affliction, ill health could take on multiple spiritual meanings: it could be an indicator of salvation, a reminder of death, a test of faith, a providential warning, and so on. In the above quotation, Rich connects her inability to pray to a "distemper then upon me." She does this again and again in the diary, describing physical infirmity in terms of its effects on her ability to carry out devotional duties. Another example is from 1668: "by reason of my bodely distemper I was somthing duller then useall yet I fond the deasires of my heart went out after God."[19] Rich's ailing body, it seems, was a sort of gauge of her spirituality. I can only make this claim – a link between the religious nature of her journal and her resulting constructions of illness – when I account for how her writing was a formulaic mode of spiritual self-monitoring.

Thistlewood wrote within the frame of financial rather than religious account keeping. Meticulous record keeping was key to being a successful enslaver, a way to track output and expenses most efficiently. Such aims informed how Thistlewood recorded non-work-related aspects of his life, too, from the type of game he shot to the locations where he forced himself on enslaved women. He wrote, it seems, as an exercise in recording daily transactions for his own needs and self-satisfaction. His diary documents interesting gossip to remember, barters so he might hold others accountable, and work performed (or not) on the plantation to track who to fire and who to hire. Resulting entries tend to read like collections of mundane transactions. Unsurprisingly, so do his accounts of health: "In ye Euening Rec:d by Clara a Vomit ffor Robert, & a blanket, a Purge ffor Luacoo and some Basilicon ffor my self, also a Potte ffrom Mrs Joseph Borloche." This entry focuses mostly on remedies provided by an enslaved woman named Clara and the wife of a local doctor named Joseph Borloch. Much like the rest of the diary, it is a list of matter-of-fact exchanges: who provided what and to whom. Entries tracking venereal symptoms are similarly quantifiable and brief: "running much as before," "continue growing rather worse," "continues much the same."[20] Here Thistlewood records the ebbs and flows of his venereal emissions, comparing each day to the one that came before. This form of writing, while terse, still offers useful information, including the financial implications of illness, relationships with healers, and treatments.

A wigmaker and book trader from Manchester named Edmund Harrold did not have venereal disease, but accounting informed his life writing in similar ways. His diary is filled with calculations of his spiritual development, business transactions, and all kinds of other intimate details: "on ye 9th at night I did wife 2 tymes couch and bed in an hour an 1/2 time." Harrold's accounts of illness are likewise terse and comparative, as they too were shaped by his approach to diary writing as a form of daily accounting: "[Sept.] 3 I was Extream ill & 4 as so and 5th worst of all." Similarly, a man named Giles Moore wrote in 1668:

> Finding my selfe distempered I swet myselfe 3 or 4 houres, which day & the next I was tolerably well. On the 14th Beeing Friday I had an high feaver & was very sick all that day & the forepart of the night On Sunday the 16th Beeing my Feaver day I tooke Physick & was mighty sicke. About 4 post meridiem I began to swete & grew better On Tuesday the 18th my feaver held mee strong from 3 in the Morning till about 1 in the afternoone which day I purging by Sirop of Roses very gratly & frequently On Thursday the 20th the Feaver did Sensebly abate. On Saturday the 22th I lost my Feaver (Deo gratias).[21]

For Moore, much like Thistlewood and Harrold, a diary was not a place to ruminate on spiritual matters so much as to tabulate daily activities. These men might have been pious. There are hints of faith, for example, in the quick thanks to God ("Deo gratias") at the end of the above passage. But the dominant mode in that excerpt is quantification rather than spiritual reflection: the length of a sweat, the duration of a fever, the frequency of a purge. The intentions and conventions of life writing informed the ways these men recorded life events, illness included. Exposing the links between form and content, as I do here (and above with Rich), is the work of analysis. It involves close reading, picking apart illustrative examples, and connecting disparate sources to expose patterns.

Another way of connecting form and content is by way of an author's audience. Determining readership might shed light on surprising aspects of a source, such as why one diarist seemed to document more information about the health of his horse than about himself or his family. Another author, Dionys Fitzherbert, penned an account of a six-month-long delusional state in an attempt to convince her friends and family that she suffered from a spiritual trial rather than physical melancholy.[22] Her motive and intended audience are connected and both are crucial to understanding the resulting narrative. A different but no less illustrative example is an autobiographical account by a woman named Alice Thornton. She organized her writing around significant accidents and events, such as swallowing a pin or life-threatening childbirth. She also was religious, and writing afforded her a way to consider her own spiritual journey. But she wrote with a specific audience in mind. Thornton was writing to her community and posterity to salvage her reputation from vicious slander. Her imagined readers clearly informed her self-portrayals, which tended to involve overcoming near-continual hardship. In 1666, she describes her "daily decay and dieing condittion." She was not simply ill, but "exceeding feeble and weake" for weeks on end. She endured "continuall faintings upon the reneuall of the extreamity" and she referred to her malady as a "terrible visitation and languishing condition." She documents numerous similar episodes, as well. In 1654, she explains how her "deare mother and aunt and friends did not expect my life" and in 1665, she describes "beeing soe weake … that all gave me for dead."[23] Thornton was not fabricating these brushes with death nor their severity. Yet the number and nature of them are noteworthy. Extreme physical infirmity seemed to provide her a way to demonstrate distress as virtue. For Thornton, physical suffering was a site of self-constitution and her imagined audience made such self-presentations possible.

So far, I have suggested several approaches to analyzing life writing that require reading sources fully rather than cherry-picking episodes on discrete themes. One strategy involves asking analytical questions, either about content or about how authors' biographical details might have shaped constructions of themselves and medical matters. Another strategy is attending to genre conventions, authorial motivations, and intended readerships, and examining how those various factors might have informed resulting accounts in writing. A final strategy is to read for patterns. I have tried to model this last approach throughout this chapter. For example, I noted Mary Rich's tendency to refer to her illnesses as "afflictions" and to conceptualize her health as a measure of her own spiritual capacity. Noticing that pattern and explaining its meaning is the work of analysis.

I also noted a pattern in the above discussion of Harrold, Thistlewood, and Moore. All three men wrote about health in similarly transactional ways. Now that I see this pattern, I can use it to interpret other similar sources like William Byrd's diary, which I introduced at the outset of this essay. He, too, traced venereal symptoms in systematic, quantifiable ways: "My running began again," he wrote one day. Then the next, "My running was violent," followed by, "My running was extremely bad." Situating Byrd within the larger pattern I found in men's writing can help me extract meaning from his otherwise unremarkable entries. Did Byrd record the appearance and disappearance of venereal symptoms in order to take stock of his body and perhaps also take control of it? Exposing the pattern among these men is the work of analysis. And making sense of that pattern – for example, by linking it to men's shared writing practices, overlapping occupational roles, or common approaches to collecting and distributing medical knowledge – uses analysis to support an original argument.[24]

The approaches to analysis outlined in this chapter are by no means the only ones available. Early modern life writing encompasses an incredibly varied set of sources that document a broad range of potential medical matters. Surely methods vary depending on specific sources and research interests. The focus here has been on illness narratives, but I could have framed this chapter instead around reproductive health or emotional well-being or any other number of themes. Perhaps, most obviously, these sources are so useful to historians of medicine because they offer first-person accounts, cover long stretches of time, and record intimate, detailed information about past lives. By reading them in their entirety, historians are able to see authors before and after an incident, as an episode ramps up and as it recedes.

So, too, an enormous virtue of life writing is that it allows historians to place medical events in non-medical contexts – a world view, a belief system, a marital dispute, and so on. Considering the constructions, productions, aims, and conventions of these sources enables us to connect accounts of particular medical topics to larger lives, anxieties, beliefs, imaginations, and writing practices. Some forms of life writing are terse and opaque, and others still may not mention anything relevant to medicine. But those that offer glimpses of what we want to know – whether it is the smell of a hospital ward or the sensation of pain – can expose both vivid details of past lives, as well as the assumptions, hopes, and dreams that shaped constructions of those details on the page.

Notes

1 Beinecke Rare Book & Manuscript Library, Yale University, New Haven, CT, OSB MSS 176, Thomas Thistlewood Papers (hereafter cited as "Thistlewood Papers"), digitized at https://collections.library.yale.edu/catalog?f%5BcallNumber_ssim%5D%5B%5D=OSB+MSS+176. I am grateful to Amanda Herbert, who first brought this source to my attention, and to Claire Gherini for sharing her knowledge and transcription of it.

2 Thistlewood Papers, 1752, box 1, folder 3, no. 3, pp. 98, 105, 108; 1755, box 2, folder 6, no. 6, p. 89; 1756, Box 2, Folder 7, no, 7, pp. 96, 111.

3 William Byrd, *The London Diary (1717–1721) and Other Writings*, ed. Louis B. Wright and Marion Tinling (New York: Oxford University Press, 1958), 140.

4 Roger Chartier, "Languages, Books, and Reading from the Printed Word to the Digital Text," *Critical Inquiry* 31 (2004): 133–52.

5 For a few (of many) examples, see Sharon Howard, "Imagining the Pain and Peril of Seventeenth-Century Childbirth: Travail and Deliverance in the Making of an Early Modern World," *Social History of Medicine* 16 (2003): 367–82; Leah Astbury, "Being Well, Looking Ill: Childbirth and the Return to Health in Seventeenth-Century England," *Social History of Medicine* 30 (2017): 500–19; Elaine Leong, "Making Medicines in the Early Modern Household," *Bulletin of the History of Medicine* 82 (2008): 145–68; Olivia Weisser, "Grieved and Disordered: Gender and Emotion in Early Modern Patient Narratives," *Journal of Medieval and Early Modern Studies* 43 (2013): 247–73. For classic work on the early modern patient's perspective based on life writing, see Roy Porter and Dorothy Porter, *In Sickness and in Health: The British Experience, 1650–1850* (New York: B. Blackwell, 1988); Roy Porter and Dorothy Porter, *Patient's Progress: Doctors and Doctoring in Eighteenth-Century England* (Stanford, CA: Stanford University Press, 1989); Lucinda McCray Beier, *Sufferers & Healers. The Experience of Illness in Seventeenth-Century England* (London: Routledge, 1987).

6 Thistlewood Papers, 1751, box 1, folder 2, no. 2, pp. 264, 239, 250; 1752, box 1, folder 3, no. 3, pp. 193, 197, 255; 1753, box 1, folder 4, no, 4, p. 3; 1755, Box 2, Folder 6, no, 6, pp. 80, 71, 63.

7 Thistlewood Papers, 1757, box 2, folder 8, no., 8, pp. 179, 187; 1756, Box 2, Folder 7, no., 7, p. 179.

8 Olivia Weisser, *Ill Composed: Sickness, Gender, and Belief in Early Modern England* (New Haven, CT: Yale University Press, 2015).

9 For example, see Stephen Greenblatt, *Renaissance Self-Fashioning: From More to Shakespeare* (Chicago, IL: University of Chicago Press, 1980); Felicity Nussbaum, *The Autobiographical Subject: Gender and Ideology in Eighteenth-Century England* (Baltimore, MD: Johns Hopkins University Press, 1989); Henk Dragstra, et al., *Betraying Our Selves: Forms of Self-Representation in Early Modern English Texts* (New York: St. Martin's Press, 2000).

10 Roger Lowe, *Diary of Roger Lowe, of Ashton-in-Makerfield, Lancashire, 1663–74*, ed. William L. Sachse (New Haven, CT: Yale University Press, 1938), 22. On life writing by middling and lower status early modern individuals, see James S. Amelang, *The Flight of Icarus: Artisan Autobiography in Early Modern Europe* (Stanford, CA: Stanford University Press, 1998); Brodie Waddell, "Writing History from Below: Chronicling and Record-Keeping in Early Modern England," *History Workshop Journal* 85 (2018): 239–64.

11 On the public nature of private writing, see Elspeth Graham, "Women's Writing and the Self," in *Women and Literature in Britain 1500–1700*, ed. Helen Wilcox (Cambridge: Cambridge University Press, 1996), 209–33; Andrew Cambers, "Reading, the Godly, and Self-Writing in England, Circa 1580–1720," *Journal of British Studies* 46 (2007): 796–825.

12 Nicholas Blundell, *The Great Diurnal of Nicholas Blundell*, eds. Bagley, J.J. and Frank Tyrer, The Record Society of Lancashire and Cheshire (Liverpool: C. Tinling & Co. Ltd., vol. 1, 1968, vol. 2, 1970, vol. 3, 1972); see also Samuel Pepys, *The Diary of Samuel Pepys. A New and Complete Transcription*, eds. Robert Latham and William Matthews, vols. 1–11 (Berkeley: University of California Press, 1970–1983).

13 For a published edition of two (at times) conflicting life narratives, see Elizabeth Freke, *The Remembrances of Elizabeth Freke 1671–1714*, ed. Raymond A. Anselment (Cambridge: Cambridge University Press, 2001).

14 Thomas Tyldesley, *The Tyldesley Diary: Personal Records of Thomas Tyldesley (Grandson of Sir Thomas Tyldesley, the Royalist), During the Years 1712–13–14*, eds. Joseph Gillow and Anthony Hewitson (Preston: A. Hewitson, 1873). On this hybrid form of life writing, see Karen Harvey, *The Little Republic: Masculinity and Domestic Authority in Eighteenth-Century Britain* (Oxford: Oxford University Press, 2012), 88–98.

The hybrid diary-commonplace book is by Sarah Cowper, reproduced on microfilm in *Women's Language and Experience 1500-1940*, ed. Amanda Vickery (Marlborough: Adam Matthew Publications, 1994), Part 1, reels 5–7. A digitized version is available from "Perdita Manuscripts 1500–1700": https://www.amdigital.co.uk/primary-sources/perdita-manuscripts-1500-1700.

15 Adam Smyth, "Almanacs, Annotators, and Life-Writing in Early Modern England," *English Literary Renaissance* 38 (2008): 200–44; Elaine Leong, *Recipes and Everyday Knowledge: Medicine, Science, and the Household in Early Modern England* (Chicago, IL: University of Chicago Press, 2018), esp. ch 5.

16 Samuel Jeake, *An Astrological Diary of the Seventeenth Century: Samuel Jeake of Rye 1652–1699*, eds., Michael Hunter and Annabel Gregory (Oxford: Clarendon Press, 1988), title page.

17 Sir Walter Calverley, "Memorandum Book of Sir Walter Calverley, Bart," in *Yorkshire Diaries & Autobiographies in the Seventeenth and Eighteenth Centuries,* ed. S. Margerison (Durham: Andrews, 1886), 43.

18 British Library, London (hereafter cited as BL), Add. MS 27353, Mary Rich, Diary, f. 160v; Add. MS 27355, Mary Rich, Diary, f. 87r. On motives for diary keeping more generally, see Robert A. Fothergill, *Private Chronicles: A Study of English Diaries* (London: Oxford University Press, 1974), esp. 64–94

19 BL, Add. MS 27351, Mary Rich, Diary, ff. 189r, 189v, 190v.

20 Thistlewood Papers, 1751, box 1, folder 2, no. 2, p. 243; 1752, box 1, folder 3, no. 3, pp. 98, 105, 108.

21 Chetham's Library, Manchester, MS. Mun. A.2.137, Edmund Harrold, Wigmaker of Manchester, His Book of Remarks and Observations (1712–16), ff. 2v, 15r. This diary has been published as Edmund Harrold, *The Diary of Edmund Harrold, Wigmaker of Manchester 1712–15*, ed. Craig Horner (Aldershot: Ashgate, 2008). Giles Moore, *The Journal of Giles Moore*, ed. Ruth Bird, vol. 68. (Lewes: Sussex Record Society, 1971), 139.

22 The horse example is from Adam Eyre, "A Diurnall, or Catalogue of All My Accounts and Expences from the 1st of January, 1646-(7)," in *Yorkshire Diaries and Autobiographies in the Seventeenth and Eighteenth Centuries,* ed. H.J. Morehouse (Durham: Andrews, 1877), 1-118. For Dionys Fitzherbert, see *Women, Madness and Sin in Early Modern England: The Autobiographical Writings of Dionys Fitzherbert*, ed. Katherine Hodgkin (Farnham: Ashgate, 2010).

23 Alice Thornton, *The Autobiography of Mrs. Alice Thornton*, ed. Charles Jackson (London: Andrews, 1875), 152, 153, 92, 149. On the complex production of this text, see Alice Thornton, *My First Booke of My Life: Alice Thornton*, ed. Raymond A. Anselment (Lincoln: University of Nebraska Press, 2014); Cordelia Beattie, "The Discovery of Two Missing Alice Thornton Manuscripts," *Notes and Queries* 66 (2019): 547–53. For similar findings, see Harriet Blodgett, *Centuries of Female Days: Englishwomen's Private Diaries* (New Brunswick: Rutgers University Press, 1988), 27–30; Paul Delany, *British Autobiography in the Seventeenth Century* (London: Routledge & Kegan Paul, 1969), 5.

24 Byrd, *The London Diary*, 153. Here I summarize my own argument that explains this pattern in Weisser, *Ill Composed*, Ch. 2.

Bibliography

Manuscript Sources

Beinecke Rare Book & Manuscript Library, Yale University, New Haven, CT, OSB MSS 176, Thomas Thistlewood Papers.

British Library, London, UK, Add. MS 27351-5, Mary Rich, Diary.

Chetham's Library, Manchester, UK, MS. Mun. A.2.137, Edmund Harrold, Wigmaker of Manchester, His Book of Remarks and Observations (1712–1716).

Cowper, Sarah. Daily Diary, 7 vols., in *Women's Language and Experience 1500–1940*, ed. Amanda Vickery. Marlborough: Adam Matthew Publications, 1994. Part 1, reels 5–7.

Print Primary Sources

Blundell, Nicholas. *The Great Diurnal of Nicholas Blundell*, edited by J.J. Bagley and Frank Tyrer. Liverpool: C. Tinling & Co. Ltd., vol. 1, 1968, vol. 2, 1970, vol. 3, 1972.

Byrd, William. *The London Diary (1717–1721) and Other Writings*, edited by Louis B. Wright and Marion Tinling. New York: Oxford University Press, 1958.

Calverley, Sir Walter. "Memorandum Book of Sir Walter Calverley, Bart." In *Yorkshire Diaries & Autobiographies in the Seventeenth and Eighteenth Centuries*, edited by S. Margerison, 43–148. Durham: Andrews, 1886.

Eyre, Adam. "A Diurnall, or Catalogue of All My Accounts and Expences from the 1st of January, 1646-(7)." In *Yorkshire Diaries and Autobiographies in the Seventeenth and Eighteenth Centuries*, edited by H.J. Morehouse, 1–118. Durham: Andrews, 1877.

Fitzherbert, Dionys. *Women, Madness and Sin in Early Modern England: The Autobiographical Writings of Dionys Fitzherbert*, edited by Katherine Hodgkin. Farnham: Ashgate, 2010.

Freke, Elizabeth. *The Remembrances of Elizabeth Freke 1671–1714*, edited by Raymond A. Anselment. Cambridge: Cambridge University Press, 2001.

Harrold, Edmund. *The Diary of Edmund Harrold, Wigmaker of Manchester 1712–15*, edited by Craig Horner. Aldershot: Ashgate, 2008.

Jeake, Samuel. *An Astrological Diary of the Seventeenth Century: Samuel Jeake of Rye 1652–1699*, edited by Michael Hunter and Annabel Gregory. Oxford: Clarendon Press, 1988.

Lower, Roger. *Diary of Roger Lowe, of Ashton-in-Makerfield, Lancashire, 1663–74*, edited by William L. Sachse. New Haven, CT: Yale University Press, 1938.

Moore, Giles. *The Journal of Giles Moore*, edited by Ruth Bird, vol. 68. Lewes: Sussex Record Society, 1971.

Pepys, Samuel. *The Diary of Samuel Pepys. A New and Complete Transcription*, edited by Robert Latham and William Matthews, vols. 1–11. Berkeley: University of California Press, 1970–1983.

Thornton, Alice. *The Autobiography of Mrs. Alice Thornton*, edited by Charles Jackson. London: Andrews, 1875.

Thornton, Alice. *My First Booke of My Life: Alice Thornton*, edited by Raymond A. Anselment. Lincoln: University of Nebraska Press, 2014.

Tyldesley, Thomas. *The Tyldesley Diary: Personal Records of Thomas Tyldesley (Grandson of Sir Thomas Tyldesley, the Royalist), During the Years 1712–13–14*, edited by Joseph Gillow and Anthony Hewitson. Preston: A. Hewitson, 1873.

Secondary Sources

Amelang, James S. *The Flight of Icarus: Artisan Autobiography in Early Modern Europe*. Stanford, CA: Stanford University Press, 1998.

Astbury, Leah. "Being Well, Looking Ill: Childbirth and the Return to Health in Seventeenth-Century England." *Social History of Medicine* 30 (2017): 500–19.

Beattie, Cordelia. "The Discovery of Two Missing Alice Thornton Manuscripts." *Notes and Queries* 66 (2019): 547–53.

Beier, Lucinda McCray. *Sufferers & Healers. The Experience of Illness in Seventeenth-Century England.* London: Routledge, 1987.

Blodgett, Harriet. *Centuries of Female Days: Englishwomen's Private Diaries*. New Brunswick: Rutgers University Press, 1988.

Cambers, Andrew. "Reading, the Godly, and Self-Writing in England, Circa 1580–1720." *Journal of British Studies* 46 (2007): 796–825.

Chartier, Roger. "Languages, Books, and Reading from the Printed Word to the Digital Text." *Critical Inquiry* 31 (2004): 133–52.

Delany, Paul. *British Autobiography in the Seventeenth Century*. London: Routledge & Kegan Paul, 1969.

Dragstra, Henk, et al., *Betraying Our Selves: Forms of Self-Representation in Early Modern English Texts*. New York: St. Martin's Press, 2000.

Fothergill, Robert A. *Private Chronicles: A Study of English Diaries.* London: Oxford University Press, 1974.

Graham, Elspeth. "Women's Writing and the Self." In *Women and Literature in Britain 1500–1700*, edited by Helen Wilcox, 209–33. Cambridge: Cambridge University Press, 1996.

Greenblatt, Stephen. *Renaissance Self-Fashioning: From More to Shakespeare*. Chicago, IL: University of Chicago Press, 1980.

Harvey, Karen. *The Little Republic: Masculinity and Domestic Authority in Eighteenth-Century Britain.* Oxford: Oxford University Press, 2012.

Howard, Sharon. "Imagining the Pain and Peril of Seventeenth-Century Childbirth: Travail and Deliverance in the Making of an Early Modern World." *Social History of Medicine* 16 (2003): 367–82.

Kugler, Anne. *Errant Plagiary: The Writing Life of Lady Sarah Cowper (1644–1720)*. Stanford, CA: Stanford University Press, 2002.

Leong, Elaine. "Making Medicines in the Early Modern Household." *Bulletin of the History of Medicine* 82 (2008): 145–68.

———. *Recipes and Everyday Knowledge: Medicine, Science, and the Household in Early Modern England.* Chicago, IL: University of Chicago Press, 2018.

Nussbaum, Felicity. *The Autobiographical Subject: Gender and Ideology in Eighteenth-Century England.* Baltimore, MD: Johns Hopkins University Press, 1989.

Porter, Roy and Dorothy Porter. *In Sickness and in Health: The British Experience, 1650–1850*. New York: B. Blackwell, 1988.

———. *Patient's Progress: Doctors and Doctoring in Eighteenth-Century England.* Stanford, CA: Stanford University Press, 1989.

Smyth, Adam. "Almanacs, Annotators, and Life-Writing in Early Modern England." *English Literary Renaissance* 38 (2008): 200–44.

Waddell, Brodie. "Writing History from Below: Chronicling and Record-Keeping in Early Modern England." *History Workshop Journal* 85 (2018): 239–64.

Weisser, Olivia. "Grieved and Disordered: Gender and Emotion in Early Modern Patient Narratives." *Journal of Medieval and Early Modern Studies* 43 (2013): 247–273.

———. *Ill Composed: Sickness, Gender, and Belief in Early Modern England.* New Haven, CT: Yale University Press, 2015.

13 Family Letters

Sandra Cavallo

In spring 1669, Marquis Orazio Spada, engaged in the management of his landed properties in Castel Viscardo, wrote almost daily letters to his wife Maria (in Rome) that contain minute accounts not only of his own health but also the ailments affecting the employees of his household. We learn that, in the space of two months, the accountant Benigno was troubled for several days by an intermittent fever that Orazio reckoned to be "catarrhal," and for which the doctor was summoned. The coachman, meanwhile, was in bed with "tertian double fever." Orazio recommended him to the hospital's governor in nearby Orvieto, and he was transferred and treated there with bloodletting. The same coachman would soon also suffer from a painful abscess to his gums. Meanwhile, the valet Felice was troubled by his usual flank pain (*dolori di fianco*), but fortunately only for a couple of days, whereas another servant, nicknamed Sciampagna, could not eat or drink due to a severe inflammation of the throat, for which the surgeon prescribed gargling. Marquis Orazio, by contrast, was feeling reinvigorated by the countryside air and by the walking he was doing there, and, apart from one episode of vomiting that resolved quickly with a light diet, was in a great shape. He was worried, however, about the prospect of returning to Rome, since both Maria and their chaplain warned him that three members of the family were in bed with a catarrhal flu (*influenza catarrale*) reckoned to be contagious. He was also anxious for his wife, affected by a flux at the eyes (*flussione agli occhi*) that he attributed to the unseasonal hot weather, and for the enduring poor health of his daughter-in-law Vittoria, which different cures seemed incapable of resolving.[1]

The frequency and richness of Orazio's missives are not exceptional but epitomize patterns of epistolary exchange that were common between temporarily separated family members: with no other way of maintaining contact they recreated through these minute – and at times trivial – details, a shared quotidian. As a genre, family letters offer a vivid image of the significant place that health concerns occupied in people's lives in an age marked by high levels of morbidity and mortality. For us, they provide precious insight into early modern understandings of disease, the vocabulary employed to describe it, and the measures taken to fight and prevent it.

As suggested by studies that have interrogated this material since the 1980s, family letters also have the merit of documenting the roles played by laypeople in the

DOI: 10.4324/9781003094876-17

management of their health, their independence of judgment, and self-determination, thus rebalancing the picture of uncontested authority that other sources still tend to attribute to medical practitioners.[2] Even if the history of healing is no longer as physician-centered as in the 1980s, much of the evidence employed by historians of medicine still conveys the perspectives of medical professionals. Indeed, medical treatises, private consultation notes, hospital records, and the medical advice books so popular in scholarship in the last few years elucidate how medical practitioners understood the body and its pathologies, how they reached their diagnoses, and the therapies they prescribed. Some of these sources also give voice to the patients, expected to describe their symptoms and brief the practitioner about their constitution and the life habits possibly responsible for their pathologies. Such information, however, was then filtered by the medical editor based on what he thought was worth recording. By depicting sufferers and those tending to them as actors in the medical event, family letters offer a more accurate picture of early modern medical practice.

Additionally, while the sources produced by medical professionals tend to focus on disease and cures, letters document the significant efforts made by healthy people to maintain their physical well-being. In so doing, they illustrate practices largely ignored by the medical literature, such as the harsh preventive therapies seasonally adopted by healthy people (see Section "Maintaining Health"). Inevitably, moreover, sources authored by doctors for other doctors – *consilia*, *curationes*, casebooks – focus on rare and complicated health conditions rather than everyday ones.[3] Hence, they fail to document how minor and more common disorders of the kind that troubled Marquis Orazio were managed in the household, and, conversely, what was considered a serious ailment and when qualified healers were asked to intervene (see Section "Perceptions of Disease"). In other words, the study of letters makes it possible to ascertain the extent to which lay people and medical professionals shared the same interpretative medical framework, as recent scholars have suggested. Whether the cures applied independently by householders diverged from those prescribed by medical practitioners (see Section "Treatment") and previous distinctions between learned and popular or lay and professional medicine now appear obsolete.[4]

The way in which correspondents understood pathogenic states and their causes and the working of the adopted therapies also offers precious insights into the conceptual bases of early modern medical culture and the timing of its transformations. Was disease increasingly seen as an ontological entity that attacks the body from outside rather than an internal alteration of the body's humoral physiology?[5] Was the view of the individual body as a unique being replaced by the idea of a universal body that functions according to uniform laws and therefore requires standardized rather than personalized treatment? Letters may help us address these debated questions.[6]

Cautions in the Use of Letters

Despite its significant value, the evidence provided by correspondence cannot be taken as a direct reflection of reality.[7] All types of letters are a form of self-presentation: the sufferer may feel and portray themselves as more vulnerable to disease than they really are or over-emphasize their ability to manage their health independently (an example will be offered by Eugenia Spada later on). Those tending to the patient may also perceive and thus represent the situation as more or less critical than it is. Writing a letter is a relational act and its contents are inevitably influenced by the image that one more or less unconsciously wishes to present of oneself, as well as the expectations of the recipient. These drawbacks, however, also concern the production of sources whose transparency is doubted to a much lesser extent, such as the various types of medical writing in which practitioners engaged. Like letters, medical casebooks, treatises, and *consilia* were forms of self-fashioning since they played a key role in the construction of a career and in maintaining and reinforcing one's professional reputation.[8]

All accounts are subjective to an extent. However, compared with other types of correspondence, we can expect more transparency from the letters exchanged by members of a household. Often, the same matter was the subject of various letters written to a person simultaneously by different members of the family. This criss-crossing of information tends to increase its authenticity. Indeed, these letters differ considerably from those in which there is just one source of information and news is reported unchecked by one person to another, since the facts narrated by, say, a wife to her husband were often also dealt with in the letters he received from his sons and daughters, or, as in the case of Orazio Spada, even recounted to him in person while his children were visiting.

An additional factor to consider is that these types of letters were implicitly directed to the whole household – indeed, they were often read aloud to all present. They had no private character, multiplying the possibilities for further checks.[9] The same servant who had delivered the letter had also often witnessed the facts reported or had been informed of them by the other household servants. Thus, he was often interrogated by the recipients to obtain further details.

Family correspondence tends therefore to offer straightforward and often corroborated description of both illness and treatments. Moreover, many of the items that matter to us – such as the vocabulary employed to describe disease and the treatment administered to the patient (which provide rare insights into the therapies used to fight specific pathologies) – are unlikely to be affected by individual feelings.

Letter-writing was to some extent dictated by the conventions of the early modern period, and the manuals that established specific rules for this practice were very popular.[10] Traces of these conventions can also be found in the correspondence I consulted, especially in the order in which the various subjects are presented. A letter typically started with a detailed account of one's journey, how long, smooth, or complicated it was, and how it had affected the well-being of the correspondent. News of the weather and its potential impact upon the health, as well as the movements and activities of the sender, tended to come second (or first, if there was no recent travel). Other information, however, including updates on the health of the letter-writer and their household, did not follow a predetermined order. The structure of family letters is not as rigid as that of complimentary or petitionary letters, and they are also less formal than the latter, being prevalently hand-written by the sender rather than dictated to a secretary or scribe trained to adapt the text to conventions.

A frequent objection to the value of these sources is that family correspondence in the early modern period only concerns well-off, educated individuals, and that the medical culture they express is therefore an exclusive one. Yet, as we have seen in the letters that Marquis Orazio addresses to his wife, these accounts often deal with the health of *all* household members: the humble domestic servants and their complaints are understood and treated in the same ways as those of kin. It may even be argued that, characterized by the close intermingling of social classes, the affluent, extended household might have favored the stabilization of a common language of the body, its pathologies, and its needs.

The discussion that follows is based on my analysis of hundreds of letters exchanged between members of the Spada family – a recently ennobled family living in Rome – between 1641 and 1680.[11] They concern the health status of Orazio Spada, his wife Maria, their daughter-in-law Vittoria, and their children: the adult Eugenia, Fabrizio, and Virginia, and the younger Bartolomeo, Ciriaco, and Guido.

Maintaining Health

Family letters have the merit of highlighting the central role – often obscured in other sources and therefore long underestimated in the history of medicine – that the purpose of preserving health occupied in the everyday. Even if the technical term "non-naturals" was not employed, references to the need to protect oneself from what medical theory considered the six main risk factors for health (air, food and drink, sleep, exercise, evacuations, and passions) abound.[12]

The importance that correspondents attribute to these different elements holds, however, some surprises: concerns about air quality and temperature prevail, followed by those about exercise. Much less attention is paid to the other non-naturals, with no mention of evacuations, which are central to the therapies adopted to combat disease.

The minimal concern for diet is particularly striking, given the space that guides to healthy living – highly popular at the time – devoted to foods. Their extensive presence in these texts has led many to assume that diet was considered the most relevant among the six non-naturals. Yet, in the sizeable Spada correspondence, I have found only a few recommendations about avoiding foods and drinks deemed unsuitable for health, such as chocolate, fruit, and fresh water. Otherwise, there are no more specific instructions concerning food unless when one is ill. In those occasions, a restricted diet – broths, eggs, or soup of almond milk – is regularly adopted, either independently or following doctor's advice, and is regarded as an integral part of the cure.

Letters therefore act as a corrective to the picture obtained from the printed medical advice literature. In those tracts, the length of the sections on foodstuffs is probably ascribed to the fact that, having different properties, each of them had to be discussed individually, rather than a supposed primacy of their role in health.

The negative impact of intense passions upon health is also mentioned relatively rarely in the Spada letters, although these seem to acquire greater importance toward the end of the century.[13] Certainly, melancholy is seen as a possible cause of disease, and so are the upsetting feelings prompted by family conflict or by the loss of a loved one. In September 1657, for example, the *alterazione* (low-grade fever) of Eugenia's husband is seen as a reaction to the death of his powerful aunt Olimpia. Conversely, the illness of the bishop of Sulmona is dismissed as not too serious precisely because "being more melancholic humor than anything else," it is of little consequence.[14]

The most dangerous factor affecting health is undoubtedly represented by atmospheric conditions. Previous studies had already noted, in relation to Samuel Pepys' diary – an invaluable source for the history of lay perceptions of disease – that most of his health complaints were ascribed to "the cold" caught from the negligence of forgetting to wear a wig, underdressing, or imbibing exceedingly cool drinks.[15] This concern also recurs in the Spada correspondence. Here, however, the hot temperature, the sun, and the bad quality of the air are also described as harmful agents. The Prince of Palestrina is even said to be near death for getting too overheated: "he just confessed and has been blood-let, and they attached six vesicants to him and we are very fearful, they say that his affliction derives from having *preso caldo* [taken the heat] on the eight day of the Stigmata."[16] And from Castel Viscardo, Orazio Spada encourages his wife to:

> Keep in good heart because there is no danger that I will catch the sun whilst the weather carries on like this and I am already feeling the effects of this good air which serves to purge me without resorting to medicines and syrups which make me nauseous.[17]

Places characterized by good air have, therefore, a beneficial effect upon one's health. By contrast, the arrival of bad airs, produced by unhealthy winds such as *scirocco* or *tramontana*, are a sufficient motive for refraining from travelling or even from leaving the house.[18] Hence, travel plans always need to consider whether the move is toward a better or worse air. We thus learn that "signor Lorenzo Roberti, having gone to Naples, even if before the arrival of the blazing sun [*Sol Leone*], none other than for the ordeal of the journey and the change of air has lost his life."[19] Airs are clearly understood as localized. The decision to leave is often a matter for extensive discussion in which many express their opinions and frequently entails strategies of diversion through intermediate localities to slowly adapt the body to the change of air. In 1678, Maria informs her husband:

> Many are of the opinion that Bartolomeo [their son, aged 21 and currently in Castel Viscardo] should not go to Viterbo so soon because its air is similar to that of Rome [i.e., notoriously bad], all the more so since he is coming from places with perfect airs, such as Perugia and Castello. He could first go to Giove and then carry on to Viterbo … and the Duchess [Bartolomeo's sister] says that … the airs of Perugia and Castello are too perfect.[20]

Regular exercise (which in this period corresponds to taking walks) is also of great importance for keeping in good health. Orazio frequently encourages his wife to resume walking "since exercise does her more good than any kind of medicine" and tells her that "ever since I have been walking every morning I am much better."[21] Meanwhile, there is almost no reference to the benefits of sleep. Here moral preoccupations seem to override health concerns: the correspondents are eager to represent themselves as perennially busy and needing only few hours of sleep per night.

Contrary to the balanced representation of the importance of the six non-naturals found in the medical advice literature, family letters show that everyday preoccupations concentrated on just two of them. This source offers therefore the opportunity to ascertain how far medical texts that enjoyed considerable popularity can be taken as a mirror of practice.

The importance assigned to one's lifestyle and to the environment in preventing disease that emerges from family letters has wider implications: it suggests that health was perceived as being largely under laypeople's control rather than that of practitioners. Often, in fact, a health complaint appears to be generated by disregarding the rules of healthy living: typically, having over-tired oneself, having ignored adverse weather conditions, or having neglected exercise. Maria's malaise, which obliges her to rely on pills for her lack of appetite and great thirst, is attributed by her husband to having discontinued her regular walks.[22] Meanwhile, the flux at the eye of their son Bartolomeo is explained by his disorderly eating and drinking.[23]

The corollary of this link continuously established between disease and the neglect of the rules for healthy living is that one's health could be maintained by regularly taking the right precautions and acknowledging that, although every person is born with a distinct constitution, this is something that can be controlled and modified. We get a pleasant example of this way of thinking in the love affair that Orazio establishes with onions. He discovers by experience that they are ideal for his stomach and prevent any digestion problems. In three different letters, he praises the merits of this food for his constitution, suggesting that everyone should try and understand what is good for them by studying their own reactions to certain foods. As he declares elsewhere, when attacking chemical practitioners who treat specific ailments irrespective of individual constitutions: "what has proved beneficial to one person will not work on another person, even if affected by the same illness."[24] We begin to see how beliefs in the individuality of bodies still had considerable currency.

The Annual Purge

Another practice discussed in letters much more frequently than current scholarship might predict is the annual purge. Routinely performed by healthy people (presumably those who could afford spending a few days away from absorbing occupations), the practice confirms the importance that early moderns attributed to preventative healthcare. Despite its universally acknowledged benefits, however, the operation was dreaded by the Spadas and various ploys were utilized to postpone, dilute, or avoid it all together.

The topic is often discussed minutely in letters, and we learn that the procedure sometimes took place in the autumn but more often in April or May, aiming to free the body from any waste (what some today would call toxins) accumulated in winter and during the strenuous period of Lent. It consisted of a thorough intestinal purging, stimulated by the oral ingestion of substances such as absolute serum, rhubarb, Angelica water, *manna*, and rose syrup. This operation was always accompanied by complete rest and the adoption of a strict diet, followed by bloodletting. A full day spent in bed marked the end of the purge, but only if the quality of the blood extracted was considered acceptable. This blood was carefully examined, and if it appeared too watery, the purge was deemed ineffective and was therefore prolonged, administering at the same time medicaments aimed to "sweeten" or "refresh" the blood and therefore ease the removal of impurities.[25] Eugenia Spada's purge once lasted for 22 days![26]

We can appreciate people's reluctance to submit to this torture. Members of the family nevertheless encouraged each other to overcome reservations and do the purge. Orazio reminds Maria:

> we are in the last quarter of the May's moon and it is time to do the purge and do it well … this is what matters the most to me … and I would like to hear that you have discussed it with the doctor.[27]

Even if persuaded of its benefits, people found ways of escaping the unpleasant obligation. Adverse climatic factors, which had acquired so much relevance in the discourse about health, were often used as an excuse to postpone it: Maria, for example, says that she cannot because the weather is still unusually cold.[28] One of her sons, Cardinal Fabrizio, acknowledges his need to undergo the annual purge and associated bloodletting at the beginning of April, but then decides to defer it to a warmer period, given that the flux that troubled him during Lent is improving and the weather is still cold.[29] He hopes instead to derive similar benefits from the air of the countryside and the exercise he can do there. Indeed, it was thought that taking walks and breathing pure air also had a purgative effect. Often, these activities integrated the operations of purging but were sometimes proposed as an alternative to it: Virginia "is continuing the purge but does not see any benefits, it is reckoned that changing air by moving to some places nearby may do the trick."[30]

The prospect of the purge seems therefore to have inspired patients to take care of their health in their own ways. Eugenia, who had recently given birth in Viterbo, manages to postpone it by two months, arguing first that she wants to hear a second opinion and consult the doctor in Rome, and then that it is unnecessary since "her breast almost does not leak" and she would rather take walks.[31] Her liver, she argues, does not trouble her and she does not want to upset her stomach. Given that she can wait until the end of May, she "will watch whether her liver causes any discomfort, and will do it if she sees the need for it."[32] A month later, she writes that, in consultation with her husband (not the doctor, "since he would certainly have agreed"), she has finally made up her mind and will proceed with the purge, but first will wait until her period is over.[33]

The patient's will emerges very strongly in this case. Eugenia's defiant statements aim perhaps to showcase her particularly obstinate personality, but it is in any case significant that rather than on the doctor's opinion and customary practice, her decisions were based on feeling and observing her body – a practice in which patients were encouraged by the humoral paradigm. The idea that individual bodies were distinct physiological entities enhanced the self-determination of sufferers: Eugenia exploits this view to her favor, supporting the conviction that patients are the best interpreters of what is going on in their bodies. In the end, she adheres to prescription, but in her own time and terms.

Perceptions of Disease

How did early modern people recognize disease, and what did they consider minor ailments or more worrying symptoms? Who took care of these patients and how was the working of disease conceptualized? Letters provide helpful evidence for addressing these questions.

Lack of appetite, restlessness at night, thirst, coldness, and shivering were seen as alarming signs of malaise and closely monitored. Having a bitter taste in one's mouth or a knot in one's stomach required intervention, and "*incordatura di collo*" (presumably a stiff neck) was also taken seriously.[34] Usually, these ailments were treated in the household without calling the doctor, through lean eating, resting in bed, and – even when the disorder did not affect the bowels – with enemas.

Fever was considered more worrisome and required close oversight to determine its origins and possible evolution. Yet this complaint, too, was initially managed independently. Interestingly, in the Spada letters, we do not always encounter the idea that fever was understood as an illness in its own right (rather than a symptom of disease), nor the concept that fevers shift around the body from one organ to the other.[35] These views have been found to characterize patients' narratives in other European countries but were clearly not universal. In Rome, people searched for the causes of fever in the sufferer's recent experiences, trying to establish the kind of fever and how dangerous it might be. Was it just an "*alterazione*," a low-grade fever that generally did not rise further? Or was it a "*febbre catarrale*," a temperature rise accompanied by some sort of "*flussione*" (flux), another disorder that appears easily recognizable by laypeople, and not particularly worrying.

These types of fever might be caused by a simple cold, indigestion, or exposure to cold weather. They could also originate from exhaustion (following, for example, a long journey in a jolting carriage), or, in the case of children, from an excess of movement, all activities that caused an "agitation of the blood" and an over-heating of the body.[36] These disorders, too, often resolved without a doctor's intervention, treated with just rest, light meals, and the inevitable enema: "the fever came with the cold and he had an headache but with a bit of diet and a clyster he was cured."[37]

In children, however, fever may signal the presence of measles or rubella, and this suspicion persuaded the family to summon the doctor. The same occurred if the symptom persisted in an adult, since it could be the sign of a "malign fever," which might lead to death. In these cases, an affluent family like the Spadas would rely on the opinions of more than one doctor and this would make the medical encounter at the sickbed a much more complex affair than we often tend to assume.[38] Indeed, the various practitioners did not always speak with one voice, and their professional opinions might diverge. Paradoxically, therefore, it was often up to the family and the patient – if the latter's condition allowed – to solve the dispute and decide which of the advised treatments should be applied.

An enduring fever sparked considerable anxiety in the patient and those attending to them. The prognosis also became uncertain. In these cases, the convention still applied that even when there was an improvement, one should wait for the seventh day of illness, and then for the fourteenth to be sure that there would not be a relapse.[39] These beliefs betray the vestiges of an ancient understanding of feverish states as regulated by rigid cycles, a concept documented as common in the fifteenth and sixteenth centuries and clearly still fully credited in the late seventeenth century.[40]

At the same time, we find that prognoses once again reflected the idea that bodies are individualized and react differently to pathogenic attacks: Maria Spada's daughter, for example, did not take the news that her mother was in bed with fever lightly, since "when she has fever, it never lasts for a short time."[41] Fever was supposed to behave in specific ways in Maria's body, and not according to more universal models.

How alarming a disease seemed also depended on which area was affected: in the case of the eyes (considered "a noble part"), for example, there was maximum concern.[42] Obviously an illness of the eyes sparked apprehension since sight could be at risk, but the distinction between more and less noble body parts was also key and seems to reflect a hierarchical distinction between the upper and the lower body. Orazio, for example, rejoiced to hear that the flux that had afflicted his son Guido in the previous year had now descended to his heel: "I believe this is good, since it has moved away from the noblest part." Likewise, Maria was glad that the swelling and redness of her knee had moved "below," to her foot.[43]

These passages suggest that, as already observed by other scholars, rather than viewing bodily disorders as localized, early modern people tended to see them as shifting within the body.[44] In the case of Guido, it is assumed that a disease may relocate to a different body part even months after its first appearance. Two terms, *flussioni* (fluxes) and *flati* (vapors), signaled pathogenic manifestations that may circulate through a body. The first term seems to refer to something visible, a swelling deriving from an inflammation or an internal bleeding or fluid leakage into the body cavity (as in the cases cited above). But the term may also relate to an external discharge: Bartolomeo Spada, for example, is affected by a *flussione* from the eye. *Flati*, by contrast, seems to refer to an internal pain, perceived only by the patient and invisible from outside: Signora Lorenza, for instance, "feels a torment of *flati*, having caught humidity this evening in the cold living room."[45] Orazio attributes the pain he feels at his right shoulder, near the neck, to *flati*. This pain prevents him from turning in the bed during the night as each movement provokes a stitch so acute that, in the morning, he cannot lift his arms and must be dressed by the valet: "and one knew they were *flati*, since they were moving around."[46]

Letters advance, therefore, our understanding of the ways in which early modern people conceptualized disease. However, there are no signs that, as some have argued, a view of disease as an independent entity that attacks the body from outside was becoming dominant, replacing the idea that pathogenic states derive from an alteration in the physiology of the body.[47] When correspondents mention the supposed cause of disease, this always appears to originate from an excessive concentration of certain humoral qualities (cold, hot, dry, or humid) in parts of the body. Such a change could be induced by external factors (like the weather or unsuitable food), but also by a defect in the regular working of the body, especially in its normal excretory functions, rather than by a foreign morbid agent. Likewise, therapies aim to restore normal physiological processes by removing such excess and thus creating a refreshing, warming, moisturizing, or exsiccating function. For example, after Maria deems the treatment adopted to cure her eyes ineffective, Orazio explains to her that:

> medicaments need time to work, it has been said that the disorder proceeds from excessive heat in the liver and you have started to refresh it, one needs to wait that the liver stops transmitting heat to the head and at that point you will begin to feel the benefit to the eyes.[48]

The abnormal heating of the liver affects the eyes, and it is therefore the health of the liver than needs to be restored, not that of the eyes directly.

Treatment

The Spada correspondence also provides rare insights into the treatments they adopted. These sometimes include a detailed description not only of the medicaments used but even of their quantities. The method used by barber-surgeons to bleed patients with different pathologies is often specified (cups, leeches, cutting the vein, even which vein is cut) as is the part of the body where the procedure is applied (shoulder, foot, arm, and so on). Even the ounces of blood let are sometimes mentioned, offering an indication of how these varied across age and gender.

As we have already seen, treatment was multifaceted: it relied on the use of topical preparations (applied also in the case of internal afflictions), oral medications, clysters, cauterization, and sometimes bloodletting. Domestic baths – a therapy that, unlike thermal baths, has received little attention – were also employed.[49] Moreover, diet and absolute rest were a regular component of treatment. We find no divergence between therapies prescribed by learned doctors (allegedly relying on diet) and more popular therapies (based on evacuative treatment), as postulated by previous scholars.[50] Diet and forced evacuation were regularly used together; they were inseparable both when the treatment was ordered by a physician and when adopted independently.

The letters discussing the inflammation of the breast afflicting Eugenia for over a year offer an example of the amount of detail that correspondence may offer about the cures administered. They also highlight how, in difficult cases, treatments derived from an indistinguishable mix of laypeople's recommendations, different doctors' prescriptions, and the patient's resolution. Having tried (on her mother's advice) a vinegar with roots of *romici* (a common medicinal plant also used for skin disorders) that proved ineffective, then serum (also unhelpful), in July Eugenia decides to try Nocera water (coming from the thermal springs in Central Italy) as recommended by both her mother and doctors. At the same time, she takes freshwater baths and anoints her breast with an infusion of *litargirio* (litharge: pulverized lead oxide).[51] The first morning, she drinks four *fogliette* (two liters) of Nocera water mixed with four ounces of rose syrup. Then she continues with just Nocera water for 12 days, eating only soup and boiled meat. In the evening, she takes freshwater baths.[52] Interestingly, the doses and duration of the treatment – as well as the accompanying diet – correspond exactly to those recommended in print.[53] In this case, there is total accord between practice and the instructions on how to use Nocera water found in the printed advice literature also available to patients. However, Eugenia is not healed, and in September, she chooses a different treatment: she will take a spoon of preserve of borage flowers every morning together with a glass of Nocera water and will avoid any food with a hot humoral quality that may worsen the inflammation. Moreover, the doctors want her to try seawater baths.[54]

Nocera water and the other oral remedies used by Eugenia have laxative properties, hence the therapy adopted to treat her breast was essentially evacuative. This type of treatment was employed to cure most ailments. At first, oral preparations that induce intestinal evacuation were attempted. Depending on the look of the feces, this could be followed by enemas. If the stools seemed full of "undigested matters" a clyster was deemed necessary. Bloodletting was also conceived as an evacuative procedure performed however less regularly than purging. It was part of the annual internal cleansing undergone by healthy people, but not necessarily when treating specific ailments. To complete the removal of morbid matter, cauterization was often employed, even in infants.[55]

It is interesting that curative remedies aimed at healing specific disorders are never mentioned here. The objective of both topical and oral preparations was to stimulate the evacuation of substances in excess, or to refresh or sweeten the liver or the blood and ultimately favor such evacuation.[56] This characteristic of the treatment normally adopted both independently by laypeople or on professional prescription is at odds with the picture that emerges from recipe books and medical domestic manuscripts, whose organization by ailments and their cures seems to imply that an intense recourse to curative medicine was the norm. This contrast between different representations of medical practice is intriguing and deserves further investigation.

Therapies were in any case entirely pharmacological, dietetic, and mechanical. While recourse to religious and magical healing was often encountered in epistolary exchanges in previous centuries, it is completely marginal in the seventeenth-century Spada correspondence. Similarly, any references to the influence of stars and their movements upon diagnosis and the timing of treatment, prominent in earlier narratives of illness, are totally absent from our letters.[57]

The psychological element, by contrast, is also a component of treatment, especially in the case of sick children. An adult always keeps them company and they receive repeated visits from reassuring female figures, like grandmothers and aunts. Much is done to keep their morale high: hence the Spada children Guido and Ciriaco (eight and ten years old) are first allowed to exchange written messages from one room to the other while sick. Once both are diagnosed with rubella (and thus unable to infect each other), they are allowed to share the bed so that "they can be cheerful together."[58] While her young son Andrea is slowly recovering from a long and serious illness, and still unable to stand on his own, Eugenia decides to dress him to the nines "to cheer him up."[59]

Conclusion

Family letters are one of the few sources capable of providing vivid descriptions of everyday medical practice, thus offering a wealth of rare information about the perception of serious and less serious disorders, the way in which pathogenic logics were conceptualized, and how the various ailments were treated. They also help us reconstruct the medical vocabulary in use and what early modern people meant with expressions such as "fluxes," "vapors," or "alteration." In these accounts, it is often impossible to distinguish the voice of medical professionals from those of sufferers. Clearly, as far as the working of the body and disease are concerned, laypeople and practitioners spoke a common language and shared the same conceptual framework. Indeed, even if discrepancies sometimes emerge between the doctors' opinions and the patients' decisions, these do not concern the fundamental explanatory premises but exemplify the role of active participants in making a diagnosis and deciding on treatment that humoral physiology granted to patients.

The frequency with which certain topics are discussed in letters has been a key indicator of the priorities in people's attitudes to health. We have learned that the preservation of health was a quotidian concern, and even induced healthy people to regularly endure the discomforts of a thorough evacuative procedure to preserve their bodies from disease. Another theme unexpectedly prominent in letters are the pathologies of the breast, especially the months-long painful inflammation that often tormented women who decided not to breast-feed their newborns.

Focusing on everyday practice epistolary exchanges also reveals the limitations of textual genres which, due to their popularity among a non-professional audience, have been seen as reflecting the behavior of laypeople. The image of an intense consumption of curative remedies emerging from recipe books appears incompatible with the composite nature of treatment documented in letters; more likely these preparations were just one component of therapies that included balneological (bathing in therapeutic springs), surgical, dietary, and (above all) evacuative therapies – all of which were not normally mentioned in recipe books. Likewise, while guides to healthy living tend to assign equal importance to the six behavioral factors on which health was seen to depend, letters provide a more irregular and dynamic picture of their significance, showing, for example, the importance that concerns about climate had assumed in a period strongly influenced by Hippocratic thinking on the environment.

Comparison with earlier epistolary exchanges, such as the late fifteenth-century letters about the final illness of the Visconti Duchess, is also fruitful. It highlights how medical theory and its vocabulary are far from static and how, for example, recourse to religious healing has become entirely marginal and astrological medicine has disappeared altogether – a subject that has not been possible to address here.

Finally, comparison with studies conducted on similar sources in other countries highlights both similarities and discrepancies in ideas concerning the functioning of the body and disease. Italian correspondents seem to have remained immersed in a humoral medical culture for longer than their English counterparts and, unlike English and other European correspondents, persisted in believing in the diversity of bodies and their differential reactions to pathologies and medicines. In mid-seventeenth-century Rome, the view of disease as an independent agent foreign to the body does not seem to have taken root, suggesting that the timing of changes in medical culture may have varied in different parts of Europe and that we must therefore refrain from generalizing from individual cases.

Notes

1 Twenty-two of the 42 letters sent by Orazio to Maria between early March and early May 1669 contain instances of poor health in the household. Like all the other letters considered in this essay they are held in Archivio di Stato di Roma, Fondo Spada-Veralli.

2 Lucinda M. Beier, "In Sickness and in Health: A Seventeenth-Century Family Experience" and Joan Lane, "'The Doctor Scolds Me': The Diaries and Correspondence of Patients in Eighteenth-Century England," both in *Patients and Practitioners: Lay Perceptions of Medicine and Pre-Industrial Society*, ed. Roy Porter (Cambridge: Cambridge University Press, 1985), 101–128, 205–248; Marilyn Nicoud, "L'Expérience de la maladie et l'échange épistolaire: les derniers moments de Bianca Maria Visconti," *Mélanges de l'École française de Rome* 116, no. 2 (2000): 85–101; Alfonso Zarzoso, "Mediating Medicine through Private Letters: The Eighteenth-Century Catalan Medical World," in *Cultural Approaches to the History of Medicine: Mediating Medicine in Early Modern and Modern Europe*, ed. Willem de Blécourt and Cornelie Usborne (Basingstoke: Palgrave Macmillan, 2004), 108–126.

3 Alessandra Quaranta, "The *Consilia* of Learned Physicians Pietro Andrea Mattioli and Francesco Partini: Doctrine, Empirical Knowledge, and Use of the Senses in Sixteenth-Century Europe," *Social History of Medicine* 35 (2021): 20–48.

4 On the shared medical world between medical practitioners and laypeople, see Michael Stolberg, *Experiencing Illness and the Sick Body in Early Modern Europe* (Basingstoke: Palgrave Macmillan 2011), 14, 79–82.

5 Michael Stolberg, *Learned Physicians and Everyday Medical Practice* (Berlin and Boston: de Gruyter, 2023), esp. 221–25.

6 Harold Cook, "Markets and Cultures: Medical Specifics and the Reconfiguration of the Body in Early Modern Europe," *Transactions of the Royal Historical Society* 21 (2011): 123–45.

7 E.g., Hannah Newton, *The Sick Child in Early Modern England, 1580–1720* (Oxford: Oxford University Press, 2012), 20–24; Willemijn Ruberg, "The Letter as Medicine: Studying Health and Illness in Dutch Daily Correspondence, 1770–1850," *Social History of Medicine* 23, no. 3 (2010): 492–508; Nicoud, "L'expérience de la maladie." Useful are also the observations in Stolberg, *Experiencing Illness,* 14–18 (which deals however with the correspondence between patients and their doctors).
8 Newton, *The Sick Child*, 25.
9 Hence a letter written by Eugenia Spada to her mother begins with the warning: "do not read aloud." Later she explains that "as I know that when letters arrive they are publicly read, I will add at the top: 'do not read aloud.'" October 2, 1669, B.1115.
10 On which, see Peter Mack, "Letter-Writing Manuals," in *A History of Renaissance Rhetoric, 1380–1620*, ed. Peter Mack (Oxford: Oxford University Press, 2011), 228–56.
11 For further information on this family, see Sandra Cavallo and Tessa Storey, *Healthy Living in Late Renaissance Italy* (Oxford: Oxford University Press 2013), chapter 2.
12 On the six non-naturals, see Sandra Cavallo and Tessa Storey, eds., *Conserving Health in Early Modern Culture: Bodies and Environments in Italy and England* (Manchester: Manchester University Press, 2017).
13 Sandra Cavallo, "The Role of Medicinal Remedies in Seventeenth-Century Medical Treatment: The Case of Rome," in *Medicine in Early Modern Italy: Between Theory and Practice,* ed. Sandra Cavallo and John Henderson (Turnhout: Brepols, forthcoming).
14 September 30, 1657, B.410; October 15, 1654, B.619.
15 Roy Porter, "The Patient's View: Doing Medical History from Below," *Theory and Society* 14, no. 2 (1985): 178–79; Olivia Weisser, "Disease," in *A Cultural History of Medicine in the Renaissance*, ed. Elaine Leong and Claudia Stein (London: Bloomsbury, 2021), 72–74.
16 September 28, 1678, B.618.
17 April 23, 1658, B.607.
18 See the letters cited in Cavallo and Storey, *Healthy Living*, 109.
19 July 8, 1660, B.619. The expression *Sol Leone* denotes the hottest part of the summer.
20 September 21, 1678, B.618.
21 August 2, 1661, B.607.
22 March 15, 1659, B.607.
23 June 7, 1661, B.607.
24 November 2, 1666, B.607.
25 E.g. June 18, 1662, B.1115.
26 June 25, 1662, B.1115.
27 May 4, 1664, B.607.
28 May 13 and May 17, 1664, B.607.
29 April 6, 10 and 13, 1678, B.618.
30 April 7, 1679, B.618.
31 April 9 and 26, 1662, B.1115.
32 April 30, 1662, B.1115.
33 May 31, 1662, B.1115.
34 March 5, 1678 and May 3, 1679, B.618; October 16, 1669, B.1115.
35 Weisser, "Disease," 70–72; Stolberg, *Experiencing Illness*, 144; Nicoud, "L'experience de la maladie," 333.
36 October 8, 1672, B.1115; October 3, 1651, B.619.
37 October 3, 1657, B.410.
38 June 2, August 12, 13 and 14, 1662, and October 2, 1669, B.1115.
39 August 2, 1661, B.607; October 5 and October 9, 1669, B.1115.
40 See Nicoud, "L'expérience de la maladie." 333; Stolberg, *Learned Physicians*, 238.
41 October 8, 1672, B.1115.
42 June 1, 1661, B.607.

43 May 31, 1661, B.607; September 23 and September 27, 1642, B.619.
44 Weisser, "Disease;" Stolberg, *Experiencing Illness*, 95–100.
45 February 23, 1662, B.607.
46 June 15, 1665, B.607.
47 Stolberg, *Experiencing Illness*, 24–26.
48 May 15, 1660, B.607.
49 Baths were used, for example, by Maria to treat her swollen knee. September 27, 1642, B.619.
50 Gianna Pomata, *Contracting a Cure: Patients, Healers, and the Law in Early Modern Bologna* (Baltimore, MD: Johns Hopkins University Press, 1998).
51 July 26 and 30, 1662, B.1115.
52 August 2 and 9, 1662, B.1115.
53 Annibale Camilli, *Del bagno di Nocera nell'Umbria, potentissimo ai morsi velenosi, detto acqua santa overo acqua bianca* (Perugia: Angelo Bartoli, 1627).
54 September 7 and 13, 1662, B.1115.
55 E.g., March 9, 1666, B.607.
56 I develop this point in Cavallo, "The Role of Medicinal Remedies."
57 Compare the late fifteenth-century letters published in Nicoud, "L'expérience de la maladie," 234–58.
58 May 6 and May 7, 1661, B.607.
59 July 23, 1662, B.1115.

Bibliography

Camilli, Annibale. *Del bagno di Nocera nell'Umbria, potentissimo ai morsi velenosi, detto acqua santa overo acqua bianca*. Perugia: Angelo Bartoli, 1627.

Cavallo, Sandra. "The Role of Medicinal Remedies in Seventeenth-Century Medical Treatment: The Case of Rome." In *Medicine in Early Modern Italy: Between Theory and Practice*, edited by Sandra Cavallo and John Henderson. Turnhout: Brepols, forthcoming.

Cavallo, Sandra and Tessa Storey. *Healthy Living in Late Renaissance Italy*. Oxford: Oxford University Press, 2013.

Cavallo, Sandra and Tessa Storey, eds. *Conserving Health in Early Modern Culture: Bodies and Environments in Italy and England.* Manchester: Manchester University Press, 2017.

Cook, Harold. "Markets and Cultures: Medical Specifics and the Reconfiguration of the Body in Early Modern Europe." *Transactions of the Royal Historical Society* 21 (2011): 123–45.

Mack, Peter. "Letter-Writing Manuals." In *A History of Renaissance Rhetoric, 1380–1620*, edited by Peter Mack, 228–56. Oxford: Oxford University Press, 2011.

Newton, Hannah. *The Sick Child in Early Modern England, 1580-1720*. Oxford: Oxford University Press, 2012.

Nicoud, Marilyn. "L'Expérience de la maladie et l'échange épistolaire: les derniers moments de Bianca Maria Visconti." *Mélanges de l'École française de Rome* 116 (2000): 85–101.

Pomata, Gianna. *Contracting a Cure: Patients, Healers, and the Law in Early Modern Bologna*. Baltimore, MD: Johns Hopkins University Press, 1998.

Porter, Roy, ed. *Patients and Practitioners: Lay Perceptions of Medicine and Pre-Industrial Society*. Cambridge: Cambridge University Press, 1985.

Porter, Roy. "The Patient's View: Doing Medical History from Below." *Theory and Society* 14 (1985): 178–79.

Quaranta, Alessandra. "The Consilia of Learned Physicians Pietro Andrea Mattioli and Francesco Partini: Doctrine, Empirical Knowledge, and Use of the Senses in Sixteenth-Century Europe." *Social History of Medicine* 35 (2021): 20–48.

Ruberg, Willemijn. "The Letter as Medicine: Studying Health and Illness in Dutch Daily Correspondence, 1770–1850." *Social History of Medicine* 23 (2010): 492–508.

Stolberg, Michael. *Experiencing Illness and the Sick Body in Early Modern Europe*. Basingstoke: Palgrave Macmillan 2011.

Stolberg, Michael. *Learned Physicians and Everyday Medical Practice*. Berlin and Boston, MA: de Gruyter, 2023.

Weisser, Olivia. "Disease." In *A Cultural History of Medicine in the Renaissance*, edited by Elaine Leong and Claudia Stein, 72–74. London: Bloomsbury, 2021.

Zarzoso, Alfonso. "Mediating Medicine through Private Letters: The Eighteenth-Century Catalan Medical World." In *Cultural Approaches to the History of Medicine: Mediating Medicine in Early Modern and Modern Europe*, edited by Willem de Blécourt and Cornelie Usborne, 108–126. Basingstoke: Palgrave Macmillan, 2004.

14 Newspaper Advertisements from the Eighteenth-Century Caribbean

Elise A. Mitchell

> To be Sold
>
> A Negroe Man Boy, named Monmouth, who has been brought up under a Surgeon for Three Years past, aged about 20. Whoever has a mind to Buy him, may apply to his Master, Mr. Michael Diore, Surgeon at the Plantation of Daniel Gotier Esqe. in Liguanea, he intending to go off the island.[1]

In 1719, Monmouth, an enslaved man in Linguanea, Jamaica, faced an uncertain future. He had "been brought up under" a surgeon, Michael Diore, for three years. He assisted Diore while he treated enslaved people on Daniel Gotier's plantation and likely treated enslaved people on his own. In the eighteenth century, apprenticeships were a crucial part of young free men's training to become surgeons and physicians.[2] However, for enslaved men and boys, like Monmouth, training under physicians and surgeons did not lead to a career. They often found themselves back in the fields or sold into the internal Jamaican slave trade when their slaveowners died or left the island.[3] Diore's advertisement in *The Weekly Jamaica Courant* reveals that Monmouth faced such a fate. His future was in the hands of "whoever ha[d] a mind to Buy him."

When Diore scrawled the advertisement on a small piece of paper, he did not imagine that it would ever find its way into the pages of a medical history book, such as the one you are reading now. When he submitted it to the printers, Mary and Robert Baldwin, Diore was not trying to create a historical record. He intended for his advertisement to serve a short-term purpose. Ephemera, such as newspapers, notes, letters, and other sorts of paper documents designed to serve short-term purposes, are an indispensable source for historians interested in popular and everyday histories of medicine. Over 300 years later, the advertisement for Monmouth is evidence of the roles enslaved medical practitioners played in Caribbean societies, the nature of their training, and their precarious circumstances.

This chapter focuses on eighteenth-century British and French Caribbean newspaper advertisements and how we can mine them as sources for the history of medicine and everyday life. By the eighteenth century, people of African descent vastly outnumbered Europeans in the Caribbean. The majority of these people were enslaved. Though they did not produce many printed records themselves,

DOI: 10.4324/9781003094876-18

newspapers demonstrate their influence on early Caribbean medicine. Though most collections have significant gaps, the surviving newspaper collections constitute a rich but uneven record of everyday life in the Caribbean. Collaborative digitization projects have made eighteenth-century and nineteenth-century Caribbean newspapers available to a wider audience than ever before.[4] This essay references eighteenth-century collections that are now available digitally as well as those that are still only available on microfilm or original copies in Caribbean, North American, and European archives. The first section will discuss the history of Caribbean periodicals. The second section will delve into how medical historians can use advertisements to understand everyday histories of medicine in the Caribbean. The surviving newspaper collections provide us with glimpses of the past that help us understand the everyday social relations of medicine and healing in the eighteenth-century Caribbean.

Caribbean Newspapers: A Historical Overview

When the ad for Monmouth appeared in *The Weekly Jamaica Courant*, newspapers were still a new media in the Caribbean islands. We find precursors to eighteenth-century gazettes as early as the sixteenth century. In 1542, the Spanish colonists in Mexico City printed the first *hoja volante* (flyer or newsletter). These *hojas* functioned as vehicles for the dissemination of news and current events in the sixteenth and seventeenth centuries, even though they were not printed regularly. The Spanish did not begin printing newspapers in the Caribbean until the nineteenth century, despite printing *gacetas* (gazettes) in North, Central, and South America in the early eighteenth century. Although Spanish printers were active in Jamaica before the English wrested the island from them in 1655, the first newspapers to leave a Caribbean island press were printed by English colonists and followed to the conventions of their metropolitan papers. *The Weekly Jamaica Courant* was the first periodical printed in the Caribbean and the second in the British American colonies. Before the 1760s, British Caribbean printers produced most of the periodicals in the Caribbean islands. British Caribbean printers also published other materials, chiefly almanacs, government meeting minutes, and treatises on disease and medicine. In 1764, the French established presses in Saint Domingue (present-day Haiti), Martinique, and Guadeloupe for the first time. By the late eighteenth century, the French joined the British as the leading producers of Caribbean periodicals.[5]

British and French newspapers, known as "gazettes," "couriers" (or "courants" and "*courriers*"), "*feuilles*," or "advertisers" and "*affiches*," circulated well beyond their respective colonial and imperial borders. Most printers operated out of port cities, including Kingston and Spanish Town (Jamaica), Cap-François and Port au Prince (Saint Domingue), Bridgetown (Barbados), Rousseau (Dominica), and Basseterre (Saint Christopher). These ports were all hubs for the intra-American and transatlantic circulation of news, goods, and people.[6] Printers' proximity to the ports and commercial thoroughfares ensured that their newspapers gained wide circulation. A combination of local government sponsors and subscribers funded the earliest newspapers. Subscribers included slaveowners, slave traders, medical practitioners, local politicians, tradesmen, sailors, and soldiers.

Newspapers connected colonists on the peripheries of empires to each other and the metropole. Printers typically devoted several pages to news about Europe, recycled from papers printed in London, Paris, and other metropolitan European cities.[7] This included reports of diseases on ships, epidemics, and medical successes and failures near and far. They also sometimes contained official summaries of local news often based on vestry, assembly, or council minutes. However, as one historian noted, there was "little of local interest beyond the advertisements" in eighteenth-century Caribbean newspapers.[8] The advertisements call our attention to the local context. Subscribers and local merchants submitted ads for imported foods, textiles, books, and medicines, people seeking employment, properties and businesses for sale, the sale of enslaved people, and advertisements for escaped enslaved and indentured people. Advertisements also provide detailed information about the range of drugs, medical treatments, medical literature, services, and practitioners in the Caribbean.

As the French and British vied for geopolitical control of the Caribbean, printers increasingly published bilingual newspapers. When the French ceded the islands of Dominica, Saint Vincent, and Grenada to the British in the Treaty of Paris 1763, British presses continued to publish sections of their newspapers in French with English translations. For example, a 1767 advertisement for Michael, an enslaved man from Martinique who escaped after working in a tavern in Dominica, appeared in English and French in the *Freeport Gazette*, published in Rousseau. Both advertisements describe a man named Michael/Michell who was "much pitted with the smallpox" ("*boucoup marque dans le verole*").[9] French and English readers understood what it meant to be "pitted with the smallpox." Scars revealed one's history and could also communicate or betray one's identity. Advertisements publicizing descriptions of enslaved people's bodies served as reminders of their enslaver's claims to their bodies and labor and evidence enslaved people's deft pursuits of reprieve, resistance, and freedom.[10] The advertisement for Michael/Michell also demonstrates the porous borders in the Caribbean, where people from French and British colonies moved across colonial boundaries and communicated across linguistic ones. Even after the British took over some formerly French islands in 1763, French presses continued to operate under British rule. For example, the French paper, *Courrier des Petites Antilles*, first published in British Dominica during the early 1790s, continued to print news for French audiences throughout the Caribbean.[11] Printers frequently printed material for audiences in neighboring colonies. Information printed in Caribbean newspapers circulated throughout the region as travelers carried the periodicals, clippings, handwritten copies, and translations across borders.[12]

A relatively small number of African and Native people in the Caribbean read and later published newspapers, even though Africans and Native people vastly outnumbered Europeans in the Caribbean region during the era of slavery. People of African and Indigenous Caribbean descent typically learned European languages in the context of enslavement, colonization, and missionary activity. Some free children of color received educations with European children abroad. Though few people of color could read European languages, many could read and write in other languages. For example, literate Muslims, who could read and write in Arabic, were among the enslaved Africans in the Caribbean. Native people in North and South America possessed complex writing systems and produced and circulated written, and later printed, documents. Nevertheless, town criers made public announcements and residents relied on oral communication. Knowledge, news, rumor, and gossip flowed across the aural landscape of the Caribbean region. Taverns, docks, and other places where gatherings took place served as conduits for information. In short, most eighteenth-century Caribbean inhabitants did not read the news. They heard it.[13]

Spaces where locals came together and read aloud, heard, discussed, clipped, copied, printed, and otherwise produced or reproduced news and public discourse shaped the public sphere. Social historians and historians of print culture have long argued that newspapers were a crucial part of the public sphere in early American where imperialism and slavery shaped much of the cultural and political activity.[14] Thus, these papers provide a window into local popular discourses about all sorts of topics, including medicine, health, and disease. Sometimes the discourse in the "counterpublic" spheres, in which the non-literate masses defined culture and politics for themselves, made its way into the papers too. For example, in 1779, a medical journal in Saint Domingue, *Gazette de Médecine pour les Colonies* published an essay by its founder, Duchemin de l'Étang, promoting smallpox inoculation that referenced enslaved Africans' knowledge and parlance for the practice. Étang noted, "the *Negres* also remember its utility, and they call it among themselves *buying* the smallpox."[15] Though the *Gazette de Médecine* primarily featured essays, letters, and excerpts written by and for elite, white, literate medical practitioners, historians can still find fragmentary evidence of non-elite practices and oral traditions in these journals.

Étang's reference also demonstrates local beliefs about inoculation. His essay appeared nearly two decades after smallpox inoculation was formally adopted in France.[16] It suggests that French colonists remained skeptical of inoculation. On the other hand, enslaved Africans "remember[ed] its utility." Étang alluded to a West African history of smallpox inoculation that predated the practices' introduction in Western Europe in the early eighteenth century. Examining this source in the context of other contemporary descriptions of West Africans performing smallpox inoculations brings a broader African Atlantic history of the medical practice into view.[17] Sources like this lay bare the local and global dimensions of the history of medical practices and the circulation of medical knowledge.

Like medical gazettes, general gazettes also contained valuable information about popular medical discourses. Historians have argued that *Affiches Américaines*, a general advertiser founded in Saint Domingue in 1764, exposed colonists to "the wider world of science and learning" and "fostered public conversation" about colonists' needs, including their health and medical concerns.[18] *Affiches Américaines* was geared toward a general audience and included many advertisements and excerpts from printed texts and newspapers abroad. In the 1770s, debates about the legitimacy of the *Gazette de Médicine* unfolded in the pages of the supplement to *Affiches Américaines*.[19] Members of the Cercle des Philadelphes, a prominent learned society based in Saint Domingue, felt that the *Gazette de Médicine* posed a threat to their authority. Accustomed to the censorship of the press in France, some members of the Circle de Philadelphes, notably Charles Arthaud, sought to delegitimize the journal. Arthaud's attacks were ultimately successful. The *Gazette de Médicine* only printed eight issues.[20] In contrast, eighteenth-century general gazettes ran for decades and became important sites for public debate and the circulation of medical knowledge. Though they only represent a fraction of the public discourse about medicine, health, and healing in the early modern Caribbean, they remain indispensable sources for the history of medicine and the everyday.

Advertisements and Medical History: Sources, Methods, and Approaches

Newspaper advertisements typically featured goods services, people for sale or for hire, and enslaved or indentured people who evaded bondage. Eighteenth-century Caribbean newspaper advertisements reveal the region's medical marketplace, local therapeutics and expertise, and diseases. Making sense of these advertisements requires deeper inquiry into the local and historical context. Students and scholars must read advertisements within their historical context and read beyond the text of a single advertisement to fully understand its significance and any historical actors represented in it.[21] Advertisements reveal everyday histories of medicine when we employ a method known as triangulation. This method involves approaching the advertisement from multiple angles and reading it in context with other types of contemporary sources.

Some advertisements reveal how the printer's office functioned as an information hub and node in transatlantic and local networks of the trade in medicines. For example, in September 1765, the *St. Christopher's Gazette* included the following advertisement for "Doctor Nelson's Antiscorbutic Drops."[22]

> IMPORTED from LONDON
> And to be sold at the Printing-Office
> DOCTOR NELSON'S
> Antiscorbutic Drops;
> Which are an effectual cure for the Scurvy, Rheumatism, Yaws, Venereal Diseases, Gleets and Seminal Weaknesses, and Ulcers of All Kinds. – Price 15s. a bottle, with a printed Bill of Directions.[23]

The advertisement demonstrates how printers published and participated in the sale of imported medicines. The drops were advertised as "an effectual Cure for the Scurvy, Rheumatism, Yaws, Venereal Diseases, Gleets, and Seminal Weaknesses, and Ulcers of all kinds." Ambitious doctors, like Nelson, may have advertised cures for "venereal diseases" and "seminal weakness" as panaceas with broad applications to reach sufferers, who might have been ashamed to seek treatment.[24]

All of the ailments listed in the advertisement were common among mariners in the Caribbean.[25] Slaveowners routinely complained that yaws (a contagious disease characterized by skin eruptions, sores, and eventually joint pain), venereal diseases, and rheumatism plagued enslaved people.[26] By reading this advertisement alongside other sources, such as plantation manuals and medical treatises on disease in the Caribbean, we can deduce that this ad targeted seamen and slaveowners.

European and Euro-Caribbean physicians also used the local paper to advertise their services. For example, in 1773 as smallpox epidemics spread across the Caribbean region, the British physician, Micah Broun, advertised his plans to perform smallpox inoculations in the French colony of Saint Domingue in *Affiches Américaines*.[27]

> Le Sieur Micah Broun, Médecin Anglois, ayant obtenu du Gouvernement la permission d'exercer ses talens pour l'opération de l'Inoculation, il a débuté par opérer une Négritte de M. Tardieu, Négociant au Cap. Cette enfant n'a eu qu'un seul accès de fievre la veille que la petite vérole est sortie, & n'a pas eu d'autres accidens: elle a été parfaitement guérie en trois semaines. Ledit Sieur Broun va sur l'Habitation des Héritiers Bordes, au Bonnet, Paroisse de la Petite-Anse, pour y faire la même operation aux enfans de ladite Habitation, à la requisition d'un des Cohéritiers. Il donnera avis au Public du succès qu'il ose se flatter d'avoir de ses operations à ladite Habitation.
>
> The English doctor, Sr. Micah Broun, has obtained permission from the Government to exercise his talents for the operation of inoculation, he began by operating on a *Nègritte* of Mr. Tardieu's, a business man of Cap-François. This child had only one bout of fever the day before the smallpox broke out, & had no other issues; she was perfectly healed in three weeks. The said Sr. Broun heads to the plantation of the Heirs of Bordes, at Bonnet, Parish of Petite-Anse, to carry out the same operation on the children of the said plantation at the request of the heirs. He will notify the public of the success he dares to boast of having with his operations at the said plantation.[28]

Broun's advertisement demonstrates how medical practitioners worked across the permeable colonial and imperial borders in the Caribbean. The advertisement also shows that physicians needed permission from the government in Saint Domingue to perform inoculations. In the late eighteenth century, colonial authorities increasingly regulated inoculation. Slaveowners employed European surgeons and physicians to perform inoculations that would preserve their labor force.[29] Physicians exploited the system of slavery to prove their skills and expand their businesses.

Every source has its limitations. Like most early modern sources, newspapers were written from the perspectives of white propertied colonists, physicians, and slaveowners, not the middling and poor whites and not the enslaved Black majority. Broun's advertisement represents his interests, not those of the enslaved. Broun performed these inoculations for his benefit and the benefit of Tardieu and the Bordes, not the enslaved children and their families. The advertisement describes Broun's inoculations as a "success." Success to whom? And by what standard? We cannot know whether Broun's practice aligned with the inoculation techniques enslaved Africans used among themselves or whether the children's parents approved. Enslaved people's representation in early Caribbean newspaper advertisements was never within their control. Their appearances in advertisements as test subjects, chattel for sale, fugitives, or missing property were representations constructed by their enslavers. Nevertheless, historians have still been able to use these sources to deepen our understanding of the social and cultural history of the Caribbean, including elite, middling, poor, bound, and enslaved people.

Enslaved and indentured people appear most frequently in advertisements for runaways. Using these advertisements, historians have constructed rich intellectual, social, and cultural histories of slave societies.[30] Some have aggregated and analyzed thousands of runaway slave advertisements to produce detailed histories of emerging racial discourses, the incidence of injuries, diseases, and disabilities, and histories of the surveillance and violence used against the enslaved.[31] For example, in this volume, Stefanie Hunt-Kennedy uses these types of ads to examine the history of disability. Historians have also consulted these runaway advertisements to write social, cultural, and demographic histories of enslaved people, enslaved people's modes of self-fashioning, histories slave resistance, and histories of slavery-era visual culture. In contrast, other historians have taken a microhistorical approach to these sources and used them to probe the individual, local histories of the enslaved. More recently digital humanists have used these advertisements to develop databases of advertisements and mapping projects that locate the origins and destinations of fugitive slaves. Ads for runaways with medical training or expertise expand our knowledge and concepts of what it meant to be a healer in the eighteenth-century Caribbean.

Ads for the sale of enslaved people, like Monmouth, or the return of escaped enslaved and indentured people demonstrate the range of medical expertise in the region. To historicize subjects like Monmouth, historians must read against the grain and perform triangulation using additional sources. Considering multiple sources together can yield a richer understanding of individual subjects and their wider worlds. For example, in the summer of 1718, while Monmouth was still assisting Diore in Linguanea, his neighbor, a "White-servant Boy," named John Braddas "Absented himself" from the service of the doctor who held him in bondage as an indentured servant. Though indentured servants endured forms of bondage, exploitation, and violence that were similar to enslaved people, their status was not hereditary, and, by the eighteenth century, colonial assemblies increasingly passed legislation that shielded them from the degree of brutal punishment, labor, and exploitation that enslaved people endured.[32] Less than a year after the Baldwins founded *The Weekly Jamaica Courant,* Doctor Smithell Maison submitted an advertisement seeking Braddas' capture and return.

> Absented himself the 30th of July, from his Master Doctor Smithell Maison's Service, a White Servant-Boy, named John Braddas, aged about 16 Years, well set, fair Complection, has Short Yellow Hair, wears a Pair of Oznabrig Breeches, Speckled Shirt, and Blew striped Jacket, with an old black Hat,

> Shoes and Stockings; he speaks good English and Dutch and can Read and Write, Bleed, Sing and Dance; on Each of his Arms is the sign of Jerusalem Arms, and several blew Spots, on his Hands. Whoever Secures him for his said Master, in Liguanea, shall have 20 s. Reward and whosoever Entertains him be it at their Peril.[33]

The scholar Stefanie Hunt-Kennedy explained that ads for runaway indentured servants typically focused on their skills and the physical appearances of their hands and faces – body parts that were visible when a person was fully clothed. In contrast, advertisements for runaway enslaved people often commented on their full bodies, especially their skin, marks in areas that would usually be covered with clothing and their legs and feet.[34] The symbols on Braddas arms may suggest his religious background. Like his skills, these marks were used to identify him and suggest the types of communities and activities he might have been engaged in during his "absence." Maison mentioned that Braddas could "Bleed," meaning bloodletting, or the practice of cutting a vein or artery to rid the body of a disease or ailment, was one of his skills. Maison may have hoped others would identify him if he sought employment as a medical assistant.

Runaway advertisements sometimes contained detailed descriptions of indentured and enslaved peoples' bodies, ailments, disabilities, and health as well as their expertise as barbers, medical assistants, nurses, or midwives. Nevertheless, bound people's avenues to practice medical skills varied according to their race and gender. Indentured men and boys with some medical skills, like Braddas, sometimes found opportunities to apprentice with local surgeons and physicians and eventually begin small and middling practices of their own once they were free. Enslaved men and boys of African descent, who often trained side-by-side with free white medical assistants, were not afforded the same opportunities. Most men and boys of African descent were enslaved in early eighteenth-century Jamaica. According to historians, in the first decades of the eighteenth century, there were fewer than 1,000 free people of color in Jamaica, most of whom were women.[35] Through the late eighteenth century, free women of color outnumbered free men of color. This gender imbalance persisted in the medical profession. Jamaican free men of color typically worked in the agricultural economy or as artisans, clerks, tradesmen, tavern keepers, sailors, pilots, and shopkeepers. There is little evidence of free men of color working for pay in medical professions in the British Caribbean, despite their presence as healers in enslaved and maroon communities. Similarly, in the French Caribbean male medical practitioners of African descent tended to be enslaved in urban areas rather than free.[36]

Women of African descent were more likely than men to get paid for medical labor. Enslaved and free women of African descent frequently performed medical labor in the domestic sphere, plantation sick houses, military barracks, and parish almshouses and charitable hospitals.[37] Freed women, who previously performed medical labor while they were enslaved, sometimes continued to their work in proximity to their former slaveowners or assumed the ranks of "negro nurses" laboring in hospitals. We tend to learn more about their labor as nurses, midwives, healers, and obeah practitioners from plantation records, slaveowners' diaries, local vestry minutes, hospital inventories, medical treatises, and planation manuals. Though enslaved women appear in runaway advertisements less frequently than enslaved and indentured men and boys, we occasionally find evidence of their medical labor in these advertisements as well.[38]

The following advertisement for Télémaque and Anna, a nurse, appeared in *Les Affiches Americaines* in 1783, roughly two decades after the inaugural issue of the advertiser.

> Télémaque, nation Mesurade, venu enfant dans le pays, étampé PESCAY & FPF, âgé de 38 ans, parlant bon français, de petite taille, replet & trapu, le visage noir, barbu & gravé de petite vérole, le front ouvert, les yeux petits, enfoncés, la bouche grande, les levres grosses, de belle dents, les cuisses pleines, la jambe bien faite, charnue & velue, la démarche prompte, est parti maron le 9 de ce mois avec son linge & armé d'une manchette. Anna, hospitaliere, étampée VDPY & FPF, sachant très bien saigner, âgée de 52 ans, de petite taille, la peau rouge, le visage un peu ridé, les yeux petits & enfoncés, les dents gâtées, les cheveux longs, grisonnans, les reins courts & arqués, les hanches hautes, est partie maronne le 4 de ce mois. Ceux qui en auront connaissance, sont priés d'en donner avis à M. Pescay fils, sur son habitation, au Piment. Il y aura deux portugaises de récompense pour chaque negre.
>
> Télémaque, Kanga nation, came to the country as a child, branded PESCAY & FPF, 38 years old, speaks good French, small stature, plump & stocky, black face, bearded and pitted with the smallpox, broad forehead, deep set, small eyes, big mouth, big lips, nice teeth, full thighs, well-made legs, fleshy & hairy, quick gait, escaped on the 9th of this month with his linen & cuffs. Anna, *hospitaliere*, branded VDPY & FPF, can bleed very well, 52 years old, small stature, red skin, slightly wrinkled face, small deep-set eyes, bad teeth, long gray hair, small curvy waist, high hips, escaped the 4 of this month. Those who know of them are requested to give notice to Mr. Pescay's sons, at their plantation, in Piment. There will be two Portuguese reward for each *négre*.[39]

In the description of Anna, we learn that she was a *hospitalière,* or nurse in charge of the hospital on a plantation, who could "bleed very well."[40] *Hospitalières* possessed a valuable skillset and played a crucial role as the primary caretakers of enslaved people on plantations.[41] Pescay likely viewed Anna's escape as an economic loss as well as a disciplinary matter. Slave owners valued *hospitalières* at a high price. The advertisement also mentioned that Anna was "52 years old." French and British plantation manuals from this era recommended that the *hospitalière* or "Hospital Matron or Doctress must be a woman of middling age, of a compassionate disposition [with] the skill to dress ordinary wounds and sores."[42] One slaveowner from Saint Domingue claimed that their skills "set some of those women, in many respects, above surgeons."[43] Anna's skills may have represented multiple strands of medical expertise. In Saint Domingue, she could have learned from a variety of sources. Bloodletting was a standard medical practice among European surgeons and plantation managers in the Caribbean. West Africans also practiced bloodletting and were known as skilled barbers in the Americas. European sources dating to the sixteenth century describe West Africans bleeding one another to treat diseases and seasonal afflictions. The advertisement seeking Anna provides an entry point into a deeper history of Black Atlantic medicine and healing.[44]

The advertisement also tells us about Anna and Télémaque's bodies. Eighteenth-century popular descriptions of bodies are not necessarily commensurate with our modern notions of phenotype. For example, the references to Télémaque's "black" face and Anna's "red skin" may not necessarily have been indicative of their skin tones, but rather observers' ideas about their humoral balance and physiognomic observations about their bodies.[45] The description of Télémaque includes a detailed description of his body, noting that he was "pitted with the smallpox." Smallpox outbreaks were common along slave trading routes to the Caribbean in the late eighteenth century. The advertisement notes that Télémaque was African-born and of the *Mesurade* or, in English, Kanga "nation." These terms were French and British ethnonyms that referred to enslaved people from the Upper Guinea region and the Bight of Benin in West Africa.[46] He may have had scarification or other bodily markings that locals associated *Mesurade*/Kanga people, making him more identifiable.

The little we gather about Anna, Télémaque, John Braddas, Monmouth, and legions of other people represented in early Caribbean newspapers are precious glimpses of everyday histories that would otherwise be beyond our reach. They leave us with unanswered questions about these enslaved people's inner lives. How did Anna and John Braddas learn to bleed? Why did Anna and Télémaque flee together? Was Télémaque also a healer? Why did John Braddas have those tattoos on his arms? What were the enslaved people's reactions to Micah Broun? Who wandered into the printer's office to buy Dr. Nelson's drops? What did Monmouth do after Diore left? These and myriad other questions demand that we look beyond individual advertisements, speculate, and probe other sources for possible answers. Nevertheless, the newspapers provide fruitful starting points.

Conclusion

Like medical journals and medical treatises, the pages of eighteenth-century Caribbean newspapers evidence the circulation of people, healing knowledge, and drugs in the early modern Caribbean and wider Atlantic World. The advertisements in these papers reveal the convergence of local and global forced, free, and fugitive migrations, trade, and knowledge production that was integral to the formation of Caribbean medical practices. These newspapers simultaneously evidence the expertise of enslaved and indentured healers, like Monmouth, John Braddas, and Anna, and the ways colonialism and bondage circumscribed their ability to practice. These sources are not without their limitations. Early Caribbean newspapers were first and foremost produced by and for elites and small-scale property-owning Europeans living in the Caribbean, most of whom were slaveowners.

This population constituted a shrinking minority in the eighteenth century. As the slave trade reached its zenith in the mid-eighteenth century, enslaved Africans and their descendants vastly outnumbered Europeans and Euro-Caribbeans. African and Indigenous Caribbeans' medical and healing knowledge circulated by word of mouth, experience, and demonstrations more often than in print. We can glimpse their knowledge in mediated accounts written by predominantly white medical men and advertisements describing their knowledge or seeking to capture or sell enslaved healers. Nevertheless, despite the inherent biases of these sources and their fragmentary state, historians can use newspapers to reconstruct rich histories of medicine and everyday life in the early Caribbean.

Notes

1 "[To be Sold]," *The Weekly Jamaica Courant*, April 15, 1719, The National Library of Jamaica, Newspaper Collection.

2 Sheridan, *Doctors and Slaves*, 42–47, 111; Hogarth, *Medicalizing Blackness*, 93, 111; Weaver, "Surgery, Slavery, and the Circulation," 108–09.

3 For examples of skilled enslaved medical laborers who were sent back to field after their enslavers died, see: "Galen" in Alexander Johnston's papers in The Powel Family Papers (Col. 1582), Historical Society of Pennsylvania.

4 Levi and Inniss, "Decolonizing the Archival Record about the Enslaved."

5 The first Spanish American newspaper, *La Gaceta de México*, was printed in Mexico City in 1722, followed by gazettes published in Guatemala and Lima. Uribe-Uran, "The Birth of a Public Sphere in Latin America," 425–57. The French, like the Dutch and Portuguese, were reticent to permit printing presses in the Americas. Popkin, "A Colonial Media Revolution," 3–25. On English predecessors of British Caribbean papers see: Newman, *Freedom Seekers:* xxviii–xxix On the history of the press in the Caribbean see: Hester, "Newspapers and Newspaper Prototypes," 73–88; Cave, "Printing Comes to Jamaica," 11–17; Steele, *The English Atlantic*, 153; Cave, "Printing Comes to Jamaica," 11–17; Steele, *The English Atlantic*, 153; Shilstone, "Some Notes," 19–33; Cundall, "The Press and Printers of Jamaica," 290–354; Cundall, *A History of Printing in Jamaica from 1717 to 1834,* 1–32; Cundall, "The Press and Printers of Jamaica," 290–354; Cundall, *A History of Printing in Jamaica from 1717 to 1834,* 1–32.

6 Scott, *The Common Wind*, 15, 44.

7 Steele, *The English Atlantic*, 132–67; Copeland, *Colonial American Newspapers,* 15–16.

8 Cundall, "The Press and Printers of Jamaica," 334.

9 "[Runaway]," *The Freeport Gazette or the Dominica Advertiser*, July 18, 1767, *Caribbean Newspapers: Series 1, 1718–1876.*

10 Waldstreicher, "Reading the Runaways," 245; Fuentes, *Dispossessed Lives,* 13–21; Hunt-Kennedy, *Between Fitness and Death,* 95–126.

11 *Courrier des Petites Antilles*, July 24, 1790–December 6, 1790, Bibliothèque National de France.

12 Cave, "Early Printing and the Book Trade in the West Indies," 163–92; Robertson, "Eighteenth-Century Jamaica's Ambivalent Cosmopolitanism," 607–31; Scott, *The Common Wind*, 129–30; Steele, *The English Atlantic*, 132–67; Soriano, *Tides of Revolution*, 15–46.

13 For examples of people of African descent who published see: Scott, *The Common Wind*, 135–36; Johnson, *The Fear of French Negroes*, 157–87. On free children of color's education: Peabody, *"There Are No Slaves in France,"* 80–81; Livesay, *Children of Uncertain Fortune*. On Muslim literacy: Diouf, *Servants of Allah*, 25, 203–09, 254. On

Native writing systems: Tavárez, "Zapotec Time, Alphabetic Writing, and the Public Sphere," 73–85. Town criers throughout the Caribbean islands were often of African descent. Along the South American coast many were Native or African. For example, see: Cundall, "The Press and Printers of Jamaica," 291. On the circulation of news in the Caribbean see: Scott, *The Common Wind.*

14 Foundational work on the public sphere, see: Habermas, *The Structural Transformation of the Public Sphere*; Calhoun, *Habermas and the Public Sphere*; Anderson, *Imagined Communities*; Waldstreicher, "Reading the Runaways," 243–72; Brooks, "The Early American Public Sphere and the Emergence of a Black Print Counterpublic," 67–98.

15 Duchemin de l'Etang, "Inoculation," in *Gazette de Médecine Pour Les Colonies*, January 1, 1779, Archives Nationales d'Outre Mer, 87 MIOM/63.

16 Miller, *The Adoption of Inoculation for Smallpox*, 195–240.

17 Herbert, "Smallpox Inoculation in Africa," 539–59; Weaver, "Surgery, Slavery, and the Circulation," 105–17.

18 McClellan, *Colonialism and Science,* 171; Taber, "*Le Sens Commun,*" 569–83.

19 *Supplément aux Affiches Américaines*, 2–4, Archives Nationales d'Outre Mer, 87 MIOM/63.

20 McClellan, *Colonialism and Science,* 141–140.

21 Waldstreicher, "Reading the Runaways"; Block, *Colonial Complexions*, 143–49; Hunt-Kennedy, *Between Fitness and Death*, 96.

22 "Antiscorbutic" referred to a range of treatments used against scurvy, often acidic liquids. "antiscorbutic, adj. and n." OED Online. December 2021. Oxford University Press. https://www-oed-com.ezproxy.princeton.edu/view/Entry/8845?redirectedFrom=antiscorbutic (accessed January 3, 2022).

23 "Doctor Nelson's Antiscorbutic Drops," *The St. Christopher's Gazette*, September 4, 1765, *Caribbean Newspapers.*

24 On shame and venereal disease see: Paugh, "Yaws, Syphilis, Sexuality, and the Circulation," 225–52.

25 Harrison, *Medicine in an Age of Commerce and Empire*, 237–53.

26 Grainger, *An Essay on the More Common West-India Diseases*; On the incidence of these diseases among enslaved people in the Caribbean and the racialization of disease in the Caribbean: Sheridan, *Doctors and Slaves*; Kiple, *The Caribbean Slave*; Hogarth, *Medicalizing Blackness*; Seth, *Difference and Disease*; Schiebinger, *Secret Cures of Slaves*.

27 Smallpox was endemic in the Caribbean by the 1770s. For example, in 1772 and 1773 outbreaks raged in Saint Domingue, Antigua, and Martinique. See: McClellan, *Colonialism and Science*, 29; Sheridan, *Doctors and Slaves*, 258.

28 "Avis Divers," *Les Affiche Américaines*, May 15, 1773, The Digital Library of the Caribbean. All translations my own unless otherwise noted.

29 Weaver, *Medical Revolutionaries*, 51.

30 In short, most eighteenth-century Caribbean inhabitants did not read the news. They heard it.

31 Block, *Colonial Complexions*; Hunt-Kennedy, *Between Fitness and Death*, 95–125; Hogarth, *Medicalizing Blackness*, 133–58, 173; Scott, *The Common Wind*; Gomez, *Exchanging Our Country Marks*; Waldstreicher, "Reading the Runaways," 243–72; Wood, *Blind Memory*, 87–99; Morgan, *Laboring Women,* 178–83; Read and Zimmerman, "Freedom for Too Few," 404–26; Eddins, *Rituals, Runaways, and the Haitian Revolution*; Fuentes, *Dispossessed Lives*, 13–21. See also "Selected Bibliographies, Directories, and Databases" at the end of this chapter.

32 Paton, "Punishment, Crime, and the Bodies of Slaves in Eighteenth-Century Jamaica," *Journal of Social History* 34, no. 4 (2001): 923–54; Amussen, *Caribbean Exchanges*, 129–35; Shaw, *Everyday Life in the Early English Caribbean*, 15–42; Jennifer L. Morgan, "*Partus Sequitur Ventrem,*" 1–17; Hunt-Kennedy, *Between Fitness and Death*, 39–68.

33 "[Absented, John Braddas]," *The Weekly Jamaica Courant*, July 30, 1718, The National Library of Jamaica, Newspaper Collection.
34 Hunt-Kennedy, *Between Fitness and Death*, 95–125.
35 Mair, *A Historical Study of Women in Jamaica*, 87.
36 Free and enslaved men of African descent rarely joined the medical professions in Jamaica and other British Caribbean territories. However, in the Spanish and Portuguese Americas, free and enslaved men often gained admittance or continued to labor as respected popular healers. On free people of color's professions in Jamaica see: Braithwaite, *The Development of Creole Society in Jamaica*, 172–74; On Black healers in the Caribbean: Sheridan, *Doctors and Slaves*, 72–97; Paton, *The Cultural Politics of Obeah*; Hogarth, *Medicalizing Blackness*, 85–93. On Black healers in the French Caribbean: Weaver, "Surgery, Slavery, and the Circulation," 105–17.
37 Paugh, *The Politics of Reproduction*, 122–153; Turner, *Contested Bodies*, 112–50; Moitt, *Women and Slavery*, 63–68; Weaver, *Medical Revolutionaries*.
38 Bush, *Slave Women in Caribbean Society*, 63–65; Enslaved men were also more likely than enslaved women to run away in groups. See: Morgan, *Laboring Women*, 178–83.
39 "[Télémaque and Anna]," *Affiches Américaines*, October 15, 1783, The Digital Library of the Caribbean; See also: "Télémaque" and "Anna," Saint-Domingue, *Affiches américaines*, 1783-10-15, *Le Marronage dans le monde Atlantique: Sources et trajectoires de vie*, http://www.marronnage.info/fr/document.php?id=11468 (accessed November 1, 2021).
40 Weaver, *Medical Revolutionaries*, 2.
41 Weaver, "Surgery, Slavery, and the Circulation," 110–13.
42 Laborie, *The Coffee Planter of Saint Domingo*, 166–67.
43 Laborie, *The Coffee Planter of Saint Domingo*, 166–67.
44 On bloodletting see: Weaver, "Surgery, Slavery, and the Circulation," 109; Kananoja, *Healing Knowledge in Atlantic Africa*, 121–29; Hicks, "Blood and Hair," 61–82; Anonymous, "Description of a Voyage from Lisbon," 164–65.
45 Block, *Colonial Complexions*, 60–83.
46 Africans called Kanga/*Mesurade* may have hailed from Sierra Leone or the Gold Coast region. Hall, *Slavery and African Ethnicities in the Americas*, 31–32.

Bibliography

Amussen, Susan. *Caribbean Exchanges: Slavery and the Transformation of English Society, 1640–1700.* Chapel Hill: University of North Carolina Press, 2007.

Anderson, Benedict. *Imagined Communities: Reflections on the Origin and Spread of Nationalism.* New York: Verso, [1983] 2006.

Blake, John William, ed. *Europeans in West Africa, 1540–1560.* London: The Hakluyt Society, 1942.

Block, Sharon. *Colonial Complexions: Race and Bodies in Eighteenth-Century America.* Philadelphia: University of Pennsylvania Press, 2018.

Braithwaite, Kamau. *The Development of Creole Society in Jamaica, 1770–1820.* Kingston: Ian Randle Publishers, [1971] 2005.

Brooks, Joanna. "The Early American Public Sphere and the Emergence of a Black Print Counterpublic." *The William and Mary Quarterly* 62 (2005): 67–98.

Bush, Barbara. *Slave Women in Caribbean Society, 1650–1838.* Bloomington: Indiana University Press, 1990.

Calhoun, Craig ed., *Habermas and the Public Sphere.* Cambridge: Massachusetts Institute of Technology, 1992.

Cave, Roderick. "Printing Comes to Jamaica." *Jamaica Journal* 9, no. 2–3 (1975): 11–17.

———. "Early Printing and the Book Trade in the West Indies." *The Library Quarterly* 48, no. 2 (1978): 163–92.

Copeland, David. *Colonial American Newspapers: Character and Content.* Newark: University of Delaware Press, 1997.

Cundall, Frank. "The Press and Printers of Jamaica Prior to 1820." *Proceedings of the American Antiquarian Society* 26 (1916): 290–354.

Cundall, Frank. *A History of Printing in Jamaica from 1717 to 1834.* Kingston: The Institute of Jamaica, 1935.

Diouf, Sylviane. *Servants of Allah: African Muslims Enslaved in the Americas.* New York: New York University Press, 1998.

Eddins, Crystal. *Rituals, Runaways, and the Haitian Revolution.* New York: Cambridge University Press, 2021.

Fuentes, Marisa. *Dispossessed Lives: Enslaved Women, Violence, and the Archive.* Philadelphia: University of Pennsylvania Press, 2016.

Gomez, Michael. *Exchanging Our Country Marks: The Transformation of African Identities in the Colonial and Antebellum South.* Chapel Hill: University of North Carolina Press, 1998.

Grainger, James. *An Essay on the More Common West-India Diseases.* London: T. Becket and P.A. De Hondt, 1764.

Habermas, Jürgen. *The Structural Transformation of the Public Sphere: An Inquiry into a Category of Bourgeois Society*, translated by Thomas Burger. Cambridge: Massachusetts Institute of Technology, [1962] 1989.

Hall, Gwendolyn Midlo. *Slavery and African Ethnicities in the Americas: Restoring the Links.* Chapel Hill: University of North Carolina Press, 2005.

Harrison, Mark. *Medicine in an Age of Commerce and Empire: Britain and Its Tropical Colonies, 1660–1830.* New York: Oxford University Press, 2010.

Herbert, Eugenia. "Smallpox Inoculation in Africa." *The Journal of African History* 16, no. 4 (1975): 539–59.

Hester, Al. "Newspapers and Newspaper Prototypes in Spanish America, 1541–1750." *Journalism History* 6, no. 3 (Autumn 1979): 73–88.

Hicks, Mary. "Blood and Hair: Barbers, Sangradores, and the West African Corporeal Imagination in Salvador da Bahia, 1793–1843." In *Medicine and Healing in the Age of Slavery*, edited by Christopher Willoughby and Sean Morey Smith, 61–82. Baton Rouge: Louisiana State University Press, 2021.

Hogarth, Rana. *Medicalizing Blackness: Making Racial Difference in the Atlantic World, 1780–1840.* Chapel Hill: University of North Carolina Press, 2017.

Hunt-Kennedy, Stefanie. *Between Fitness and Death: Disability and Slavery in the Caribbean.* Urbana: University of Illinois Press, 2020.

Johnson, Sara. *The Fear of French Negroes: Transcolonial Collaboration in the Revolutionary Americas.* Berkeley: University of California Press, 2012.

Kananoja, Kalle. *Healing Knowledge in Atlantic Africa: Medical Encounters, 1500–1850.* New York: Cambridge University Press, 2021.

Kiple, Kenneth. *The Caribbean Slave: A Biological History.* New York: Cambridge University Press, 1984.

Laborie, Pierre-Joseph. *The Coffee Planter of Saint Domingo.* London: T. Cadell and W. Davies, 1798.

Levi, Amalia and Tara Inniss. "Decolonizing the Archival Record about the Enslaved: Digitizing the Barbados Mercury Gazette." *Archipelagos* 4 (2020): http://archipelagosjournal.org/es/issue04/levi-inniss-decolonizing.html (accessed November 1, 2021).

Livesay, Daniel. *Children of Uncertain Fortune: Mixed-Race Jamaicans in Britain and the Atlantic Family, 1733–1833*. Chapel Hill: University of North Carolina Press, 2018.

Mair, Lucille Mathurin. *A Historical Study of Women in Jamaica, 1655–1844*, edited by Hilary McD. Beckles and Verene A. Shepherd. Kingston: University of the West Indies Press, 2006.

McClellan, James. *Colonialism and Science: Saint Domingue in the Old Regime*. Chicago, IL: University of Chicago Press, [1992] 2010.

Miller, Genevieve. *The Adoption of Inoculation for Smallpox in England and France*. Philadelphia: University of Pennsylvania Press, 1957.

Moitt, Bernard. *Women and Slavery in the French Antilles, 1635–1848*. Bloomington: Indiana University Press, 2001.

Morgan, Jennifer. *Laboring Women: Reproduction and Gender in New World Slavery*. Philadelphia: University of Pennsylvania Press, 2004.

———. "*Partus Sequitur Ventrem*: Law, Race, and Reproduction in Colonial Slavery." *Small Axe: A Caribbean Journal of Criticism* 22, no. 1 (2018): 1–17.

Newman, Simon P. *Freedom Seekers: Escaping from Slavery in Restoration London*. London: University of London Press, 2022.

Paton, Diana. "Punishment, Crime, and the Bodies of Slaves in Eighteenth-Century Jamaica." *Journal of Social History* 34, no. 4 (2001): 923–54.

———. *The Cultural Politics of Obeah: Religion, Colonialism and Modernity in the Caribbean World*. New York: Cambridge University Press, 2015.

Paugh, Katherine. "Yaws, Syphilis, Sexuality, and the Circulation of Medical Knowledge in the British Caribbean and the Atlantic World." *Bulletin of the History of Medicine* 88, no. 2 (2014): 225–52.

———. *The Politics of Reproduction: Race, Medicine, and Fertility in the Age of Abolition*. New York: Oxford University Press, 2017.

Peabody, Sue. *"There Are No Slaves in France": The Political Culture of Race and Slavery in the Ancien Régime*. New York: Oxford University Press, 2002.

Popkin, Jeremy. "A Colonial Media Revolution: The Press in Saint-Domingue, 1789–1793." *The Americas* 75, no. 1 (2018): 3–25.

Read, Ian, and Kari Zimmerman. "Freedom for Too Few: Slave Runaways in the Brazilian Empire." *Journal of Social History* 48, no. 2 (2014): 404–26.

Robertson, James. "Eighteenth-Century Jamaica's Ambivalent Cosmopolitanism." *History* 99, no. 337 (2014): 607–31.

Schiebinger, Londa. *Secret Cures of Slaves: People, Plants, and Medicine in the Eighteenth-Century Atlantic World*. Stanford, CA: Stanford University Press, 2017.

Scott, Julius. *The Common Wind: Afro-American Currents in the Age of the Haitian Revolution*. New York: Verso, 2020.

Seth, Suman. *Difference and Disease: Medicine, Race, and the Eighteenth-Century British Empire*. New York: Cambridge University Press, 2018.

Shaw, Jenny. *Everyday Life in the Early English Caribbean: Irish, Africans, and the Construction of Difference*. Athens: University of Georgia Press, 2013.

Sheridan, Richard. *Doctors and Slaves: A Medical and Demographic History of Slavery in the British West Indies, 1680–1834*. New York: Cambridge University Press, 1985.

Shilstone, E.M. "Some Notes on Early Printing Presses and Newspapers in Barbados." *The Journal of the Barbados Museum and Historical Society* 26, no. 1 (November 1958): 19–33.

Soriano, Cristina. *Tides of Revolution: Information, Insurgencies, and the Crisis of Colonial Rule in Venezuela.* Albuquerque: University of New Mexico Press, 2019.

Steele, Ian Kenneth. *The English Atlantic, 1675–1740: An Exploration of Communication and Community*. New York: Oxford University Press, 1986.

Taber, Robert. "'*Le Sens Commun*': Atlantic Pathways and Imagination in Saint-Domingue's *Affiches Américaines*." *The Latin Americanist* 61, no. 4 (December 2017): 569–83.

Tavárez, David. "Zapotec Time, Alphabetic Writing, and the Public Sphere." *Ethnohistory* 57, no. 1 (2010): 73–85.

Turner, Sasha. *Contested Bodies: Pregnancy, Childrearing, and Slavery*. Philadelphia: University of Pennsylvania Press, 2017.

Uribe-Uran, Victor. "The Birth of a Public Sphere in Latin America during the Age of Revolution." *Comparative Studies in Society and History* 42, no. 2 (April 2000): 425–57.

Waldstreicher, David. "Reading the Runaways: Self-Fashioning, Print Culture, and Confidence in Slavery in the Eighteenth-Century Mid-Atlantic." *The William and Mary Quarterly* 56, no. 2 (1999): 243–72.

Weaver, Karol. *Medical Revolutionaries: The Enslaved Healers of Eighteenth-Century Saint Domingue.* Urbana: University of Illinois Press, 2006.

———. "Surgery, Slavery, and the Circulation of Knowledge in the French Caribbean." *Slavery and Abolition* 33, no. 1 (March 2012): 105–17.

Wessels, Julianna. "The Fugitive Barbados Mapping Project: Speculative Knowledge and Movement in the Archive." *The Fugitive Barbados Mapping Project*, April 12, 2021, https://storymaps.arcgis.com/stories/78af50ed1ebb4c8993f1086c1f0e0ce9.

Wood, Marcus. *Blind Memory: Visual Representations of Slavery in England and America, 1780–1865.* New York: Routledge, 2000.

Selected Bibliographies, Directories, and Databases

"Caribbean Newspapers, 1718–1876: From the American Antiquarian Society." *Readex*. https://www.readex.com/products/caribbean-newspapers-series-1-1718-1876-american-antiquarian-society.

"CariDiScho: A Directory of Caribbean Digital Scholarship." *Caribbean Digital,* NYC. https://caribbeandigitalnyc.net/caridischo/.

"Dictionaire des journaux, 1600–1789." *Voltaire Foundation*. https://dictionnaire-journaux.gazettes18e.fr/.

Eddins, Crystal. "On the Lives of Fugitives: Runaway Slave Advertisement Databases." *Humanities, Arts, Science, and Technology Alliance and Collaboratory: Blog.* March 30, 2017. https://www.hastac.org/blogs/crystal-eddins/2017/03/30/lives-fugitives-runaway-slave-advertisement-databases.

Le Marronnage dans le monde Atlantique: Sources et trajectoires de vie, 1760–1848. http://www.marronnage.info/fr/index.html.

Menier, Marie-Antoinette, and Gabriel Debien. "Journaux de Saint-Domingue." *Outre-Mers: Revue d'histoire* 36, no. 127 (1949): 424–75.

Pactor, Howard. *Colonial British Caribbean Newspapers: A Bibliography and Directory.* New York: Greenwood Press, 1990.

"Seventeenth and Eighteenth-Century Burney Newspapers Collection." *Gale Primary Sources.* https://www.gale.com/intl/c/17th-and-18th-century-burney-newspapers-collection.

15 Disability History in Slavery's Archive

Stefanie Hunt-Kennedy

When I first set out to study disability among the enslaved, very little work had been done on the lived experience of enslaved people with disabilities in the British Caribbean.[1] Scholars had long discussed health and slavery, as well as the violence of slavery with death as the exemplary image of slavery's brutality.[2] There was good reason for the attention that death received in the scholarship, for the total life span of an enslaved person on a Caribbean plantation was a mere seven years. While premature, painful, and often violent death was an integral aspect of slavery, I was struck by the absence of those who must have survived the hostile world of enslavement but whose bodies and psychologies were permanently marked with slavery's violence. Who were the individuals who became disabled through legally sanctioned punishments or the chance violence of an overseer and how did their experiences of enslavement change with physical impairment? Who were the individuals born with congenital disabilities and how were their disabilities perceived among the enslaved and the white plantation authorities? What about those who acquired disabilities due to disease or aging? How did disabled bondspeople make their way in a virulently racist, ableist, and violent world that was based on white freedom and Black enslavement? I set out to uncover a disability history from the archives of British Caribbean slavery and along the way I discovered that such a history did not depend on finding new or underused sources but rather reading familiar sources through a disability lens – to read slavery's archive anew.

This chapter illustrates how to analyze primary sources in slavery's archive through a disability lens. Using three sources from the eighteenth-century Caribbean and Atlantic World – slave ship surgeon records, runaway advertisements, and European travelogues – it seeks to highlight the kinds of questions historians of disability ask the archive and what the archive reveals and conceals about disability. I chose these three sources because they offer insights into the place of disability at different stages and locations of enslavement, the lived experience of disabled bondspeople, and the ways in which notions of disability were used to justify African dispossession in the Atlantic World. The sources illustrate that slavery produced disability among the enslaved through violence, labor accidents, and disease and malnutrition, and that racism and ableism worked in tandem to create interlocking forms of oppression for Africans and their descendants. Slavery's archive also reveals that several different and often contradictory understandings of

DOI: 10.4324/9781003094876-19

physical fitness and ability existed at once in the Atlantic world economy. Physical ability and disability meant different things to slave merchants at sea than they did to slaveowners on plantations. And, of course, perceptions and responses to disability among an unfree, non-wage-earning labor force often ran counter to broader societal understandings of labor and fitness.

Scholars of disability emphasize that disability is not fixed, natural, nor stable, but rather socially constructed and particular to time and place. This chapter begins with a brief discussion about the kinds of questions asked and approaches taken by disability historians. It then explores sources from the British Caribbean and Atlantic World to illustrate that, despite being a universal human condition, disability must be understood in specific historical contexts. This chapter aims to illustrate that disability history is both a topic and an analytic. It is the study of disabled people as historical actors and it is also a lens or a perspective through which we look at the past, akin to gender, race, and class.[3] The sources we explore in this chapter show both of these modalities at work – the lived experience of disability among the enslaved and the cultural meanings of disability in the British Atlantic World. Throughout this discussion, we consider what the sources reveal and what they conceal, and how to read the silences and piece together the life-worlds of enslaved people whose voices are seldom found in the archives of the British Atlantic World.

What Do Historians Talk About When They Talk About Disability?

The field of disability history emerged, in part, as a response to the scholarship on the history of medicine, which had traditionally relegated the lives of disabled individuals to their medical diagnoses and treatments.[4] Medical histories focused on the physicians and medical knowledge of the day which perceived disability as something to be prevented and cured if possible.[5] By considering disabled people as historical actors and not just diagnoses and treatments or as so-called heroes who "overcome" their disabilities, historians of disability have recentered disabled people in their dialogues with the past. Over the past three decades, historians have explored what disabled people have long known: that there are many different ways to think about disability and disabled people.[6] As David M. Turner explains,

> deformed, disabled, or otherwise anomalous bodies have been subject to a variety of interpretations and responses throughout history: as omens or prodigies, visitations of sin, freaks and curiosities, as inducing mockery, embarrassment or compassion, and as the subjects of disciplining, institutionalisation or charitable provision.[7]

Although, historically speaking, societal responses to disability have been overwhelmingly negative, historians have shown that disabled individuals are never just the "other." Like their able-bodied/minded counterparts, disabled people have complex personhoods and social worlds that reflect that vast spectrum of human experience and that the lives of people with disabilities intersect and are shaped by gender, class, race, place, and time.

Until recently, archives did not include disability-related indexes because the persistent social stigma of the medical view of disability compelled individuals and groups who collected historical artifacts to deem disability-related topics outside the purview of historians. Much research on disability history consists of historians looking at traditional sources but through a disability lens. For instance, historians have re-examined the Western suffrage movement to illustrate how opponents of women's equality frequently claimed that women were weak, irrational, and overly emotional, accusations which are in essence, physical, intellectual, and psychological disabilities. Historians of disability consider not only the wrong in denying rights to people based on perceived defect but also *why* the trope of disability holds so much power to exclude people from the benefits of what it means to be human.[8] It is with these two modalities – historical topic and analytic – that we will approach slavery's archive.

Atlantic Slavery: A (Very) Brief Introduction

Slavery has existed since time immemorial but Atlantic slavery, which emerged in the fifteenth century and expanded in the seventeenth century, constituted the largest and most intense system of slavery in history. There were commonalities to all systems of slavery including legal subordination; denial of lineages and genealogies – what scholar Orlando Patterson has termed "natal alienation"; forced labor; and a loss of control over one's own migration.[9] But several factors made Atlantic slavery distinct from the systems of enslavement that preceded it. First, Atlantic slavery involved the greatest number of people enslaved in history, with an estimated 12.5 million people, forcibly taken from sub-Saharan Africa to the Americas (and to a lesser degree Europe). Also unique to Atlantic slavery was its eventual identification with specific racialized groups of people (first Indigenous and African peoples, then primarily Africans and their descendants).

In contrast to other systems of slavery, manumission – the legal freeing of enslaved individuals – was rare in Atlantic World slavery.[10] Atlantic slavery was hereditary, based as it was on the principle of maternal inheritance, which meant that the legal status of the mother dictated the status of her child.[11] This legal principle was used to expand and sustain slavery by making all children born of enslaved women the property of the mother's owner, irrespective of the legal status or skin color of the father. The enslaved Black woman's womb, therefore, determined the legal status of enslavement and served to expand slavery.[12] Atlantic slavery generated incredible amounts of wealth for Western slaveholding states and was also the longest running system of slavery – the total time span of the transatlantic slave trade in Africans to the Americas was from the early sixteenth century to the mid-nineteenth century.[13] The distance traveled and utter loss of personal contact with home was also unprecedented.

Slavery in the British Caribbean consisted of incredible levels of violence, hostile living conditions, and the physically destructive labor demanded of sugar production. There is sometimes a misconception of the colonial Caribbean as a place that existed outside the law because of its culture of violence; however, British

Caribbean slavery was a carefully governed institution. Lawmakers legally sanctioned disabling punishments, and plantation authorities ordered them at the cost of reducing the enslaved person's ability to perform labor. But perhaps most importantly, slavery legislation granted slaveowners almost sovereign power to punish bondspeople however they saw fit and privately on plantation grounds. Caribbean bondspeople were vulnerable to disabilities and deformities caused by the violence meted onto their bodies, as well as through malnutrition, disease, and labor accidents. Sugarcane, which was the predominant crop grown in the Caribbean, was one of the most physically destructive crops to produce in the Americas. As "landmark experiments in modernity," sugar plantations were precociously industrial, and, like their nineteenth-century European counterparts, enslaved laborers became severely injured and disabled in the factory-like settings of sugar production.[14] Sugar production entailed an intricate and vast labor organization that was unlike any other industrial enterprise in the early modern Atlantic. The process of sugar cultivation – land preparation, planting, weeding, and cutting – was teamed with grinding canes, boiling the cane juice, curing and refining the sugar, and distilling the molasses into rum. As a consequence of the materially deprived world of Caribbean slavery, the enslaved population did not reproduce itself by natural means.[15] British Caribbean slaveowners, therefore, relied on the slave trade to grow their enslaved labor force until the legal end of the slave trade in 1807.

Despite the violence, trauma, and hostile environment that characterized Caribbean slavery, enslaved people used a variety of means to challenge authority and transform their circumstances. In so doing, their goals were complex: sometimes they aimed to escape slavery individually; sometimes they sought to undermine the system of slavery as a whole; and sometimes they had more short-term or focused concerns, like escaping a situation of extreme cruelty or demanding better working conditions. Reading slavery's archive reveals a range of acts of opposition in which the enslaved engaged, ranging from small, everyday acts of covert, nonviolent, and individual resistance, to the massive, collective, and violent explosions of slave insurrections. The archive also reveals the often-conflicting place of disability in the lives of enslaved people. On the one hand, the disabilities produced by slavery and endured by the enslaved became a sign of slaveowner power and a physical marker of Africans' enslaved status. On the other hand, such marks also told a narrative of enslaved people's personhood, survival, and their refusal to accept their enslavement. As we will see, disability in slavery's archive emerges not only as a sign of victimization but also a self-fashioning tool that enslaved people utilized to powerfully negotiate the terms of their bondage.

A Disability Analysis of Slavery's Archive

When I teach the history of Caribbean slavery, my students are often puzzled at the fact that although slave merchants and slaveowners desired young, healthy, and physically able captives who they estimated could survive the Middle Passage – the notorious transatlantic journey from sub-Saharan Africa to the Americas – and labor on the plantations, slavery worked to undermine and destroy the health and fitness of African captives at every stage of their enslavement. The economic logic of Atlantic capitalism determined that it was more efficient to work enslaved people to death and replace them, than to treat them well so that they might survive. Although both traders and planters wanted physically able bondspeople, they placed different value on the bodies of forced laborers. Slave ship merchants, for instance, desired captives whose bodies could survive the traumas of the Middle Passage and then secure the highest bid on the open market in the Caribbean. This meant that merchants often rejected captives who showed any signs of incurable disabilities and infirmities, such as "lameness" and "old age."[16] Caribbean planters, in contrast, had a different economic context in which they valued enslaved laborers. On the plantations, enslaved laborers were worked in some capacity until they literally could not contribute to plantation production at all. Impairment, therefore, did not necessarily exempt one from hard labor, nor diminish their value as laborers. Unlike merchants, planters did not reject the ill and the disabled but found new ways to obtain profit from such bodies through any means necessary.[17]

By the late eighteenth-century, the law required that each British slave ship be accompanied with a surgeon, a medical man hired to treat the inevitable illnesses and maladies that plagued both the crews and human cargo of slave ships.[18] Ship doctors were responsible for helping ship captains weed out the sick, the physically and intellectually impaired, and the otherwise compromised – the aged for instance – from the able bodied to secure the very best laborers. According to Alexander Falconbridge, a slave ship surgeon (1780–1787) who later became an abolitionist,

> if they [Africans] are afflicted with any infirmity, or are deformed, or have bad eyes or teeth; if they are lame, or weak in their joints, or distorted in the back, or of a slender make, or are narrow in the chest; in short, if they have been, or are afflicted in any manner, as to render them incapable of much labour; if any of the foregoing defects are discovered in them, they are rejected.[19]

Slave trading was first and foremost a business and it was a "risky business" at that. The perils of the arduous journey, the financial investments, the illnesses that could easily spread among the crew meant that merchants were most concerned about their investments in the slave ship business.[20] It is within this historical context of money, human trafficking, and sickness at sea that a disability history emerges from slave ship surgeon records.

Written in scrolling early modern cursive on large sheets of paper, slave ship surgeon records were kept by the ship's surgeon and contain daily accounts of African captives' health conditions and the treatments and medicines prescribed by the ship's surgeon. Most often the page was divided into categories that recorded incoming captives and the state of their health while they remained on the ship during the passage. Although every slave ship surgeon's record is unique, they generally included the following categories at the top of the page running horizontally: Day of the Month and Year; Men; Men boys; Boys; Women; Women girls; Girls.

These age and gender designations denoted what modern readers would consider grown men and women, teenage boys and girls; and children. Next to these headings are the categories "Discharge," to record individuals who were rejected from the ship due to illness or impairment, and "Dead" followed by two categories of calculation: "Total purchased" and "total on board." On the opposite page of the folio is where the surgeon added his medical notes regarding illness among the enslaved. At the top of the page, it reads: Sick Slaves – Nature of the disorder and remedies employed. On the one hand, slave ship records can reveal a great deal about the physical, emotional, and psychological trauma of slavery at sea. On the other hand, they are frustratingly limited in the amount of information they give and the silences surrounding the lives of the enslaved. The records contain daily information about the state of individuals' health, the medicine prescribed to them, and whether they recovered. In this way, the bodies of enslaved people are at the forefront of the source itself. And yet, the records tell us very little about the enslaved themselves; captives remain voiceless objects of the white European medical gaze.

In 1792, while the *Lord Stanley* was moored on the African coast, Christopher Bowes, the ship's surgeon removed two disabled captives from the ship and returned them to the shore.[21] The first, according to Bowes' April 9, 1792 entry, was a "man that was lame in his arm…. The boy received on the 10th was in place of the man sent ashore." This limited information reveals that slave ship captains and surgeons perceived an impaired arm as a detriment to the sale of that individual. Bowes calculated that an individual with a lame arm would not fare well on the slave market in the Americas. The second disabled person rejected from the slave ship was a teenage boy. After inspecting his body for signs of disease, illness, or disability, Bowes determined that the boy was physically fit enough to survive the Atlantic crossing and the boy proceeded to the hold of the ship. However, that same day, the young boy had an "epileptic fit," which Bowes discovered. The surgeon's records only state that the boy was immediately "sent ashore" and replaced by a man, "No. 9."[22]

From this cryptic medical log, we discover that merchants and planters considered epilepsy an undesirable and unmarketable condition among newly commodified human beings. In the world of Atlantic slavery, epilepsy was a feared disease that both slave traders and slaveowners associated with insanity and uncontrollability. As a condition characterized by the uncontrolled body, epilepsy took on particular cultural relevance in slave societies, for in its disorder it threatened the very foundations of the institution of slavery – namely, whites' power and control over African bodies.[23] Bowes rejected the two individuals from the slave ship because he perceived their disabilities as a disadvantage to their worth as commodified labor units. For Christopher Bowes and the *Lord Stanley,* captives' worth was tied directly to the market, whereas slaveowners calculated bondspeople's so-called worth as both commodities on the open market and laborers on the plantation.

In their descriptions of the physical appearances of fugitives, runaway advertisements reveal the prevalence of a variety of physical, sensory, intellectual, and sometimes psychological impairments experienced by enslaved individuals. By the eighteenth century, slaveowners were legally obliged to advertise in the local newspapers "the height, names, marks, sex, and country…of each runaway in their custody."[24] Written in small paragraphs and grouped together among other paid advertisements in Caribbean newspapers, runaway advertisements were read by the white public, who shared an invested interest in defeating the threat runaways posed to the order of plantation society. All runaway advertisements were written in a similar fashion – they contained common language and sequence of information. This information often included the location from which the captives fled, the name and description of the fugitives, details about the fugitives' physical and behavioral characteristics, her or his possible whereabouts and familial connections on neighboring plantations, and other instances in which the bondsperson had run away. Almost all advertisements ended with monetary rewards offered by owners to anyone who apprehended the individuals and concluded with a warning to ship captains to not take runaways on board. Runaway notices were often accompanied by one or two stock images of a fugitive bondsperson.

Historians working with contested and fragmented archives, where the voices of the enslaved and the disabled are often silenced, are sometimes left with more questions than answers.[25] Take for example, a runaway advertisement placed in the Jamaican newspaper in 1781, advertising for a teenage boy named Tom:

> RUN AWAY, a Negro Boy named *Tom* of the Mocco country, about 17 years old, 5 feet 6 inches high, very much pitted with the small-pox, and walks with his knees bent, and appears an awkward foolish fellow; he is of a coal black complexion. He had on when he went away a long osnaburg frock, and check shirt: Whoever apprehends him and delivers him to the subscriber, shall receive TWENTY SHILLINGS reward; and whoever harbours him, will be prosecuted to the utmost rigour of the law. LEONARD WRAY jun.[26]

A lot can be said about Tom by reading the advertisement from a disability perspective. By centering Tom as the historical actor, and not his diagnosis or his slaveowner, we begin to ask questions about how Tom's physical and potential intellectual disabilities may have shaped his experience of slavery and fugitivity. We know that Tom was African born and made the forced migration from Africa to the Americas on a slave ship. We do not know the circumstances that led to his capture or when he arrived in the Caribbean. By the time he was 17 years old, Tom had survived the smallpox, a highly contagious and frequently deadly disease that was common among the enslaved due to the tight quarters in which they lived on plantations and the way the disease spread throughout the slave ship. The smallpox caused fever, fatigue, and scabs filled with pus. Disability historians have demonstrated that although disease and disability are not the same conditions, they share an overlapping history. For instance, those who survived smallpox were sometimes left with sight impairments and often disfigured, or "pitted" with scars, which could lead to disability in the form of social stigma. For slaveowners, however, the marks from smallpox in fact increased the marketable value of the enslaved individual because they were proof that the individual was now immune to the smallpox.[27] Thus, "pitted with smallpox" in one context constituted a disability, while in another (the slaveholders' perspective), it was deemed proof of immunity and therefore desirable.

Many of the diseases and malnutrition that enslaved individuals were susceptible to because of their hostile living conditions could lead to short- or long-term disability. According to the advertisement, it is likely that Tom's bent knees were caused by rickets, a disease caused by calcium and Vitamin D deficiencies due to the very high in starch diets enslaved people were fed.[28] The rickets could also cause intellectual disability. The advertisement engenders numerous questions that reflect disability as a historical topic and an analytic. Did the subscriber's description of Tom as an "awkward foolish fellow" mean that Tom was intellectually disabled or was it rather a reflection of a white man's racist assumptions about Black people's supposed intellectual deficiency? If Tom was intellectually disabled, how did this impact his experience of slavery, relationship to white authorities, kin and other relations, as well as his labor? What was Tom's experience with smallpox and how did his scars influence his "worth" on the open market?

Understanding that disability is historically constructed – that what constituted disability in one place and time may not have in another – is key to doing disability history. In modern Europe and North America, definitions of disability were tied to one's ability to labor. In other words, one became disabled when unable to participate in a productive economy. In contrast, Caribbean enslaved people continued to perform hard labor with physical disabilities which, in other historical contexts, would have excluded individuals from the productive economy. For instance, an advertisement from Jamaica in 1791 described Bob, "a stout able negro man… of the Congo country, and marked on one shoulder G.G." According to the subscriber's description, Bob was "blind of the left eye, has a large scar across his left cheek, which he got about sixteen years ago by the kick of a Mule, by which accident he came to lose his eye."[29] Blindness and missing eyes made regular appearances in runaway advertisements, though the condition did not necessarily impair one's ability to be productive on the plantation, where it was more common for bondspeople to experience a loss of vision due to environmental conditions. Despite being partially blind, Bob was a "most excellent swimmer and diver, has been occasionally employed as a fisherman and sailor negro." Enslaved individuals, like Bob, who were blind had to learn how to navigate their new reality and keep up with the demands of plantation labor. By reading this advertisement through a disability lens, we learn that Bob's impairment did not preclude him from taking up important positions in the slave labor hierarchy, nor did it prevent him from escaping the plantation.

Runaway advertisements offer more evidence of the significance of visible disabilities and deformities in determining how slaveholding authorities calculated a bondsperson's so-called worth. Concepts of "worth" and "value" would have likely impacted plantation management's decision whether or not to advertise for impaired, diseased, or permanently injured fugitives. How many impaired, permanently injured, or diseased runaways were unaccounted for in the British Caribbean press? The rewards offered in runaway advertisements for apprehending and returning fugitives can be read as a reflection of this economy of "worth." For instance, an advertisement in the Jamaican press in 1780 read:

> RUN AWAY, about 15 months ago, a Negro Man of the Mungola country, named JAMAICA, of a black complexion, about five feet three inches high, pretty stout made, his forehead very much wrinkled, and marked with the letter R or R.S. on one or both cheeks, about forty five years of age, was formerly the property of Richard Simmons, deceased, and has been used to the brick making and fishing business. Also, about two months ago, two negro men, named JAMES and SAMBO. James of the Congo country, of a vey black complexion, about about [sic] 50 or 55 years of age, walks very lame, by trade a bricklayer, he was formerly the property of Richard Reeder, deceased. Sambo, a creole, very old, his head quite white, pretends to be blind; he is supposed to be harboured by his son, who lives to windward, he was formerly the property of John Coughlan, deceased; a reward of ten pounds, for Jamaica, and a half Joe each for James and Sambo, will be given, by the subscriber, to any person or persons, that apprehends and lodges them in any of the gaols of this island, so that the proprietor may get them again, and any person proving by whom they are harboured or concealed, so as the person or persons so harbouring or concealing said negroes be convicted, shall receive TEN POUNDS for each….RICHARD LATIMER.[30]

All three bondsmen were skilled laborers; however, Jamaica's younger age and physical health and abilities likely placed his value as a laborer higher than James and Sambo, who were both older and had physical limitations. There were times when slaveowners and managers suspected that certain individuals feigned illness or impairment and were, therefore, skeptical of injuries and illnesses among the enslaved. According to the above advertisement, Sambo "pretends to be blind." Masquerading as disabled, whether on or off the plantation, provided bondspeople opportunities to self-consciously shape their appearance and allowed them to use the changing physical and environmental context of freedom to adjust and renew their bodies.[31]

So far, this chapter has illustrated disability as a historical topic that focuses on the lives of enslaved people with disabilities. But disability can also be used as an analytic framework to revisit familiar sources and recenter disability in traditional histories that have been inattentive to disability. Using disability as an analytic tool consists of examining how notions of disability, and its counterpart ability, shaped cultural, religious, social, and political understandings of the body, gender, race, citizenship, competency, and a host of other things in society. How were fitness and unfitness defined in the past and how did such definitions consequently structure power and shape social hierarchies? Disability as an analytic tool is not divorced from the familiar triad of gender, class, and race but rather intimately connected to these categories.

Early modern European travelogues about Africa illustrate how the categories of race, gender, and disability intersected and framed European perceptions of African people and how such perceptions served to determine Black people's subjugation in the Atlantic World. European travelogues have long been studied by historians of slavery for how they relate to questions of gender, ethnicity, and race.[32] However, notions of deformity and monstrosity – precursors to the modern notion of disability – underpin the racist European perceptions of Africans during the expansion of the slave trade. European travel narratives to Africa date back to the ancient period but they were revived during the Age of Exploration when the Spanish and Portuguese began their colonizing pursuits in Africa and the Americas. By the time English voyagers landed on African shores in the mid-sixteenth century, their imaginations were already full of prejudiced depictions of Africans as belonging more to the realm of the fantastic than the human. Sixteenth-century Spanish and Portuguese travel writings and English translations of ancient texts circulated among the English elite and influenced English views of Africans and their descendants. These texts told fanciful tales of races whose body parts were organized differently than those of "normal" human beings: some lacked necessary organs, whereas others were half-man, half-animal.[33]

Using disability as an analytic framework, we see that Europeans used disability as a powerful rhetorical tool to justify, or mute opposition to, the enslavement of Africans and their descendants in the Atlantic World. For instance, in the most widely read travel narrative of the medieval and early modern world, *The Voyages and travailes of Sir John Mandeville Knight* (ca. 1366, translated into English in 1496), the author described Africans as having deformed bodies, with missing or misplaced parts, and bodies that did not resemble human form. "And in one of the Iles," he wrote "are men that have but one eye, and that is in the middest of their front…And in another Ile dwell men that have no heads, and their eyes are in their shoulder, and their mouth is on their breast." Others, he claimed,

> have flat faces without nose, and without eyes, but they have two small round holes instead of eyes, and they have a flat mouth without lips. And in that Ile are men also that have their faces all flat without eyes, without mouth, and without nose, but they have their eyes and their mouth behind on their shoulders.[34]

Mandeville's description of Africans as possessing deformed and monstrous bodies suggests that Africans were not fully human like their white European counterparts. His claim that Africans had anomalous bodies justified their dispossession and enslavement in the Atlantic World. Mandeville's text illustrates the way that ableism and racism worked together as mutually constitutive forces of oppression in the world of Atlantic slavery.[35]

Through a disability lens, we can also read a history of *ability*. For instance, eighteenth-century plantation management guides, written by slaveowners as a sort of "how to" for planters, gave advice to fellow enslavers on what to look for when purchasing bondspeople. An eighteenth-century guide written by Jamaican slaveowner John Dovaston warned merchants and planters to "be careful that they [Africans] are not foolish, which you may judge by their looks and attention on you." Those from the Congo, Dovaston claimed, were more "refined" in their senses, and "well featured, straight limb'd, and more tractable and easily taught to labour." Creoles (those born in the Americas), however, were the most sought-after laborers because "they understand the language you discourse in…and being born with you and his parents with him, he doth not think his labour slavery, and having never known any other goes with cheerfulness about it." According to Dovaston, Ibo and Gold Coast Africans were supposedly the best field laborers because "their disposition is dull and stupid and only fit for labour."[36] Africans supposed intellectual deficiencies, in other words, *enabled* them to perform physically demanding hard labor. From Dovaston's text, we learn that in the context of Atlantic slavery, "ability" was not measured solely in terms of productivity; Africans' supposed acceptance or compliance with enslavement was equally important. The notion of an "obedient" labor force was a defining feature of "ability" in the capitalist economy of Atlantic slavery.

Conclusion

The majority of voices in the colonial archives belong to free white men. Finding the voices of the disabled in the early modern period is difficult under the best circumstances, and even more so when those disabled individuals were enslaved in the Caribbean. The sources discussed in this chapter were written by white Europeans or creoles and reflect the pervasive anti-Black racism of the Atlantic World. As such, they must be approached with care and criticism. Slave ship surgeon records are replete with the European colonial and medical gaze which saw Africans as, first and foremost, commodities. Although they provide one of the most detailed descriptions of bondspeople's appearances in slavery's archive, runaway advertisements still play to white fear and were part of a much broader environment of white surveillance and control over Africans and their descendants. European travelogues are particularly challenging because they unabashedly express a developing anti-Black racism that was shaped by European notions of deformity and monstrosity – in a word, disability – and gender. These travelogues were highly influential and were utilized to lend support to Africans' enslavement in the Atlantic World economy. With the proliferation of archival digitization, many of these sources are increasingly available in online databases. European travelogues, for instance, are widely published in online libraries and open-access databases. In recent years, a number of scholars and institutions have produced online databases of runaway advertisements.[37] When unearthing a disability history from slavery's archive, we must be attuned to the damaging ways in which racism, sexism, and ableism worked together to produce historically specific systems of exploitation and violence and the affective toll such material can have on contemporary readers.

The methods I describe in this chapter are widely applicable. Readers can apply disability as an analytic tool and a topic of historical inquiry to all sorts of different sources. The archive engenders many questions about how enslaved people themselves thought about and cared for their bodies, disabled or otherwise. How did Africans and their descendants understand the body in its relationship to health and labor? How did certain enslaved individuals become disabled – was the impairment congenital or acquired, permanent or temporary? What kind of treatments and aids did the enslaved create to assist their bodies? What did disabled individuals think of their marked bodies – did they see them as signs of protest and personhood, or of slavery's mastery and power? How did disability effect kin relationships? Although slavery's archive contains many silences, it offers an opportunity to uncover and piece together the lives of disabled bondspeople. If we look carefully, disabled bondspeople appear as historical actors, taking their lives and sometimes the lives of their children and other family members into their own hands. We can read against the archive and resist its silencing power to uncover the lives of people who left very few, if any, records themselves.

Notes

1 Although scholars Jerome Handler and Kenneth Kiple wrote about the disabling diseases enslaved people were prone to, they did so from a bio-medical perspective and did not consider the lived experience of disability. In recent years, only a handful of scholars have explored disability among the enslaved in the Atlantic World. For the US context, see Jenifer L. Barclay, *The Mark of Slavery: Disability, Race, and Gender in Antebellum America* (Urbana: University of Illinois Press, 2021); Dea Boster, *African American Slavery and Disability: Bodies, Property and Power in the Antebellum South, 1800–1860* (New York: Routledge, 2015). For the French Caribbean see Ashley Williard, *Engendering Islands: Sexuality: Reproduction, and Violence in the Early French Caribbean* (Lincoln: University of Nebraska Press, 2021). For the British Caribbean see, Stefanie Hunt-Kennedy, *Between Fitness and Death: Disability and Slavery in the Caribbean* (Urbana: University of Illinois Press, 2020).

2 Some examples of scholarship on slavery, health, and medicine in the British Caribbean include: Richard B. Sheridan, *Doctors and Slaves: A Medical and Demographic History of Slavery in the British West Indies, 1680–1834* (Cambridge: Cambridge University Press, 1985); Sasha Turner, *Contested Bodies: Pregnancy, Childrearing, and Slavery in Jamaica* (Philadelphia: University of Pennsylvania Press, 2017); Rana A. Hogarth, *Medicalizing Blackness: Making Racial Difference in the Atlantic World, 1780–1840* (Chapel Hill: University of North Carolina Press, 2017). For scholarship that reveals the violence of the British Caribbean, see, for instance, Vincent Brown, *The Reaper's Garden: Death and Power in the World of Atlantic Slavery* (Cambridge, MA: Harvard University Press, 2010); Marissa Fuentes, *Dispossessed Lives: Enslaved Women, Violence, and the Archive* (Philadelphia: University of Pennsylvania Press, 2016); Sowande Mustakeem, *Slavery at Sea: Terror, Sex, and Sickness in the Middle Passage* (Urbana: University of Illinois Press, 2016).

3 Kim E. Nielsen, "Historical Thinking and Disability History," *Disability Studies Quarterly* 28, no. 3 (2008).

4 Western disability scholarship emerged in the 1980s in response to a medical view of disability that had dominated scholarly discussions of disability. However, it is important to recognize that the disability rights movements that the scholarship was connected to differed in Britain, the United States, Canada, etc.

5 Over the years, there have been many debates and fruitful discussions about the relationship between medical history and disability history. See, for instance, Catherine J. Kudlick, "Disability History and History of Medicine: Rival Siblings or Conjoined Twins?" (paper, Society for the Social History of Medicine annual meeting, Glasgow, September 3, 2008). Also see the discussion prompted by Beth Linker's article: Beth Linker, "On the Borderland of Medical and Disability History: A Survey of the Fields," *Bulletin of the History of Medicine* 87, no. 4 (2013): 499–535; Catherine

Kudlick, "Comment: On the Borderland of Medical and Disability History," *Bulletin of the History of Medicine* 87, no. 4 (2013): 540–59; Daniel J. Wilson, "Comment: On the Borderland of Medical and Disability History," *Bulletin of the History of Medicine* 87, no. 4 (2013): 536–39; Julie Livingston, "Comment: On the Borderland of Medical and Disability History," *Bulletin of the History of Medicine* 87, no. 4 (2013), 560–64.

6 This includes the scholarship on race and disability in other disciplines and outside the period of slavery. For instance, Christopher M. Bell, ed., *Blackness and Disability: Critical Examinations and Cultural Interventions* (East Lansing: Michigan State University Press, 2011); Therí A. Pickens, *Black Madness: Mad Blackness* (Durham: Duke University Press, 2019); Josh Lukin, "Disability and Blackness," in *The Disability Studies Reader*, ed. Lennard J. Davis (New York: Routledge, 2013), 308–15.

7 David M. Turner, "Introduction: Approaching anomalous bodies," in David M. Turner and Kevin Stagg (eds.), *Social Histories of Disability and Deformity* (New York: Routledge, 2006), 1.

8 Douglas C. Baynton, "Disability in History," *Perspectives on History* (Nov. 1, 2006). https://www.historians.org/publications-and-directories/perspectives-on-history/november-2006/disability-in-history.

9 Orlando Patterson, *Slavery and Social Death: A Comparative Study* (Cambridge, MA: Harvard University Press, 1982).

10 The historiography on manumission in the Atlantic World is large. For a starting point, see Elsa V. Goveia, *The West Indian Slave Laws of the 18th Century* (Eagle Hall: Caribbean University Press, 1970); Keila Grinberg, "Freedom Suits and Civil Law in Brazil and the United States," *Slavery and Abolition* 22, no. 3 (2001): 66–82; Sue Peabody, *"There Are No Slaves in France:" The Political Culture of Race and Slavery in the Ancien Regime* (Oxford: Oxford University Press, 1996); Alan Watson, *Slave Law in the Americas* (Athens: University of Georgia Press, 1989).

11 The principle of maternal inheritance was applied to the English Atlantic colonies after the 1656 Elizabeth Key case in Virginia. Key sued for her freedom on the basis that she was baptized, her father was an Englishman, and her father had bound her as an indentured servant for nine years, which time had passed. Following Key's freedom suit, the Virginia Assembly declared that all children born to an enslaved mother followed the legal status of the mother, regardless of the legal status of the father. Although this custom was never written into the laws of the Caribbean, it was widely practiced as custom. Taunya Lovell, "Dangerous Woman: Elizabeth Key's Freedom Suit: Subjecthood and Racialized Identity in Seventeenth Century Colonial Virginia," *Akron Law Review* 4, no. 1 (2008): 799–837; Kathleen Brown, *Good Wives, Nasty Wenches, Anxious Patriarchs: Gender, Race, and Power in Colonial Virginia* (Chapel Hill: University of North Carolina Press, 2006); Jennifer Morgan, "Partus Sequitur Ventrem: Law, Race, and Reproduction in Colonial Slavery," *Small Axe* 22, no. 1 (2018): 1–17; Melanie Newton, "Returns to a Native Land: Indigeneity and Decolonization in the Anglophone Caribbean," *Small Axe* 17, no. 2 (2013): 108–22; Joseph C. Dorsey, "Women without History: Slavery and the International Politics of *Partus Sequitur Ventrem* in the Spanish Caribbean," *Journal of Caribbean History* 28, no. 2 (1994): 165–207.

12 The brutal labor regimes, hostile living conditions, and violence that characterized British Caribbean slavery contributed to the high mortality and low fertility rates of Caribbean slavery. For scholarship on maternal health among the enslaved in the British Caribbean see, for instance, Turner, *Contested Bodies*; Richard Follet, "Heat, Sex, and Sugar: Childbearing in the Slave Quarters," *Journal of Family History* 28, no. 4 (2003): 510–39; Diana Paton, "Maternal Struggles and the Politics of Childlessness under Pronatalist Caribbean Slavery," *Slavery and Abolition* 38, no. 2 (2017): 251–68; Kenneth F. Kiple and V. H. Kiple. "Slave Child Mortality: Some Nutritional Answers to a Perennial

Puzzle," *Journal of Social History* 10 (1977): 284–309; Jennifer L. Morgan, *Laboring Women: Reproduction and Gender in New World Slavery* (Philadelphia: University of Pennsylvania Press, 2004).

13 According to the Transatlantic Slave Trade Database, to date, the earliest recorded slave ship voyage from Africa to the Americas was to Vigo, Brazil in 1514; the last recorded voyage was to Cuba in 1866. See the Transatlantic Slave Trade Database for statistical information on more than 36,000 voyages https://www.slavevoyages.org/. The first English slave trader was John Hawkins who left England for Africa in 1562 and in 1563 sold enslaved Africans in St. Domingo. The British slave trade in the Caribbean expanded in the 1640s with the Sugar Revolution.

14 Sidney W. Mintz, "Enduring Substances, Trying Theories: The Caribbean Region as *Oikoumemé*," *Journal of the Royal Anthropological Institute* 2, no. 2 (1996): 289–311, 295.

15 For more on maternal health and the causes of the population decline see, Sasha Turner, *Contested Bodies.*

16 For a primary account describing the practice of merchants rejecting disabled captives see, Alexander Falconbridge, *An Account of the Slave Trade on the Coast of Africa* (London, 1788), 18–22.

17 Stefanie Hunt-Kennedy, *Between Fitness and Death,* 72.

18 Adam Hochschild, *Bury the Chains*: *The British Struggle to Abolish Slavery* (London: Pan Macmillan Press, 2007), 154.

19 Falconbridge, *An Account of the Slave Trade*, 22.

20 Mustakeem, *Slavery at Sea*, 22.

21 RCS MS0003. For other scholarly examinations of Bowes's journal see Sowande' Mustakeem, *Slavery at Sea*; and Elise A. Mitchell, "Unbelievable Suffering: Rethinking Feigned Illness in Slavery and the Slave Trade," in *Medicine and Healing in the Age of Slavery*, edited by Sean Morey Smith and Christopher D.E. Willoughby (Louisiana State University Press, 2021), 99–120.

22 RCS MS0003.

23 Dea Boster, "An 'Epeleptick' Bondswoman: Fits, Slavery, and Power in the Antebellum South," *Bulletin of the History of Medicine* 83, no. 2 (2009):272–73.

24 *An Abridgement of the Laws in Force and Use in Her Majesty's Plantations (Viz.) Of Virginia, Jamaica, Barbadoes, Maryland, New England, New-York, Carolina &c.* (London: Printed for John Nicholson at the King's-Arms in Little Britain, R. Parker, and R. Smith, under the Royal-Exchange, and Benj. Tooke at the Middle-Temple-Gate in Fleetstreet, 1704), 145.

25 On the challenges of piecing together enslaved people's lives from fragmentary evidence, see Saidiya Hartman, "The Dead Book Revisited," *History of the Present* 6, no. 2 (2016): 208–15; Stefanie Hunt-Kennedy, "Silence, Violence, and the Archive of Slavery," *English Language Notes* 59, no. 1 (2021): 222–24; Marisa J. Fuentes, *Dispossessed Lives.*

26 *Supplement to the Royal Gazzette*, Saturday Sept. 29 to October 6, 1781., National Library of Jamaica, Kingston, Jamaica.

27 Hunt-Kennedy, *Between Fitness and Death*, 80.

28 The enslaved were fed food such as corn, rice, sugar, and plantain, which caused severe vitamin deficiencies and consequently often permanent physical deformities. See Jerome Handler, "Diseases and Medical Disabilities of Enslaved Barbadians, From the Seventeenth Century to around 1838, Part II," *Journal of Caribbean History* 40 (2006): 183. Some white colonists believed that the deformities caused by diseases such as the rickets, were racially specific deformities. For a discussion of this see, Hunt-Kennedy, *Between Fitness and Death*, 118–20.

29 *The Daily Advertiser*, Thursday December 15, 1791., American Antiquarian Society, Worcester, MA.

30 *Supplement to the Royal Gazette Saturday* 1–8 July 1780 (Jamaica), National Library of Jamaica, Kingston, Jamaica.

31 Dea H. Boster argues that in the Antebellum South, the enslaved exaggerated and feigned disability to discourage their purchase and to avoid performing particular forms of labor. See *African American Slavery*, 42, 89, 115.

32 The historiography on early European travelogues about Africans is too extensive to cite here. For an introduction to European travelogues in the Anglo-Atlantic World, see Margo Hendricks and Patricia Parker, eds., *Women, "Race," and Writing in the Early Modern Period* (New York: Routledge, 1994); Kim F. Hall, *Things of Darkness: Economies of Race and Gender in Early Modern England* (Ithaca, NY: Cornell University Press, 1995); Winthrop Jordan, *White Over Black: American Attitudes Toward the Negro, 1550–1812* (Chapel Hill: University of North Carolina Press, 1968); Colin Kidd, *The Forging of Races: Race and Scripture in the Protestant Atlantic World, 1600–2000* (Cambridge: Cambridge University Press, 2006); Catherine Molineux, *Faces of Perfect Ebony: Encountering Atlantic Slavery in Imperial Britain* (Cambridge, MA: Harvard University Press, 2012); Jennifer L. Morgan, *Laboring Women*; Cassander Smith, *Black Africans in the British Imagination: English Narratives of the Early Atlantic World* (Baton Rouge: Louisiana State University Press, 2016).

33 For more on the links between European ableism and a developing anti-Black racism in the early years of European colonization, see Hunt-Kennedy, *Between Fitness and Death*, especially Chapter 1.

34 Sir John Mandeville, *The Voyages and Travailes of Sir John Mandeville Knight Wherein Is Set Downe the Way to the Holy Land, and to Jerusalem…* (London, 1625). Attributed to the fictional John Mandeville, this work contained information from a variety of earlier travel narratives and encyclopedias. By 1500 it had been translated from the original French into German, Italian, Dutch, Spanish, Irish, Danish, Czech, and Latin. Jonathan Burton and Ania Loomba, eds. *Race in Early Modern England: A Documentary Companion* (London: Palgrave Macmillan, 2007), 70.

35 Kim E. Nielsen has convincingly argued that historians must be careful in using disability as an analytic tool that we do not lose the body and the lived experiences of disabled people in our histories. See, "Historical Thinking and Disability History."

36 John Dovaston, *Agricultura Americana* (1774), 249, 280, 246. John Carter Brown Library, Providence, RI.

37 For instance, "Documenting Runaway Slaves Project" (runawayslaves.usm.edu), which includes collections from Arkansas, Louisiana, Mississippi, Jamaica, Bahamas, and British Guiana/Suriname; "Freedom on the Move" (freedomonthemove.org); "Borealia Early Canadian History" (https://earlycanadianhistory.ca/2016/02/29/canadian-fugitive-slave-advertisements-an-untapped-archive-of-resistance/).

Bibliography

Primary Sources

An Abridgement of the Laws in Force and Use in Her Majesty's Plantations (Viz.) Of Virginia, Jamaica, Barbadoes, Maryland, New England, New-York, Carolina &c. (London: Printed for John Nicholson at the King's-Arms in Little Britain, R. Parker, and R. Smith, under the Royal-Exchange, and Benj. Tooke at the Middle-Temple-Gate in Fleetstreet, 1704).

The Daily Advertiser, Thursday December 15, 1791. American Antiquarian Society, Worcester, MA.

Dovaston, John. *Agricultura Americana* (1774). John Carter Brown Library, Providence, RI.

Falconbridge, Alexander. *An Account of the Slave Trade on the Coast of Africa.* London, 1788.

Mandeville, Sir John. *The Voyages and Travailes of Sir John Mandeville Knight Wherein Is Set Downe the Way to the Holy Land, and to Jerusalem* ... London, 1625.

Supplement to the Royal Gazette Saturday 1–8 July 1780 (Jamaica), National Library of Jamaica, Kingston, Jamaica.

Supplement to the Royal Gazzette, Saturday Sept. 29 to October 6, 1781. National Library of Jamaica, Kingston, Jamaica.

Online Primary Source Databases

Borealia Early Canadian History, https://earlycanadianhistory.ca/2016/02/29/canadian-fugitive-slave-advertisements-an-untapped-archive-of-resistance/

Documenting Runaway Slaves Project (runawayslaves.usm.edu)

Freedom on the Move (freedomonthemove.org)

Transatlantic Slave Trade Database, https://www.slavevoyages.org/

Secondary Sources

Barclay, Jenifer L. *The Mark of Slavery: Disability, Race, and Gender in Antebellum America.* Urbana: University of Illinois Press, 2021.

Baynton, Douglas C. "Disability in History." *Perspectives on History.* Nov. 1, 2006. https://www.historians.org/publications-and-directories/perspectives-on-history/november-2006/disability-in-history

Bell, Christopher M., ed. *Blackness and Disability: Critical Examinations and Cultural Interventions.* East Lansing: Michigan State University Press, 2011.

Boster, Dea. "An 'Epeleptick' Bondswoman: Fits, Slavery, and Power in the Antebellum South." *Bulletin of the History of Medicine* 83, no. 2 (2009): 272–73.

———. *African American Slavery and Disability: Bodies, Property and Power in the Antebellum South, 1800–1860.* New York: Routledge, 2015.

Brown, Kathleen. *Good Wives, Nasty Wenches, Anxious Patriarchs: Gender, Race, and Power in Colonial Virginia.* Chapel Hill: University of North Carolina Press, 2006.

Brown, Vincent. *The Reaper's Garden: Death and Power in the World of Atlantic Slavery.* Cambridge, MA: Harvard University Press, 2010.

Burton, Jonathan and Ania Loomba. *Race in Early Modern England: A Documentary Companion.* London: Palgrave Macmillan, 2007.

Dorsey, Joseph C. "Women without History: Slavery and the International Politics of *Partus Sequitur Ventrem* in the Spanish Caribbean." *Journal of Caribbean History* 28, no. 2 (1994): 165–207.

Follet, Richard. "Heat, Sex, and Sugar: Childbearing in the Slave Quarters." *Journal of Family History* 28, no. 4 (2003): 510–39.

Fuentes, Marissa. *Dispossessed Lives: Enslaved Women, Violence, and the Archive.* Philadelphia: University of Pennsylvania Press, 2016.

Goveia, Elsa V. *The West Indian Slave Laws of the 18th Century.* Eagle Hall: Caribbean University Press, 1970.

Grinberg, Keila. "Freedom Suits and Civil Law in Brazil and the United States." *Slavery and Abolition* 22, no. 3 (2001): 66–82.

Hall, Kim F. *Things of Darkness: Economies of Race and Gender in Early Modern England.* Ithaca, NY: Cornell University Press, 1995.

Handler, Jerome. "Diseases and Medical Disabilities of Enslaved Barbadians, from the Seventeenth Century to around 1838, Part II." *Journal of Caribbean History* 40 (2006): 183.

Hartman, Saidiya. "The Dead Book Revisited." *History of the Present* 6, no. 2 (2016): 208–15.

Hendricks, Margo and Patricia Parker, eds. *Women, "Race," and Writing in the Early Modern Period.* New York: Routledge, 1994.

Hochschild, Adam. *Bury the Chains: The British Struggle to Abolish Slavery.* London: Pan Macmillan Press, 2007.

Hogarth, Rana A. *Medicalizing Blackness: Making Racial Difference in the Atlantic World, 1780–1840.* Chapel Hill: University of North Carolina Press, 2017.

Hunt-Kennedy, Stefanie. *Between Fitness and Death: Disability and Slavery in the Caribbean.* Urbana: University of Illinois Press, 2020.

______."Silence, Violence, and the Archive of Slavery." *English Language Notes* 59, no. 1 (April 2021): 222–24.

Jordan, Winthrop. *White Over Black: American Attitudes Toward the Negro, 1550–1812.* Chapel Hill: University of North Carolina Press, 1968.

Kidd, Colin. *The Forging of Races: Race and Scripture in the Protestant Atlantic World, 1600–2000.* Cambridge: Cambridge University Press, 2006.

Kiple, Kenneth F., and V. H. Kiple. "Slave Child Mortality: Some Nutritional Answers to a Perennial Puzzle." *Journal of Social History* 10 (1977): 284–309.

Kudlick, Catherine J. "Disability History and History of Medicine: Rival Siblings or Conjoined Twins?" (paper presented at the Society for the Social History of Medicine annual meeting, Glasgow, September 3, 2008).

———. "Comment: On the Borderland of Medical and Disability History." *Bulletin of the History of Medicine* 87, no. 4 (2013): 540–59.

Linker, Beth. "On the Borderland of Medical and Disability History: A Survey of the Fields." *Bulletin of the History of Medicine* 87, no. 4 (2013): 499–535.

Livingston, Julie. "Comment: On the Borderland of Medical and Disability History." *Bulletin of the History of Medicine* 87, no. 4 (2013): 560–64.

Lovell, Taunya. "Dangerous Woman: Elizabeth Key's Freedom Suit: Subjecthood and Racialized Identity in Seventeenth Century Colonial Virginia." *Akron Law Review* 4, no. 1 (2008): 799–837.

Lukin, Josh. "Disability and Blackness." In *The Disability Studies Reader*, edited by Lennard J. Davis, 308–15. New York: Routledge, 2013.

Mintz, Sidney W. "Enduring Substances, Trying Theories: The Caribbean Region as *Oikoumemé*." *Journal of the Royal Anthropological Institute* 2, no. 2 (1996): 289–311.

Mitchell, Elise A. "Unbelievable Suffering: Rethinking Feigned Illness in Slavery and the Slave Trade." In *Medicine and Healing in the Age of Slavery*, edited by Sean Morey Smith and Christopher D.E. Willoughby, 99–120. Baton Rouge: Louisiana State University Press, 2021.

Molineux, Catherine. *Faces of Perfect Ebony: Encountering Atlantic Slavery in Imperial Britain.* Cambridge, MA: Harvard University Press, 2012.

Morgan, Jennifer. *Laboring Women: Reproduction and Gender in New World Slavery.* Philadelphia: University of Pennsylvania Press, 2004.

———. "Partus Sequitur Ventrem: Law, Race, and Reproduction in Colonial Slavery." *Small Axe* 22, no. 1 (2018): 1–17.

Mustakeem, Sowande. *Slavery at Sea: Terror, Sex, and Sickness in the Middle Passage.* Urbana: University of Illinois Press, 2016.

Newton, Melanie. "Returns to a Native Land: Indigeneity and Decolonization in the Anglophone Caribbean." *Small Axe* 17, no. 2 (2013): 108–22.

Nielsen, Kim E. "Historical Thinking and Disability History." *Disability Studies Quarterly* 28, no. 3 (2008).

Paton, Diana. "Maternal Struggles and the Politics of Childlessness under Pronatalist Caribbean Slavery." *Slavery and Abolition* 38, no. 2 (2017): 251–68.

Patterson, Orlando. *Slavery and Social Death: A Comparative Study.* Cambridge, MA: Harvard University Press, 1982.

Peabody, Sue. *"There Are No Slaves in France:" The Political Culture of Race and Slavery in the Ancien Regime.* Oxford: Oxford University Press, 1996.

Pickens, Therí A. *Black Madness: Mad Blackness.* Durham: Duke University Press, 2019.

Sheridan, Richard B. *Doctors and Slaves: A Medical and Demographic History of Slavery in the British West Indies, 1680–1834.* Cambridge: Cambridge University Press, 1985.

Smith, Cassander. *Black Africans in the British Imagination: English Narratives of the Early Atlantic World.* Baton Rouge: Louisiana State University Press, 2016.

Turner, David and Kevin Stagg. *Social Histories of Disability and Deformity.* New York: Routledge, 2006.

Turner, Sasha. *Contested Bodies: Pregnancy, Childrearing, and Slavery in Jamaica.* Philadelphia: University of Pennsylvania Press, 2017.

Watson, Alan. *Slave Law in the Americas.* Athens: University of Georgia Press, 1989.

Williard, Ashley. *Engendering Islands: Sexuality: Reproduction, and Violence in the Early French Caribbean.* Lincoln: University of Nebraska Press, 2021.

Wilson, Daniel J. "Comment: On the Borderland of Medical and Disability History." *Bulletin of the History of Medicine* 87, no. 4 (2013): 536–39.

16 Reproducing Ballads[1]

Mary E. Fissell

Scholars and students interested in ordinary early modern English people's beliefs and ideas have long turned to broadside ballads for evidence. Named "broadside" for the size of paper they were printed on, these single sheets contain the lyrics to a song, or ballad. Sold in the streets for as little as a halfpenny a copy, they represent a lowest common denominator of print, with important crossover consumption by those who heard them sung but could not, or did not, read them. Ballads were composed and sold on all kinds of topics: news, from battles to gruesome crimes to politics; love affairs both happy and sad; celebrations of royalty; and moral tales abounded. Given the number devoted to love, sex, and reproduction, they offer valuable evidence for historians pursuing topics in the histories of sex, reproduction, and gender relations more broadly. In this essay, we'll explore a single ballad called *The Lass of Lynn's New Joy*, published in London in the 1680s or early 1690s.[2] We can employ a range of interpretive techniques to analyze a ballad, including a literary focus on narrative; using social history to contextualize the story; connecting it to other ballads by using intertextual references and thematic similarities; focusing on the material object including images; and exploring the performative qualities of the work, particularly in relation to the music.

The study of ballads has been revolutionized by the advent of the digital humanities. Professor Patricia Fumerton has spearheaded a project that is putting the contents of major collections of British ballads online, with rich supporting materials. At this moment, the English Broadside Ballad Archive (EBBA) holds 9,834 ballads and is adding more every week (https://ebba.english.ucsb.edu/). As we will see, it is now possible to search ballads thematically, to research the woodcut images in depth, and to trace the melodies to which the ballads were sung. The project even includes clips of modern renditions of their melodies. Ballads are songs, and they use relatively simple and highly stereotyped forms; *The Lass of Lynn* is no exception. Ballads were usually composed of quatrains that are four-line stanzas often with an ABAB or ABCB rhyme scheme. Some had a refrain repeated at the end of each stanza. *The Lass of Lynn* has an ABAB rhyme scheme, and each line usually has three stressed syllables relatively evenly spaced through the line. The rhythm is simple, but as we will discuss below, it needs to be integrated into a discussion of the music to which the ballad was sung; the melody is cheerful and lilting.

DOI: 10.4324/9781003094876-20

Fumerton's scholarship emphasizes the mobility of ballads.[3] When we look at a ballad online, it is a fixed object on a computer screen. But in its own time, it was mobile in all kinds of ways. As we will discuss, ballads were sung and sold in the streets; they traveled in peddlers' packs; when no longer of interest, they were re-purposed as linings for pie tins or even as toilet paper. What is extant today is a small fragment of early modern ballad production, and we know little about how or why these ballads survived as material objects and others did not. Ballads moved on the page. Printers and publishers re-used woodcuts and melodies and re-wrote portions of ballads to make them more appealing or timely when they re-published them. Such mobility, however, should not paralyze us as interpreters. Indeed, understanding such movement can help us analyze a ballad.

One of the primary ways to interpret a ballad is to treat it as a literary text, looking at form and content. The story line of *The Lass of Lynn* involves a woman who tricks a man into marrying her. It turns out that the ballad is the third in a series and in effect we are starting in the middle of a story. The ballad opens with an unnamed Lass in trouble.[4] She was pregnant but lacked a husband. Her distress seemed to be well-known locally: "She had wept Tears, the whole Town knows, / would fill a whole Chamber-pot." She laced her stays tight in hopes of not "showing." Her mother counseled that a husband was "the only Cloak/ to cover a great Belly." The Lass agreed and said that she thought that George, who worked at a local tavern, would marry her, "were not my Pipkin cracked before." Her mother told her to marry George anyway, and the very next day they got married. Notice how the humble figures of speech – a chamber pot and a pipkin – serve to echo the Lass's swelling belly.

On the wedding night, George was startled by the sight of her pregnant belly, "Byth' Meat in your Pot, I find, you Whore / you've had a Cook in your Kitchen," but she reassured him that she had merely eaten too much at the wedding feast. He apologized and "so fell to the Sport." After five months, while George was at work, the Lass gave birth to a son, and the midwife went to congratulate George. He was understandably startled and assumed his wife had miscarried, but the midwife assured him it was a healthy baby boy. When George did the math and asked how that could be at five months, the midwife assured him that he did not understand the arithmetic of pregnancy: "Five Months! has the man lost his Wits?…Five Months by Days and Five by Nights / sh' has gone her full time to the day." The midwife continued by assuring George that the boy looked just like him, "had it been Spit out of your mouth / more like you it could not be." Somehow this statement of similarity persuaded George, and the ballad ends with him ordering a barrel of ale and some cakes for a feast while everyone laughed and rejoiced that the Lass has indeed found a father for her child.

One way to interpret the story in this ballad is to place it in the context of reproductive knowledge of the time. Pregnancy was very difficult to determine in the early months; usually it was only at quickening, when a woman felt the fetus move inside her, that she might have good evidence she was indeed pregnant. That knowledge, derived from the experience of her own body, was hers to keep or share. Quickening usually happens in the fourth or fifth month, and the Lass would have likely been in her fourth month when she married George, as the baby followed five months later. The hearers of the ballad are assumed to see through the midwife's claim about "five months of days and five months of nights," even if George did not. The midwife's ploy makes sense given the relative paucity of knowledge about reproductive biology available to men. Needless to say, there was no "sex ed" in schools, and knowledge about reproduction was strongly gendered female. Popular medical texts like Nicholas Culpeper's best-selling *Directory for Midwives* were addressed to all married women.[5] Indeed, authors of such works worried that men were the wrong audience; they might make lewd jokes about women's bodies after reading the texts.[6]

Thus, access to knowledge about sex and reproduction was strongly gendered. In the ballad, George was pitted against the "gossips," the women who attended his wife in childbirth, who all agreed with the midwife. When a woman went into labor, a group of female friends and family gathered to support her through long hours that lay ahead. Men often worried that these women were trading stories about male sexual performance in these all-female gatherings. Indeed, our current meaning of the word "gossip" derives from such beliefs.[7] From another perspective, such events were rich sites for the exchange of reproductive knowledge, sites from which men were, by definition, barred. So while George is portrayed as repeatedly gullible, his lack of knowledge about pregnancy might speak to a larger imbalance between men and women regarding what we would call reproductive biology.

However, scholars who have looked at life-writing, such as diaries and letters, suggest that married men were not as ignorant about reproduction as ballads might imply. Some husbands knew the timing of their wives' menstrual cycles, or knew about signs of pregnancy, however uncertain.[8] Authors of midwifery guides instructed husbands to read the books aloud to their wives if their wives could not read, pointing to another potential source of reproductive knowledge for men.[9] So perhaps ballads like *The Lass of Lynn* may point to a divide between married and unmarried men's access to knowledge about women's reproductive bodies.

Another interpretive strategy contextualizes this ballad by comparing it to other ballads on related themes. Recently, Christopher Marsh has criticized historians who cherry-pick a handful of ballads to fit with their larger arguments. He is working on a project that will list the 100 ballads that seem to have been the most popular in seventeenth-century England.[10] In comparing ballads, then, we need to be expansive and consider evidence about a ballad's popularity as suggested by the number of surviving editions or copies. Such evidence can only be suggestive, since much, if not most, of the ballad corpus does not survive. However, if a ballad exists in multiple editions, we can infer that it sold well enough to make it worth a publisher's while to issue it again. Two versions of *The Lass of Lynn* are extant today, one in the British Library and one in Samuel Pepys' collection at Cambridge. While each was published by John Millet, these may be two editions, as he lists his address differently on each.[11]

The first steps here are to investigate the earlier ballads that seem to tell *The Lass of Lynn's* story; the ballad's longer title included the words "Being a Third Song of

Marry and Thank Ye Too," implying that there were two earlier ones.[12] Unlike the Hollywood movie prequels of our own day, however, the two earlier Lass of Lynn ballads are very different in tone from the rambunctious and ultimately joyful third one. Nor can we be completely confident that what I identify as the first installment of her tale was in fact such. This song, called *The Thankful Country Lass, or, The Jolly Batchelor Kindly Entertained* is told in a man's voice, the "jolly batchelor."[13] He met a "country lass" and propositioned her, "shall I lay thee up in the grass?" all in the first stanza. He was very clear that he was "loath" to live as married men do, but wanted to "enjoy the bliss," although he raised the issue of potential pregnancy explicitly. Later in the ballad, he assured her that she could come and spend the night with him any time she wished; he lived in Lynn, next door to the sign of the Blue Anchor. At the very end of the ballad, "She made not the least demur" and "took what he proffered her." From scholarship in social history about the usual plight of actual unwed mothers in seventeenth-century England, such a song seems to be male fantasy. Couples were strongly pressured into marriage if possible; if not, parishes tried to get child support from fathers lest they have to pay poor relief to support a bastard.[14] Unwed women were interrogated during labor to reveal the name of the father, unlike the female solidarity at play in *The Lass of Lynn*, where midwife and gossips conspire to hoodwink the father.

In the second ballad, the Lass of Lynn was indeed pregnant and bemoaned her fate. It is subtitled "The Lass of Lynn's sorrowful Lamentation for the Loss of her Maidenhead," and lamentation it is.[15] Here the refrain is "I cannot tell what to do" as she regretted that "I find I was too Free" and recognized the stigma that accompanied unwed motherhood, "Each Damsel will me Degrade, / and so will the young Men too, / I'm neither Widow, Wife, nor Maid." She also worried about the costs of impending motherhood, "A Cradle I must provide, a Chair, and a Possnet too; Nay, Likewise Twenty things besides."[16] The song is not narrative; no story unfolds, but rather, the Lass bemoans her fate. It is a lamentation. The song might serve as a warning to other young women to guard their virginity more carefully than she had hers.

Neither of these two "prequel" ballads bears much resemblance to the third. The first is told in the male seducer's voice and the second is told by a young woman who is very much on her own, in contrast to the third ballad where her mother and George feature, as well as the gossips and the midwife. So too, the tone of each is markedly different, despite being sung to the same melody. Each was published by a different publisher, although there may have been other editions that did not survive. The third ballad is in a different format, with woodcut illustrations, again suggesting that the connections between the three are loose indeed.

Closer connections can be drawn thematically between *The Lass of Lynn* and other ballads not in the series. In its "Advanced Search" function, EBBA offers over 50 keywords, such as crime, death, vulgar humor, news, and even procreation, which can be combined to more tightly focus a search. Obviously, these are modern analytic categories. Alternatively, we can get a glimpse of how one seventeenth-century person categorized ballads by exploring the collecting practice of Samuel Pepys, the well-known diarist. Pepys collected ballads and pasted them into books according to 13 categories, such as "Love Pleasant," "Love Unfortunate," "Marriage," and "Drinking & Good Fellowship." Pepys' ballad books are in the library of Magdalene College at the University of Cambridge and constitute a vital source for ballad research. The category he assigned a ballad is searchable on EBBA for his ballads. Pepys listed *The Lass of Lynn* as "Love Pleasant." We might wonder, given Pepys' frequent worries about his own wife's fidelity, why he thought this story of a happily deceived husband might not have been cataloged in his hybrid category, "Love Pleasant and Unfortunate" or possibly under "Marriage."[17]

A number of other ballads use the same narrative device, where a young pregnant woman tricks a man into marrying her, although none is as lively or dialogue-driven as *The Lass of Lynn*. John Millet, the publisher of *The Lass of Lynn*, also produced a similar tale, in which the focus is on the young woman bemoaning her fate. Her mother threatens to kick her out of the house, and then decides she must marry her old flame Ned, even though "And e're two Months are gone and past, / I fear he'll smell the Plot." The important thing is that "the Child a Dad has got."[18] The timeframe is even shorter in "The Blind Eat Many a Fly." The husband is presented with twins a mere three days after the wedding! Here the woman had deceived her well-to-do husband doubly, promising him that her parents were wealthy. Once he finds that they live in an almshouse, supported by the parish, he takes it philosophically, saying "I must be contented / For marriage goes by Destiny / I can in no way prevent it."[19] In both of these ballads, the narrative resolution, as in *The Lass of Lynn*, seems to be the social good of getting these women married, even as their husbands are deceived.[20] The husbands seem to accept their situations as just something that happens to men, rather than being cast as cuckolds, a frequent ballad theme. Cuckold was a term describing men whose wives had betrayed them by having sex with another man. To be technical for a moment, these men were not actually cuckolds, as the women had not been married or even in a steady relationship with them when they conceived, but they were sexually deceived.

For example, in prior research (before EBBA was founded), I identified about 140 ballads about cuckolds in major collections.[21] Being cuckolded was a big deal in early modern England. It impugned a man's masculinity very severely. A man was expected to rule his household as a little commonwealth, that is, as a miniature version of the way the king ruled his country. A woman who had an affair with another man demonstrated that her husband lacked some essential component of masculine rule.[22] Cuckolds were depicted as wearing horns, and endless jokes and puns played upon horns as a symbol of masculine inadequacy. For example, a jokester carried a basket of ram's horns, crying them as "new fruit" for sale. When a lawyer disparaged them, the jokester replied, well, you may already have a pair, but others might want them – implying that the lawyer had been betrayed by his wife.[23]

Ballads about cuckolds often played upon the common belief that women were the lustier of the sexes. For example, the ballad *Cuckold's Haven* is sung by a husband who claims that his wife would always outwit him, "Tho narrowly I do watch / and use Lock, Bolt, and Latch / my wife will me orematch."[24] He complained that all women were such, "They have so many wayes / by nights or else by dayes," seeking to deceive their husbands. If husbands complained, the wives told them that it was all lies, and they had been faithful. Other ballads allow that husbands may also be at fault; as the subtitle of one such preaches, "…Good Husbands all be loving to your wives, / For that's the way to live contented lives; / But if you'r negligent, you may be sure / They'l ne'r want that they can elsewhere procure…"[25] The ballad tells of a farmer in Somerset who neglected his wife sexually, "But the good man was so lazy in bed / that he often neglected to touch her," so she turned to a "lusty young Butcher." Initially, they "had what each other desired," but then the ballad portrays the wife's sexual desires as too much for the butcher, as he became worn out, again referring to the idea that women were the lustier of the sexes.

The Lass of Lynn is both like and unlike such "cuckold" ballads. On the wedding night, George worried that his bride was pregnant and called her a whore, a seriously demeaning accusation, but she talked him around. The narrative heart of the song resembles two additional ballads, both of which hinge upon deceptions played upon men. The first is a version of the ancient motif called "the bed trick" in which the actual identity of a sexual partner is concealed; Shakespeare used it in *All's Well that Ends Well*.[26] In "A Cuckold by Consent," a miller (millers are often sexually rapacious in ballads) told a young woman that she must stay the night because her grain could not be ground until the morning. He then propositioned her, telling her to sleep in his parlor and he would join her there later; it was not unusual to have a bed in the parlor.[27] The young woman, however, confided in his wife, and instead the wife slept in the parlor, where her husband had intercourse with her in the dark, thinking she was the young woman. He then panicked. What if he has gotten her pregnant? He offered his servant Jack a ram if he would also have sex with her, so that he could then be blamed for fathering any resulting child. Note the sexual innuendos running through the tale. A ram is a farm animal whose role is to impregnate sheep; the grinding action of the mill, one stone upon the other, could echo two bodies in bed. The miller thus inadvertently cuckolded himself, as Jack enjoyed his wife, and the young woman returned home in the morning, still a virgin, with her grain ground for free. Here the song ends with the audience laughing at the deceived miller, while in *The Lass of Lynn* all the listeners at the end are, in effect, invited to join in the feasting to celebrate the arrival of a son even as they recognize that George has been deceived. Somehow, finding a father for the Lass's child has become a social imperative that outweighs any negative connotations of deception.

It seems, to judge by *The Lass of Lynn* and related ballads, that a pregnant woman tricking a man into marrying her was much less threatening to masculinity than a married woman cuckolding her husband. Both might result in a man raising a child who was not his biologically, but one is portrayed as much more damaging to a man's reputation than the other.

A ballad from the 1630s also features a man deceived sexually, but equally ends well. The first half of the ballad features a young man importuning his sweetheart for sex, "Oh, yeeld my sweete unto me, / or else you will undoe me."[28] Eventually she gives in and "they both were well contented." The refrain, about "over and under," emphasizes the sex act. Despite earlier protestations of fidelity, the young man scampered off to France or Flanders once she was pregnant. As in *The Lass of Lynn*, the young woman's mother sorted it out; her chief goal was to help her daughter avoid shame.[29] Once the young woman gave birth, she was whisked to London, where she passed as a virgin, "No one could be demurer / nor seeme a Virgin purer." No mention was made of the baby. In London, the young woman met a tailor who "for a mayd did take her," and they got married. While some parts of the ballad are warnings to young women about the male deceitfulness (the mother intones, "these are the trickes of men"), somehow the young woman's ability to play the virgin and find a husband is a happy ending, much like *The Lass of Lynn*.

Ballads also tell the other story of young women abandoned by their lovers without such happy resolutions. Searching in EBBA for the text word "virgin" and the subject term "procreation" yields a clutch of these stories. The title "A Love-sick maids song, lately beguild, By a run-away Lover that left her with Childe" pretty much sums up the entire ballad; a young woman warns others not to have sex with men before marriage lest they end up in her situation, pregnant and alone.[30]

When we contextualize *The Lass of Lynn* with other ballads, we see that unwed motherhood and deception are themes common to a range of ballads, although they play out in a variety of ways. Few seem to match what social history tells us about the usual situation of a pregnant unmarried young woman, in which strong pressure would be brought to bear on her and the father to get married if possible. If the father had fled to Flanders or France, as in the "Northren Song," the woman might have gotten grudging financial support from the Old Poor Law to support herself and her baby, but would have been deeply stigmatized in the process. Both this ballad and *The Lass of Lynn* imply that getting such women married is socially useful, even if men are deceived. All of these ballads play upon men's fears that they can be deceived by women because they are ignorant of basic reproductive facts, unsure about virginity or the timing of pregnancy.

Thus far, we have looked at a ballad as a literary text and analyzed its content. But ballads were also material and performative; adding these dimensions can deepen our analysis. You probably first encountered a ballad online, in digital form. While digitization has revolutionized the use of ballads for social and cultural history, it transforms a piece of paper into pixels. Try taking a ballad and printing it at its actual size to explore how the work was encountered in its own day. Paper was an expensive commodity in early modern England; it might account for half of the cost of a printed work, and ballads were not printed on tiny sheets of paper.[31] The copy of *The Lass of Lynn's New Joy* pasted into one of the albums kept by Samuel Pepys was trimmed to make it fit, so the original was perhaps about 8.5 by 14 inches.[32]

Today it can be challenging to read many seventeenth-century ballads like *The Lass of Lynn* because they were printed in what is called "black letter," the earliest printed letter forms in English. Roman type, such as that in this book, derived from Italian letter forms and became widely used in England by the beginning of the seventeenth century. Certain genres, however, continued to be printed in black letter: the Bible, catechisms, ballads, and hornbooks. (Hornbooks were used in schools to teach children to read, a sheet of paper on a wooden paddle covered with a thin transparent sheet of horn, much as we would use a sheet of plastic today, to protect the paper from generations of schoolchildren's fingers.) Historian Keith Thomas suggested that because black letter was how people learned to read, and because works such as catechisms and ballads used it, the form was associated with basic literacy and implies a potential broad readership.[33] Recently Zachary Lesser has offered another layer of meaning. He suggests that in the seventeenth century, black letter connoted a traditional English past, evoking nostalgia for a simpler time.[34] Ballads were consumed by multiple audiences, so both interpretations may be helpful. Antiquarians like Samuel Pepys and John Selden collected ballads while working people could purchase a ballad for a halfpenny or see it pinned up on an alehouse wall for decoration.[35]

Ballads were printed by the thousands. From 1624, a group of men known as The Ballad Partners dominated the trade. These men produced ballads, chapbooks (small works of fiction), almanacs, and other forms of cheap print. They had a very keen sense of the market. In theory, until 1694, all printed works in England had to be produced by members of the Stationers' Company, a trade guild, but ballads often flew under the radar. One scholar estimated that up to half of all ballads may not have been registered.[36] John Millet listed himself as having "printed and sold" both extant copies of *The Lass of Lynn*; he was "at the Angel in Little-Brittain" or "next door to the Flower-de-Luce in Little-Brittain." Perhaps he moved his shop, but it is possible that these are actually the same location. Henry Plomer, the compiler of an invaluable biographical dictionary of the print trade, tells us that Millet was a printer in London from 1683 to 1692, and that he partnered with M. Haley to produce a wealth of ballads and chapbooks.[37]

Plomer, however, worked in the 1920s, long before computers. Today we can turn to the English Short Title Catalogue (ESTC) online and see what Millet was printing, in order to contextualize this ballad.[38] Searching for Millet in the "publisher" field, ESTC lists 96 of his publications. He published an eight-page sensational chapbook about a murder as early as 1674, a very typical cheap print kind of work.[39] Fifteen years later, he was still churning out murder pamphlets, along with schoolbooks, but ballads were his most common output. His address remained either the Angel, or next door to the Flower de Luce, suggesting that these may indeed have been the same location or that he had two nearby shops. He often teamed up with well-known ballad publishers such as John Blare, William Thackeray, and Philip Brooksby. Helpfully, in an imprint on a ballad from 1690, Millett described his business: "at the Angel in Little-Brittain: where countrey chapmen may be furnish'd with all sorts of new and old small books and ballads at reasonable rates."[40] Chapmen walked the countryside with a pack of goods, selling trinkets, ballads, and a host of small items to rural customers. Thus we learn that *The Lass of Lynn* was produced by a man at the heart of London's cheap print trade who had his finger on the pulse of what sold well. The fact that two versions survive suggests that the first one may have sold well enough to prompt a second round.

Most ballads were illustrated with woodblocks, as was *The Lass of Lynn*. Woodblocks were expensive and many printers had an array on hand that they re-used repeatedly. Scholars have recently suggested that this re-use created connections across ballads as readers recognized pictures from other ballads on a new one.[41]

Just as when we browse in a bookstore and judge books by their covers, they may have judged a new ballad in part by the pictures. In a 1677 London play, a character looks at a song held by a ballad seller and identifies it by the woodblock image.[42]

Using EBBA's search function, we can trace *The Lass of Lynn*'s woodblock images across other ballads and explore what kinds of connections might have been made by seventeenth-century viewers. The ballad has two woodblocks: a man and a woman holding hands and a woman with a coif that looks a bit like Mickey Mouse ears to us. Neither were new. The first illustrated seven unique ballads in the EBBA database and the second eight, but there were multiple issues and copies of these ballads such that the images appeared a total of 36 times in EBBA. Obviously, they probably were also used on ballads that have not survived.

The picture of the man and woman holding hands implied that a ballad might be about courtship or a marital relationship, and seven of the eight unique ballads that used it were indeed such. The eighth was about a Welsh fortuneteller, and consisted largely of impossible predictions, but ended with stanza encouraging young single woman,

> Tho' you lye alone, yet make not your moan,
> For here by the Stars it is very well known,
> If you will be thrifty and both get and safe,
> When you are all marry'd you Husbands shall have.[43]

The verse acknowledges female sexual desire and a young woman's frustration with chastity, and predicts marriage, so it too speaks to a theme of courtship.

The image also illustrated ballads about marriage proposals. Two such are very similar. A man proposes to his swain by listing all the material goods he can bring to the marriage. She asks about his feelings, he says he loves her, and they commit to each other.[44] Similarly, a couple of the ballads with the "mouse ears" image are what we might call "happy ever after" stories, in which a couple is united by the last stanza.[45]

Other ballads with these images suggest more troubled relationships, often raising the issue of trust or the possibility of betrayal, a theme that resonated with *The Lass of Lynn*. Philip Brooksby, who must have owned the "mouse ears" woodblock, since it was used almost exclusively by him, produced a number of issues of "A New Scotch Ballad" about Willy and Nanny's relationship. Most of the song is about their mistrust of each other, misplaced jealousy and the like, although it ends on with promise of marriage.[46] Another ballad, again in supposed Scots dialect, warns, "Swains now of late have got the knack,/ poor Damosels to betray,/ But when they once have what they lack,/ ah! then theys gang away," although it too ends with marriage.[47] Others emphasize deception more heavily. "The Doting Old DAD, Or, The Unequal Match betwixt a Rich Muckworm of Fourscore and Ten" tells of an elderly rich man who wants to marry a 19 year old. The refrain is "O fie upon Fumblers, fie," suggesting her disgust at the thought of sexual relations with him.[48] But her mother tells her to marry him for his money, and do as she herself did, and take a young lover, "For when my Old Dad would deny,/ to yield me a daily supply,/ I still had a Friend my Will to attend/for fie upon Fumblers, fie."[49] Such sexual deception, which could result in passing off one man's child as another's, is very similar to that in that in *The Lass of Lynn.*

So when a potential buyer saw these woodcuts, or someone in an alehouse saw *The Lass of Lynn* pinned up on a wall, he or she might recognize them. The connotations of these images deepened some of the ballad's central themes about relationships and issues of trust and sexual deception. The same kinds of intertextuality could happen via the music, the tune to which the ballad was sung.[50] Most ballads did not have musical notation on them, although by the later seventeenth century, an increasing number began to do so. Instead, at the top, after the title, many noted the tune to which the ballad was to be sung, with phrases such as "to the tune of Old Simon the King" or "to the tune of The Country Farmer." Some ballads are more elliptical, saying "to an Excellent new tune" or "to a new Play tune," suggesting it came from a theatrical performance; the tune would have to be sung by the ballad seller. *The Lass of Lynn* was sung "to the tune of "Marry and I Thank You Too." Twenty-nine other entries in the EBBA database also use the same tune, including four produced by John Millet.[51] Tunes went by multiple names. The tune on the first Lass of Lynn ballad is listed as "I am so sick of Love," but the refrain of "Aye, marry, and thank ye too" indicates that it too was probably sung to the same tune as the next two.[52]

Other EBBA ballads sung to this tune were overwhelmingly about sexual relations, often illicit ones, including the first two Lass of Lynn ballads. Of 15 unique "Marry and I Thank You Too" ballads in the database (besides *The Lass of Lynn*), 11 were about some kind of extra-marital sexual encounter. A master pressured his servant into giving him a kiss, only to be caught by his wife before things went any further. A cuckolded, henpecked husband was the topic of a pair of ballads. Men cheerfully seduced women but were very clear that they would not marry.[53] Even ballads that initially seem to be about legitimate courtship turn out to have a twist; a 40-year-old woman courted a younger man, assuring him of her wealth, but sealed the deal by offering, "I vow to keep a handsome Maid,/ to pleasure thee now and then."[54] In other words, if she were not attractive to her husband sexually, he would have a younger woman in the house for his pleasure. Clearly, this lilting melody was strongly associated with sex outside of marriage for ballad writers and ballad consumers alike.

Looking at a ballad's tune can thus suggest additional layers of meaning beyond the text. Thinking about the music, however, also reminds us that ballads were not consumed passively on the printed page; they were performed. While antiquarians like Selden and Pepys might enjoy reading or re-reading a ballad in the privacy of their homes, most ballad consumers encountered them in the streets or in a tavern, in a group of people. Ballads were sold in the streets, sung by ballad sellers. Obviously, the better the performance, the better the potential sales. Especially for ballads about sexual relations, there must have been gestural components to the performance which we can only imagine. For example, a whole series of ballads use men's occupations to classify them according to their sexual attractiveness or performance; the sex act was often described in terms of men's work.[55] Either a young woman compared suitors or, in a twist in the genre, a group of married women in a tavern complained about their husbands in bed.[56] In both cases, many references were made to the specific tools of the men's trades, with obvious double entendres that would have been performed with gestures for additional comic value. In the tavern scene, the shoemaker's wife complained about his short awl, the pewterer's wife said that he seldom "cast into the mould that he should," the paver's wife bemoaned her husband's one stone (i.e., testicle) and "poor rammer." Only the blacksmith's wife was happy, for he "follow'd his labor with hammer and tongs." In singing *The Lass of Lynn*, a hawker might well have used gestures to dramatize the Lass's tears, her swelling belly, and the moment when George sees her belly on the wedding night. A skilled ballad-seller would have enhanced her performance of the song with all sorts of ribald gestures. In analyzing any ballad, it is important to read it aloud or sing it to imagine the possibilities it offered for performance. If you had to sell the ballad, how would you make the most of it?

Ballads such as these, in a female voice or voices, were most likely written by men. Indeed, it is hard not to read a certain male performance anxiety into these stories of sex as work done with male tools. *The Lass of Lynn*, written in a woman's voice, was all about how a woman tricked a man sexually. The complexities of this cross-gender voicing are deepened when we realize that many ballad-sellers were female. They were referred to as "hawkers" or "mercuries." A couple of generations later, the noted artist William Hogarth depicted ballad-sellers as pregnant women in at least five different engravings.[57] While he was playing with complex metaphorical relationships between printing and reproduction, he was also reflecting the social realities that women hawked ballads in the streets. Recently, a few historians have suggested that ballad writers may also have been aiming for a female audience, that women were eager consumers of the form, and writers sought to please them.[58] If this were the case, we have a very complex chain of gender inversions: words written by men to appeal to women, written in female (and male) voices, often about gender relations, and sung by female ballad-sellers.

While ballads were sung in the streets, they were also consumed in taverns or alehouses, where they were pinned to the walls as decoration.[59] Alehouses were common sites of sociability in early modern England and it is hard to imagine that ballads on the wall might not also have been sung there. A number of ballads, such as the one where wives bemoan their husbands' sexual performance, were set in alehouses or taverns, and woodblock illustrations of such settings feature on a number of such.[60] In gatherings such as these, perhaps not everyone understood the sexual innuendos, but knowing laughs would have at least suggested which elements of the song might have sexual meanings.[61]

In conclusion, this essay has explored a number of strategies that can be used to analyze seventeenth-century ballads as sources for the histories of sex, reproduction, and the body. We have looked at a single ballad, *The Lass of Lynn*, in a number of contexts. It suggests that male distrust of female sexual fidelity was commonplace, and while in theory, a man ruled his household as the monarch did the nation, in reality such rule was often as much aspiration as achievement. While unwed motherhood was deeply stigmatizing, this ballad implies that prenuptial pregnancy was acceptable, as long as a couple made it to the altar before the birth. A relative dearth of knowledge about reproduction left men vulnerable to being tricked by women about pregnancy, but somehow the social need to marry off a pregnant woman made such trickery a relatively minor issue, especially compared with that of cuckoldry. Analyses such as these require contextualizing a ballad in multiple dimensions. Such songs can be interpreted as literary texts, in relation to themes in other ballads, but they can also be explored via the music and woodcut images that link any ballad to a host of others. Here we have seen that both music and image suggested issues of illicit sex or sexual betrayal to a savvy consumer of ballads.

Notes

1 It is a pleasure to acknowledge with thanks the comments of Sandra Cavallo and Olivia Weisser on this chapter.
2 *The Lass of Lynn's New Joy*... (London: Printed and Sold by J. Millet, next door to the Flower-de-Luce in Little-Brittain, 1682–1692?), EBBA 21315.
3 Patricia Fumerton, *The Broadside Ballad in Early Modern England: Moving Media, Tactical Publics* (Philadelphia: University of Pennsylvania Press, 2020).
4 In what follows, *The Lass of Lynn* is italicized when it refers to the ballad; the character is referred to as the Lass, or the Lass of Lynn, without italics.
5 Nicholas Culpeper, *A Directory for Midwives* (London: Printed by Peter Cole, at the sign of the Printing Press in Cornhill, near the Royal Exchange, 1651), Thomason E.1340 (1), 216.
6 Thomas Raynalde, *The Byrth of Mankynde, otherwyse named the Womans booke* (London: Tho. Ray,1545), STC 21154, sig. C2r. See Jennifer Richards, "Reading and Hearing *The Womans Booke* in Early Modern England," *Bulletin of the History of Medicine* 89, no. 3 (2015): 434–62.
7 See also David Cressy, *Birth, Marriage, and Death: Ritual, Religion, and the Life-Cycle in Tudor and Stuart England* (Oxford: Oxford University Press, 1997): 57–59.
8 Leah Astbury, "Being Well, Looking Ill: Childbirth and the Return to Health in Seventeenth-Century England," *Social History of Medicine* 30:3 (2017): 500–19; see Sandra Cavallo's essay in this volume.
9 Richards, "Reading and Hearing *The Womans Booke*."
10 Christopher Marsh, "The Woman to the Plow; and the Man to the Hen-Roost: Wives, Husbands and Best-Selling Ballads in Seventeenth-Century England," *Transactions of the Royal Historical Society* 28 (2018): 65–88.
11 To check if a ballad exists in multiple copies or editions, see the ESTC online (http://estc.bl.uk/) as well as the EBBA (https://ebba.english.ucsb.edu/).
12 It seems that the previous installment of her tale was *An Answer to I Marry and thank ye too*... (London: Printed for P. Brooksby at the Golden Ball in Pye-corner, J. Deacon at the Angel in Gilt-spur-street, J. Blare at the Looking-glass on London-bridge, near the Church, J. Back at the Black Boy on London-bridge, near the Draw-bridge. License Licensed according to Order, 1675–1696?), EBBA 22080; probably the first installment was *The Thankful Country Lass, Or, The Jolly Batchelor Kindly Entertained* (London: Printed for J. Bissel, at the Bible and Harp near the Hospital-gate in West-smithfield, 1684–1700?), EBBA 22217.
13 *The Thankful Country Lass, Or, The Jolly Batchelor kindly entertained* (London: Printed for J. Bissel, at the Bible and Harp near the Hospital-gate in West-smithfield, 1684–1700?), EBBA 22217.

14 Richard Adair, *Courtship, Illegitimacy, and Marriage in Early Modern England* (Manchester: Manchester University Press, 1996).

15 *An Answer To I Marry and thank ye too; Or, the Lass of Lyn's sorrowfull Lamentation for the Loss of her Maiden-head* (London: Printed for P. Brooksby at the Golden Ball in Pye-corner, J. Deacon at the Angel in/Gilt-spur-street, J. Blare at the Looking-glass on London-bridge, near the Church,/J. Back at the Black Boy on London-bridge, near the Draw-bridge, 1675–1696?), EBBA 22080.

16 A possnet is a small round metal pot with three feet and a handle. Perhaps the Lass thought she needed one for preparing caudle, the warm beverage traditionally drunk during labor, or this was a more general household need.

17 Claire Tomalin, *Samuel Pepys: The Unequalled Self* (New York: Alfred A. Knopf, 2002): esp. 149–55.

18 *The Innocent Maid Deceiv'd by a Dissembling Batchelor: Or, The Mothers Advice to her Wanton Daughter* (London: Printed for W. Thackeray at the Angel in Duck-Lane, I. Millet, at the Angel in Little-Britain, and A. Milbourn, at the Stationers-Arms in the Little Old-Baily, 1689–1692), EBBA 21083.

19 *The Blind Eats Many a Flye: Or, The Broken Damsel Made Whole* (London: Printed for P. Brooksby, at the Golden=Ball, in Pye=corner, 1672–1696?), EBBA 33545.

20 For other versions of this theme, see *The Buxome Lass of Bread-street; Or, A Lamentation for the Loss of her Maiden=head: Which was Stoln from Her by Twelve Several Tradesmen. Together with her Resolution, after all, to marry her old Love* (London: Printed for P. Brooksby, J. Deacon, J. Blare, J. Back, 1675–1696?), EBBA 21310; *The Sommerset-shire Damsel beguil'd; Or, The Bonny Baker Chous'd in his Bargain. The Baker Wedded her in hast, And after that was done, She brought him e're Five months space A Daughter and a Son* (London: Printed for J. Blare, at the sign of the Looking-Glass on London-bridge, 1685–1688), EBBA 21689. Like *The Lass of Lynn*, both of these women deliver babies five months after marriage.

21 Mary E. Fissell, *Vernacular Bodies: The Politics of Reproduction in Early Modern England* (Oxford: Oxford University Press, 2004): 212; see large discussion of the cultural figure of the cuckold, 211–20.

22 On this theme, see for example, Cynthia B. Herrup, *A House in Gross Disorder: Sex, Law, and the Second Earl of Castlehaven* (New York: Oxford University Press, 1999); Elizabeth A. Foyster, *Manhood in Early Modern England: Honour, Sex, and Marriage* (London: Longman,1999). For a ballad version of the theme, see *The Hen-peckt Cuckold: Or, The Cross=grain'd Wife* (London: Printed and Sold by J. Millet, next door to the Flower-de-Luce, in Little Brittain, 1685?), EBBA 21793.

23 *Coffee-house Jests. Refined and enlarged...* (London: Printed for Hen. Rhodes, next door to the Swan-Tavern, near Bride-Lane in Fleet Street, 1686), Wing (2nd ed.), H1885, 15.

24 *Cuckolds Haven: Or, the Marry'd Mans Miserie, Who Must Abide the Penaltie of Being Hornify'd: Hee unto his Neighbours doth Make his Case Knowne, And Tels Them all Plainly, the Case is Their Owne* (Printed at London by M.P. for/Francis Grove, neere the Sarazens head without Newgate, 1638), EBBA 30036.

25 *New Western Ballad, of a Butcher that Cuckolded the Farmer* (London: Printed for R. Kell at the Anchor in Pye=corner, 1685–1688?), EBBA 21789.

26 Wendy Doniger, *The Bedtrick: Tales of Sex and Masquerade* (Chicago, IL: University of Chicago Press, 2000).

27 *A Cuckold by Consent: Or, the Frollick Miller that intic'd a Maid, Ar he did think, to Lodge in his Lawless Bed; But She Deceived Him of His Intent, And in Her Room his Wife to Bed She Sent* (London: Printed for I. Wright, I. Clarke, W. Thackeray, and T. Passenger, 1681–1684?), EBBA 21788. On millers and illicit sex, see, for example, *Grist Ground at Last...* (London: Printed for J. Clark, W. Thackeray, and T. Passinger,

1684–1686?), EBBA 21115. On beds, see Laura Gowing, "The Twinkling of a Bedstaff: Recovering the Social Life of English Beds 1500–1700," *Home Cultures: The Journal of Architecture, Design and Domestic Space* 11:3 (2014): 275–304.

28 *A New Little Northren Song Called, Vnder and Ouer, Ouer and Vnder, Or a Pretty New Least, And Yet No Wonder, or a Mayden Mistaken, as Many Now Bee, View Well This Glasse, and You May Plainely See* (No Place, Publisher Listed, 1631), EBBA 20122.

29 For a similar claim about women claiming virginity, see *The Loving Chamber-maid...* (London: Printed for Phil. Brooksby at the Goen [sic] Ball in West-Smithfield, 1672–1696?), EBBA 35756.

30 *A Loue-sick Maids Song, Lately Beguild, By a Run-Away Louer that Left Her with Childe* (London: Printed at London for I. W., 1625?), EBBA 20020.

31 John Bidwell, "French Paper in English Books," *The Cambridge History of the Book in Britain*, vol. 4, eds. John Barnard and D. F. McKenzie (Cambridge: Cambridge University Press, 2002), 587.

32 The measurements of the trimmed copy are 190 × 323 mm. https://ebba.english.ucsb.edu/ballad/21315/citation, consulted March 30, 2021.

33 Keith Thomas, "The Meaning of Literacy in Early Modern England," *The Written Word: Literacy in Transition*, ed. Gerd Baumann (Oxford: Oxford University Press, 1986): 97–131.

34 Zachary Lesser, "Typographic Nostalgia: Playreading, Popularity and the Meanings of Black Letter," *The Book of the Play: Playwrights, Stationers, and Readers in Early Modern England*, ed. Marta Straznicky (Amherst: University of Massachusetts Press, 2006): 99–126.

35 Gerald Egan, "Black Letter and the Broadside Ballad" (2007). https://ebba.english.ucsb.edu/page/black-letter, consulted March 30, 2021. Egan's essay provides the basic framework for my discussion above.

36 Hyder Rollins, "The Black-Letter Broadside Ballad," *PMLA* 34:2 (1919): 281.

37 Henry Plomer, *A Dictionary of the Printers and Booksellers Who Were at Work in England, Scotland and Ireland from 1668 to 1725* (Oxford: Oxford University Press, 1922): 207.

38 It's called "Short Title" because many early modern works have very long titles and older catalogs abbreviated them for convenience; see http://estc.bl.uk/.

39 *The Full Discovery of the Late Horrid Murther and Robbery, in Holbourn, Being the Apprehension, Examination, and Commitment of Iohn Randal: Formerly Butler to Esq; Bluck, Where The Same Was Done...* (London: Printed for John Millet, 1674), Wing F2348.

40 *The Royal Salutation, or, the Courtly Greeting between K. William and Qu. Mary at His Return from the Wars in Ireland to His Royal Pallace* (London: Printed by and for J. Millet, at the Angel in Little-Brittain: where countrey chapmen may be furnish'd with all sorts of new and old small books and ballads at reasonable rates, 1690), Wing [CD-ROM, 1996], R2152C).

41 Sarah Barber, "Curiosity and Reality: The Context and Interpretation of a Seventeenth-Century Image," *History Workshop Journal* 70 (2010): 21–45. Christopher Marsh, "Best-Selling Ballads and Their Pictures in Seventeenth-Century England," *Past & Present* 233 (2016): 53–99; Christopher Marsh, "A Woodcut and Its Wanderings in Seventeenth-Century England," *Huntington Library Quarterly* 79:2 (2016): 245–62; Alexandra Franklin, "Making Sense of Broadside Ballad Illustrations in the Seventeenth and Eighteenth Centuries," in Kevin D. Murphy and Sally O'Driscoll (eds.), *Studies in Ephemera: Text and Image in Eighteenth-Century Print* (Lewisburg, PA: Bucknell University Press, 2013): 169–94.

42 William Cavendish, *The Triumphant Widow: or, The Medley of Humours: A Comedy* (London: Printed by J[ohn]. M[acock]. for H. Herringman, at the sign of the Blew

Anchor in the lower walk of the New-Exchange, 1677), Wing (CD-ROM, 1996), N891, 6–7. I owe this quote and much else to Marsh, "Best-Selling Ballads."

43 *The Welsh Fortune-Teller, Or, Sheffery Morgan's Observation of the Stars, as He Sat Upon a Mountain in Wales* (London: Printed for G. Conyers on Ludgate=Hill, 1686–1703?), EBBA 21983.

44 *The Faithful Farmer, Or, The Down-right VVooing betwixt Robin and Nancy* (London: Printed for J. Blare, at the Sign of the Looking-Glass on London-Bridge, 1685–1688), EBBA 30634; E. W., *The Down-ight VVooing of Honest John & Betty* (London: Printed for J. Deacon, at the Angel in Guiltspur-Street, 1685–1688), EBBA 33883.

45 *The Loyal Soldiers Courtship; or, Constant Peggy's Kind Answer* (London: Printed for P. Brooksby, I. Deacon, I. Blare, and I. Back, 1689?), EBBA 21869; *Loves Wound, & Loves Cure* (London: Printed for J. Wright, J. Clarke, W. Thackeray, and T. Passinger, 1681–1684), EBBA 21120.

46 *A New Scotch Ballad of Jealous Nanny: or, False-hearted Willy turn'd True* ([NP, NP]), EBBA 30681. The other eight listed in EBBA were all printed by Brooksby.

47 *Jockey's Lamentation Turn'd into Joy: or, Ienny Yields at Last* (London: Printed for J. Deacon, at the Sign of the Angel, in Guiltspur-street, without Newgate, 1671–1702?), EBBA 30919.

48 Checking the *Oxford English Dictionary*, we see that "fumbler" was a slang term used specifically in the later seventeenth century to describe men who were inadequate sexually.

49 T*he Doting Old Dad, or, the Unequal Match Betwixt a Rich Muckworm of Fourscore and Ten, and a Young Lass Scarce Nineteen* (London: Printed for P. Brooksby, at the Sign the Golden-Ball, near the Hospital Gate, in West-Smithfield, 1685–1688), EBBA 30607.

50 Christopher Marsh, "'Fortune My Foe': The Circulation of an English Super-Tune," in *Identity, Intertextuality, and Performance in Early Modern Song Culture*. Intersections: vol. 43 (Leiden: Brill, 2016): 308–30.

51 https://ebba.english.ucsb.edu/ballad/21315/recording, consulted April 1, 2021.

52 See https://ebba.english.ucsb.edu/ballad/22217/recording, consulted April 2, 2021, for the music.

53 *A Dialogue Between a Master and his Maid; or, Beautiful Susan Willing, but Loath, to V[entu]re to Kiss her Master Least her Mistriss should Chide* (London: Printed for J. Bissel, at the Bible and Harp in West-smithfield, 1684–1700?), EBBA 22059; *The Hen-peckt Cuckold: or, the Cross=grain'd Wife* (London: Printed and Sold by J. Millet, next door to the Flower-de-Luce, in Little Brittain, 1685?), EBBA 21793; *The Wife's Answer to the Hen=peckt Cuckolds Complaint* (London: Printed for I. Millet, next door to the Flower=de luce, in Little=Brittain, 1682–1692?), EBBA 21799; *The Denying Lady: or, a Travellers Frolick with a Woman that Reply'd No to all Questions and Discourses put to Her* (London: Printed by and for A. Milbourn[,] at the Stationers-[Arms in Green-Arbor.], 1684–1695?), EBBA 22083; *The Thankful Country Lass, or, the Jolly Batchelor Kindly Entertained* (London: Printed for J. Bissel, at the Bible and Harp near the Hospital-gate in West-smithfield, 1684–1700?), EBBA 22217.

54 *Nell's Humble Petition: or, the Maidens Kind and Courteous Courtship to Honest John the Joyner, Whose Love She Earnestly Desired* (London: Printed for P. Brooksby, J. Deacon, J. Blare[,] J. Back, 1675–1696?), EBBA 21080.

55 I owe this insight to Helen Weinstein, "Hammer and Anvil: Metaphors of Sex in the Seventeenth-Century English Ballad," paper presented at the Ninth Berkshire Conference on the History of Women, Vassar College, June 1993. Occupational metaphors for sexual intercourse were long-lived; see Anna Clark, *The Struggle for the Breeches: Gender and the Making of the British Working Class* (Berkeley: University of California Press, 1995), 60 for such involving tailors a century later.

56 Comparing suitors: *The Northern Ladd: Or, the Fair Maids Choice* [No imprint; 1672–1696?] R227322; *The Merry Maid of Middlesex* (London: Printed by E. Crowch,

for F. Coles, T. Vere, & J. Wright, 1663–1674), R214176; *The Lovesick Maid of Waping Her Complaint for want of Apple-Pye* [no imprint, 1685?], R228346; Married women: *The Seven Merry Wives of London* (London: Printed for J. Blare, at the Looking-glass on London-bridge, 1664–1703?), N69973. On ballads and occupational identity, see Mark Hailwood, "Broadside Ballads and Occupational Identity in Early Modern England," *Huntington Library Quarterly* 79 (2016): 187–200.

57 Margaret Hunt, "Hawkers, Bawlers, and Mercuries: Women and the London Press in the Early Enlightenment," *Women & History* 9 (1984): 41–68; Elizabeth Kathleen Mitchell, "William Hogarth's Pregnant Ballad Sellers and the Engraver's Matrix," in *Ballads and Broadsides in Britain, 1500–1800*, ed. Patricia Fumerton and Anita Guerrini (Burlington, VT: Ashgate, 2010): 229–47; Sandra Clark, "The Broadside Ballad and the Woman's Voice," in *Debating Gender in Early Modern England 1500–1700*, ed. Christina Malcolmson and Mihoko Suzuki (Basingstoke: Palgrave MacMillan, 2002): 103–20.

58 "Several Suggestive Sources Are Gathered Together," in Natascha Würzbach, *Rise of the English Street Ballad* (Cambridge: Cambridge University Press, 2011), 263–64; 266; 278–79; 280–82. Clark, "The Broadside Ballad and the Woman's Voice"; Marsh, "The Woman to the Plow."

59 See Adam Fox, *Oral and Literate Culture in England, 1500–1700* (Oxford: Clarendon, 2000): 326, 332, for examples. On alehouses, see Peter Clark, *The English Alehouse: A Social History, 1200–1830* (London: Longman, 1983).

60 See, for example, EBBA 31861; EBBA 33191; EBBA 30268.

61 See Valerie Traub, *Thinking Sex with the Early Moderns* (Philadelphia: University of Pennsylvania, Press, 2016): esp. 204, for discussion of sexual knowledge on the London stage, and the highly variable ways in which such moments might have been consumed.

Bibliography

Primary Sources

Cavendish, William. *The Triumphant Widow: or, The Medley of Humours: A Comedy*. London: Printed by J[ohn]. M[acock]. for H. Herringman, at the sign of the Blew Anchor in the lower-walk of the New-Exchange, 1677. Wing (CD-ROM, 1996), N891.

Coffee-House Jests. Refined and Enlarged... London: Printed for Hen. Rhodes, next door to the Swan-Tavern, near Bride-Lane in Fleet Street, 1686. Wing (2nd ed.), H1885.

Culpeper, Nicholas. *A Directory for Midwives*. London: Printed by Peter Cole, at the sign of the Printing Press in Cornhill, near the Royal Exchange, 1651, Thomason E.1340 (1).

The Full Discovery of the Late Horrid Murther and Robbery, in Holbourn, Being the Apprehension, Examination, and Commitment of Iohn Randal: Formerly Butler to Esq; Bluck, Where the Same Was Done.... London: printed for John Millet, 1674, Wing F2348.

The Lovesick Maid of Waping Her Complaint for want of Apple-Pye. 1685? R228346.

The Merry Maid of Middlesex. London, Printed by E. Crowch, for F. Coles, T. Vere, & J. Wright. 1663–1674. R214176.

The Northern Ladd: Or, the Fair Maids Choice [No imprint; 1672–1696?] R227322.

Patricia Fumerton, dir., English Broadside Ballad Archive (EBBA): http://ebba.english.ucsb.edu

Raynalde, Thomas. *The Byrth of Mankynde, otherwyse named the Womans booke*. London: Tho. Ray. [1545], STC 21154.

The Royal Salutation, or, the Courtly Greeting between K. William and Qu. Mary at His Return from the Wars in Ireland to His Royal Pallace. London: Printed by and for J. Millet, at the Angel in Little-Brittain: where countrey chapmen may be furnish'd with all sorts of new and old small books and ballads at reasonable rates [1690]. Wing (CD-ROM, 1996), R2152C.

The Seven Merry Wives of London. London: Printed for J. Blare, at the Looking-glass on London-bridge, 1664–1703? N69973.

Secondary Sources

Adair, Richard. *Courtship, Illegitimacy, and Marriage in Early Modern England.* Manchester: Manchester University Press, 1996.

Astbury, Leah. "Being Well, Looking Ill: Childbirth and the Return to Health in Seventeenth-Century England." *Social History of Medicine* 30:3 (2017): 500–19.

Barber, Sarah. "Curiosity and Reality: The Context and Interpretation of a Seventeenth-Century Image." *History Workshop Journal* 70 (2010): 21–45.

Bidwell, John. "French Paper in English Books." In *The Cambridge History of the Book in Britain.* Vol. 4, edited by John Barnard and D. F. McKenzie, 583–601. Cambridge: Cambridge University Press, 2002.

Clark, Anna. *The Struggle for the Breeches: Gender and the Making of the British Working Class.* Berkeley: University of California Press, 1995.

Clark, Peter. *The English Alehouse: A Social History, 1200–1830.* London: Longman, 1983.

Clark, Sandra. "The Broadside Ballad and the Woman's Voice." In *Debating Gender in Early Modern England 1500–1700,* edited by Christina Malcolmson and Mihoko Suzuki, 103–20. Basingstoke: Palgrave MacMillan, 2002.

Cressy, David. *Birth, Marriage, and Death: Ritual, Religion, and the Life-Cycle in Tudor and Stuart England.* Oxford: Oxford University Press, 1997.

Doniger, Wendy. *The Bedtrick: Tales of Sex and Masquerade.* Chicago, IL: University of Chicago Press, 2000.

Egan, Gerald. "Black Letter and the Broadside Ballad." 2007. https://ebba.english.ucsb.edu/page/black-letter

Fissell, Mary E. *Vernacular Bodies: The Politics of Reproduction in Early Modern England.* Oxford: Oxford University Press, 2004.

Fox, Adam. *Oral and Literate Culture in England, 1500–1700.* Oxford: Clarendon, 2000.

Foyster, Elizabeth A. *Manhood in Early Modern England: Honour, Sex, and Marriage.* London: Longman, 1999.

Franklin, Alexandra. "Making Sense of Broadside Ballad Illustrations in the Seventeenth and Eighteenth Centuries." In *Studies in Ephemera: Text and Image in Eighteenth-Century Print,* edited by Kevin D. Murphy and Sally O'Driscoll, 169–94. Lewisburg, PA: Bucknell University Press, 2013.

Fumerton, Patricia. *The Broadside Ballad in Early Modern England: Moving Media, Tactical Publics.* Philadelphia: University of Pennsylvania Press, 2020.

Gowing, Laura. "The Twinkling of a Bedstaff: Recovering the Social Life of English Beds 1500–1700." *Home Cultures: The Journal of Architecture, Design and Domestic Space* 11:3 (2014): 275–304.

Hailwood, Mark. "Broadside Ballads and Occupational Identity in Early Modern England." *Huntington Library Quarterly* 79 (2016): 187–200.

Herrup, Cynthia B. *A House in Gross Disorder: Sex, Law, and the Second Earl of Castlehaven.* New York: Oxford University Press, 1999.

Hunt, Margaret. "Hawkers, Bawlers, and Mercuries: Women and the London Press in the Early Enlightenment." *Women & History* 9 (1984): 41–68.

Lesser, Zachary. "Typographic Nostalgia: Playreading, Popularity and the Meanings of Black Letter." In *The Book of the Play: Playwrights, Stationers, and Readers in Early Modern England*, edited by Marta Straznicky, 99–126. Amherst: University of Massachusetts Press, 2006.

Marsh, Christopher. "Best-Selling Ballads and Their Pictures in Seventeenth-Century England." *Past & Present* 233 (2016): 53–99.

———. "'Fortune My Foe': The Circulation of an English Super-Tune." In *Identity, Intertextuality, and Performance in Early Modern Song Culture*. Intersections: vol. 43. Leiden: Brill, 2016: 308–30.

———. "A Woodcut and Its Wanderings in Seventeenth-Century England." *Huntington Library Quarterly* 79:2 (2016): 245–62.

———. "The Woman to the Plow; And the Man to the Hen-Roost: Wives, Husbands and Best-Selling Ballads in Seventeenth-Century England." *Transactions of the Royal Historical Society* 28 (2018): 65–88.

Mitchell, Elizabeth Kathleen. "William Hogarth's Pregnant Ballad Sellers and the Engraver's Matrix." In *Ballads and Broadsides in Britain, 1500–1800*, edited by Patricia Fumerton and Anita Guerrini, 229–47. Burlington, VT: Ashgate, 2010.

Plomer, Henry. *A Dictionary of the Printers and Booksellers Who Were at Work in England, Scotland and Ireland from 1668 to 1725*. Oxford: Oxford University Press, 1922.

Richards, Jennifer. "Reading and Hearing *The Womans Booke* in Early Modern England." *Bulletin of the History of Medicine* 89, no. 3 (2015): 434–62.

Rollins, Hyder. "The Black-Letter Broadside Ballad." *PMLA* 34:2 (1919): 281.

Thomas, Keith. "The Meaning of Literacy in Early Modern England." In *The Written Word: Literacy in Transition*, edited by Gerd Baumann, 97–131. Oxford: Oxford University Press, 1986.

Tomalin, Claire. *Samuel Pepys: The Unequalled Self*. New York: Alfred A. Knopf, 2002.

Traub, Valerie. *Thinking Sex with the Early Moderns*. Philadelphia: University of Pennsylvania, Press, 2016.

Weinstein, Helen. "Hammer and Anvil: Metaphors of Sex in the Seventeenth-Century English Ballad." Paper Presented at the Ninth Berkshire Conference on the History of Women. Vassar College. June 1993.

Würzbach, Natascha. *Rise of the English Street Ballad*. Cambridge: Cambridge University Press, 2011.

Part IV

Objects and Images

17 Book Illustrations

Jane Sharp's *The Midwives Book*

Rebecca Whiteley

A woman with her abdomen opened to show the anatomy of her pregnancy (Figure 17.1). A series of fetuses assuming different positions in the womb (Figure 17.2). Three scenes with people: in a chamber; walking in a procession; and having a meal (Figure 17.3). Look closely at these images and ask: What exactly do they depict? Where are they from? How were they made? How are they related? What do they tell us about early modern cultures of midwifery and childbirth?

These are the kinds of questions we ask of images when we use them as sources for history. In some ways, they are very similar to the questions we ask of textual sources when writing histories of medicine, but there are also special considerations and techniques when working with images. This chapter will demonstrate the approaches we can take to images as sources, and the insights they can give us, by focusing on printed book illustrations and, in particular, on one English midwifery manual from the late seventeenth century.

Printed images were everywhere in early modern Europe, not least as illustrations in medical books.[1] They are rich resources for histories of medicine that can offer new perspectives and provide insight into aspects of medical culture less well or frequently expressed in texts. In the past, the history of medicine has been a bit of an "iconophobic" discipline – one that shied away from using images as sources. But, in recent decades, an interdisciplinary movement sometimes called "epistemic image studies" has seen historians of science and medicine, social historians, and historians of art collaborate to address images that have informational content.[2] Looking at some core texts in this discipline will help you to see how we can study images that created, shaped, and communicated knowledge in medicine.[3]

In this chapter, we will use the example of one illustrated midwifery manual to explore how book illustrations can be sources for the history of medicine. The small but diverse set of illustrations reproduced over the three known editions of Jane Sharp's midwifery manual demonstrates the many ways in which images could shape knowledge, medical practice, and the culture of midwifery and pregnancy in early modern England. While we will be focusing on one book, the analytical strategies could be applied to any early modern image, medical or otherwise.

DOI: 10.4324/9781003094876-22

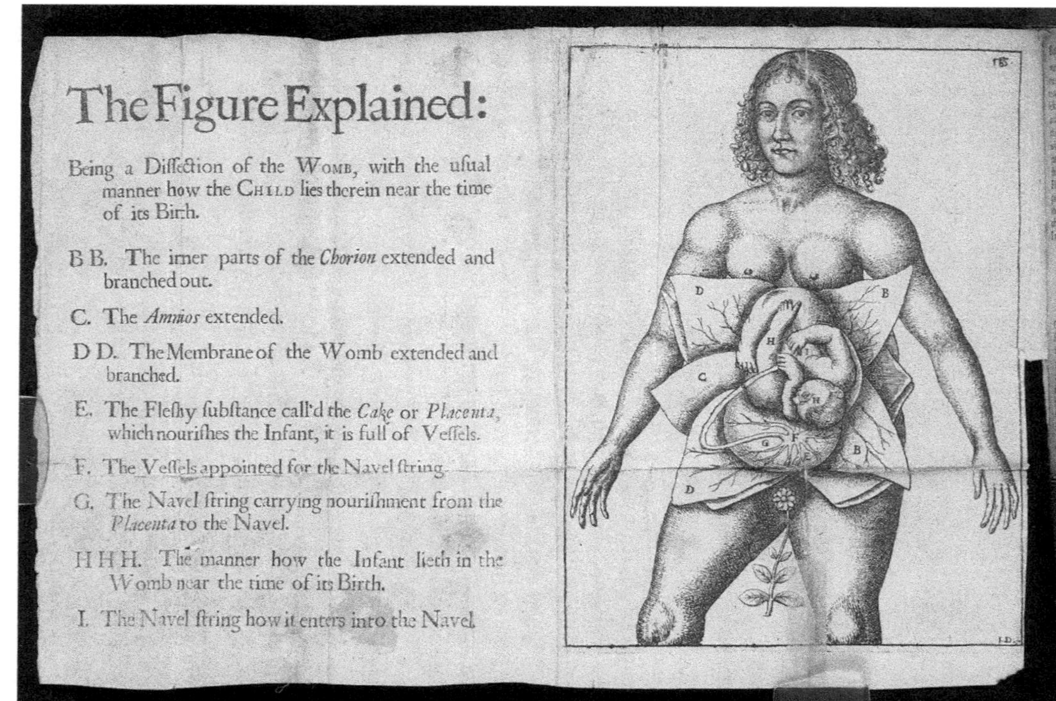

The Figure Explained:

Being a Diſſection of the WOMB, with the uſual manner how the CHILD lies therein near the time of its Birth.

B B. The iner parts of the *Chorion* extended and branched out.

C. The *Amnios* extended.

D D. The Membrane of the Womb extended and branched.

E. The Fleſhy ſubſtance call'd the *Cake* or *Placenta*, which nouriſhes the Infant, it is full of Veſſels.

F. The Veſſels appointed for the Navel ſtring.

G. The Navel ſtring carrying nouriſhment from the *Placenta* to the Navel.

H H H. The manner how the Infant lieth in the Womb near the time of its Birth.

I. The Navel ſtring how it enters into the Navel.

Figure 17.1 Anon. "[Pregnant Anatomy]," engraving, 30.2 × 20.4 cm [page]. In Jane Sharp, *The Midwives Book* (London: Simon Miller, 1671). Copyright of the University of Manchester.

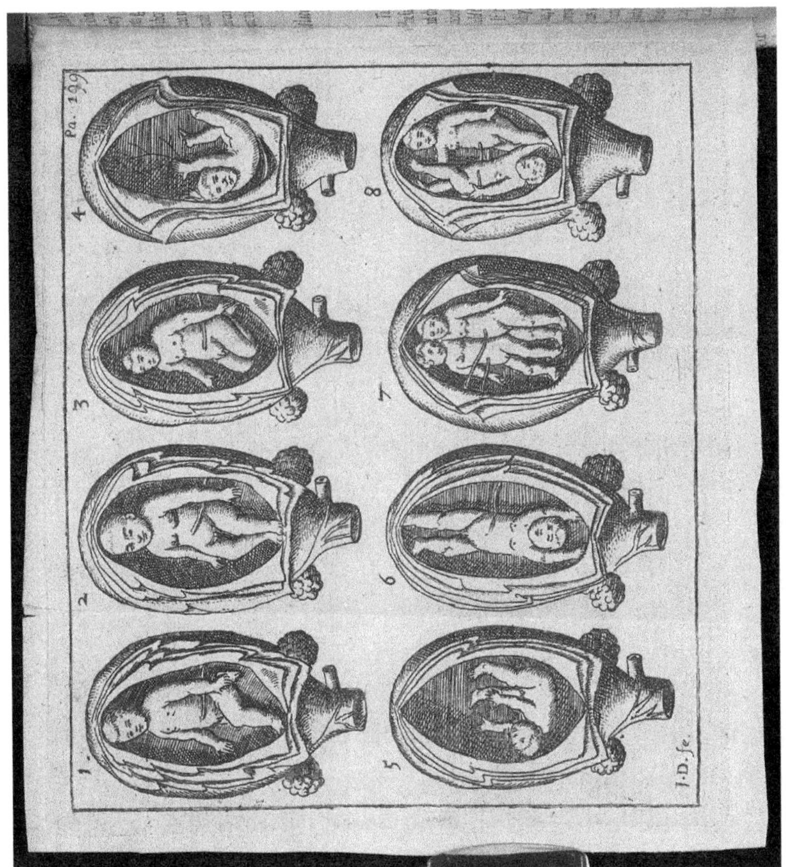

Figure 17.2 Anon. "[Birth Figures]," engraving, 14.5 × 13.2 cm [page]. In Jane Sharp, *The Midwives Book* (London: Simon Miller, 1671). Copyright of the University of Manchester.

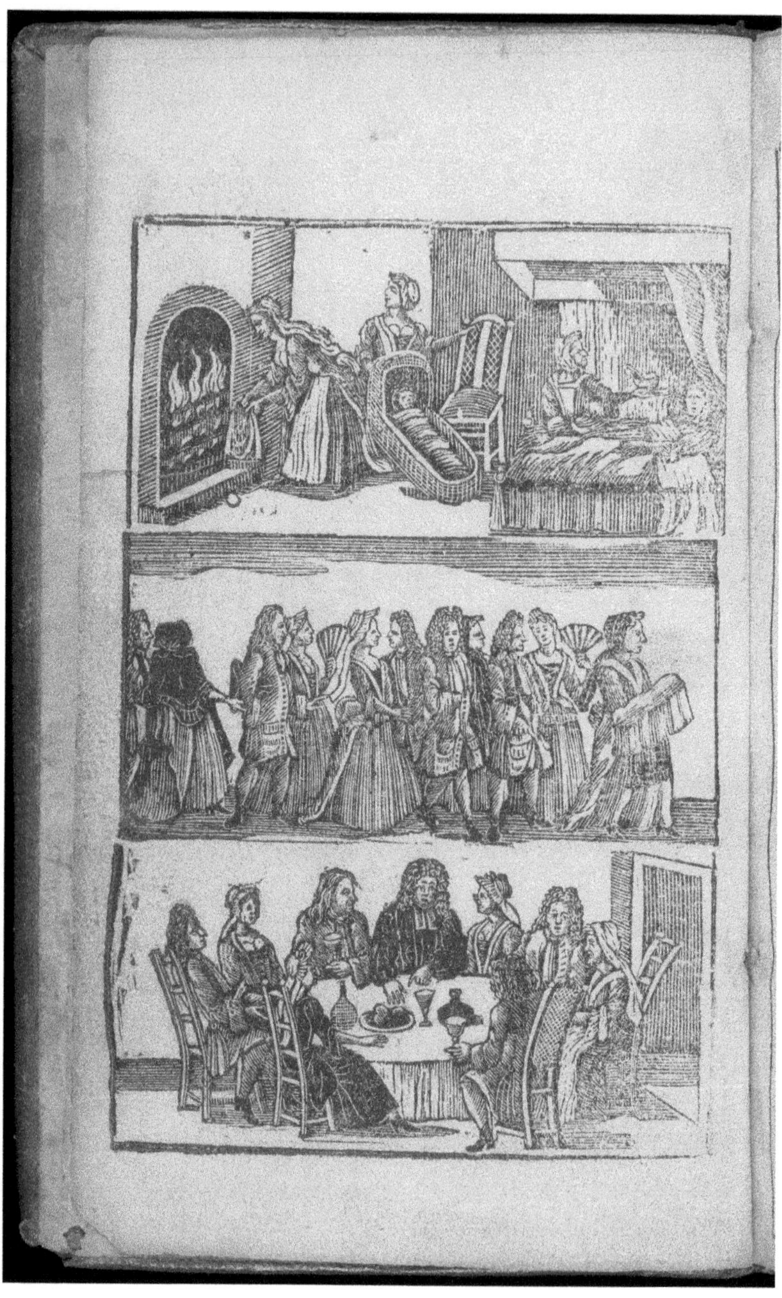

Figure 17.3 Anon. "[Childbirth Scenes]," woodcut, 9 × 15.5 cm [page]. In Jane Sharp, *The Compleat Midwife's Companion* (London: J. Marshall, 1724). Wellcome Collection.

Jane Sharp's *The Midwives Book*

This book was first published in England in 1671, and then republished several times in the 1720s.[4] It formed part of a great proliferation of print in England in the seventeenth century that covered many topics, including all branches of medicine. These vernacular books offered, on the one hand, classical and learned knowledge that had previously been restricted to the wealthy, educated, and Latin-literate, and on the other hand, the kind of empirical knowledge kept by those who worked with their hands, from midwives and surgeons to weavers and printers, which had previously been communicated verbally or kept in private manuscript notebooks.[5]

Beginning in Germany in 1513 with the publication of Eucharius Rösslin's *Der Swangern Frawen und Hebammen Roszengarten*, some male authors with medical training but little or no experience delivering women began to write vernacular texts that presented the longstanding academic knowledge on the topic of midwifery derived from the ancient authors Hippocrates and Galen, combined with Arabic sources and filtered through Medieval learned manuscripts.[6] The genre became popular all over Europe and the texts cribbed extensively from each other. In England, most midwifery manuals and illustrations published in the sixteenth and seventeenth centuries were derived from continental sources. This circulating and vernacular printed knowledge meant that cultures of midwifery in Europe could be simultaneously intensely local, and highly international.

In England, from the mid-seventeenth century, the shape of midwifery changed again as medical men began to encroach on the realm of practice. Traditionally, delivering women had been an all-female profession and midwives rarely had formal medical training. Male surgeons and physicians were only called in unusually difficult and dangerous cases. However, beginning in the seventeenth century, male practitioners began to attend a larger proportion of deliveries, charging higher fees and claiming specialist skills to save the mother and infant in difficult cases. This shift was reflected in midwifery manuals, where the mostly male authors began to combine the conventional academic knowledge with empirical knowledge derived from practice.[7] The extent to which women engaged with this book culture has been much debated. While the majority of midwifery work was still done by women, only a very few published books on the subject. Yet most of the male-authored midwifery manuals were addressed, at least rhetorically, to women midwives. The sheer number of such volumes, and the increasing levels of literacy among women during the seventeenth century, suggests that the books probably were read by both midwives and lay women, as well as doctors and surgeons.[8] What they did with the information they read is another question entirely, and one that is difficult to answer. What we can be sure about is that different readers would have reacted differently to the text and illustrations and put them to different uses.

Sharp's text, like most written in the seventeenth century, was cribbed from existing sources. In her case: *The Compleat Midwives Practice* (1656) by a collective of anonymous authors but itself borrowed from older sources; and *A Directory for Midwives* (1651) by the popular medical author Nicholas Culpeper.[9] Both of these books went through multiple editions, as well as being widely copied. Sharp's illustrations were also copied, more or less directly, from existing sources. Quite a bit has been written about Sharp's book because it appears to be the first English midwifery book to be written by a woman. Scholars such as Elaine Hobby, Eve Keller, and Caroline Bicks have argued that Sharp took an unusually pro-midwife approach to the conventional academic wisdom found in midwifery books, and added in her own expertise derived from decades of practice.[10] Others, such as Katharine Phelps Walsh, have doubted that Sharp was a real woman and argued that the text gives no special insights into women's knowledge, and that Sharp may have been a pseudonym for a male author.[11]

I do not see any evidence to say that Sharp was not a real person, though as Walsh points out there also is not much solid evidence that she *did* exist. I will refer to her as "she," but the approach of this chapter means that Sharp's gender does not really matter. Her book and the illustrations she commissioned were part of a wider and existing culture of medicine in which sharing and copying was a widely practiced technique that allowed authoritative knowledge to be agreed upon and added to within established and legible frameworks.[12] Some particularly valued epistemic images persisted for a surprisingly long time, often well after aspects of the knowledge they contained had been challenged or superseded. This is because the history of epistemic images is not linear: there was no straight "progress" in which new images replaced old as knowledge advanced. Rather, different approaches and forms of knowledge combined and clashed in a diverse culture of the body. If an image seems to us "outdated" in one way, we must ask in what other ways it was still relevant and making meaning for early modern viewers.

As well as being pluralistic in the ways they made meaning, medical illustrations were pluralistic in the way they were made. Often, we do not know the identity of the artist who drafted them, but even if we do, we almost never know the identity of every person involved in drafting, engraving, and printing them.[13] While this can be frustrating, the fact that printed book illustrations were produced by so many (often anonymous) hands, along with their prolific borrowing, makes them more generally expressive of how their culture thought about and envisioned the subject they represent.

Pregnant Anatomy

Let's begin with the anatomical illustration. In the 1671 edition of Sharp's book, it is an engraving (Figure 17.1) and in the 1720s editions, a woodcut (Figure 17.4). Identifying and understanding an image's medium, or the materials and production processes behind it, can be key to analyzing its cultural significance. Engraving is a more expensive printing technique that produces finer lines. It involves taking a sheet of copper and carving lines wherever you eventually want the ink to print. Ink is then spread over the plate and wiped away so it only remains in the carved grooves. Wetted paper is then laid over the plate and it is run through a rolling press that exerts high pressure, forcing the paper into the grooves where it picks up the ink. This is called an "intaglio" printing technique. Engravings were of higher status because they were more expensive to produce and to print.

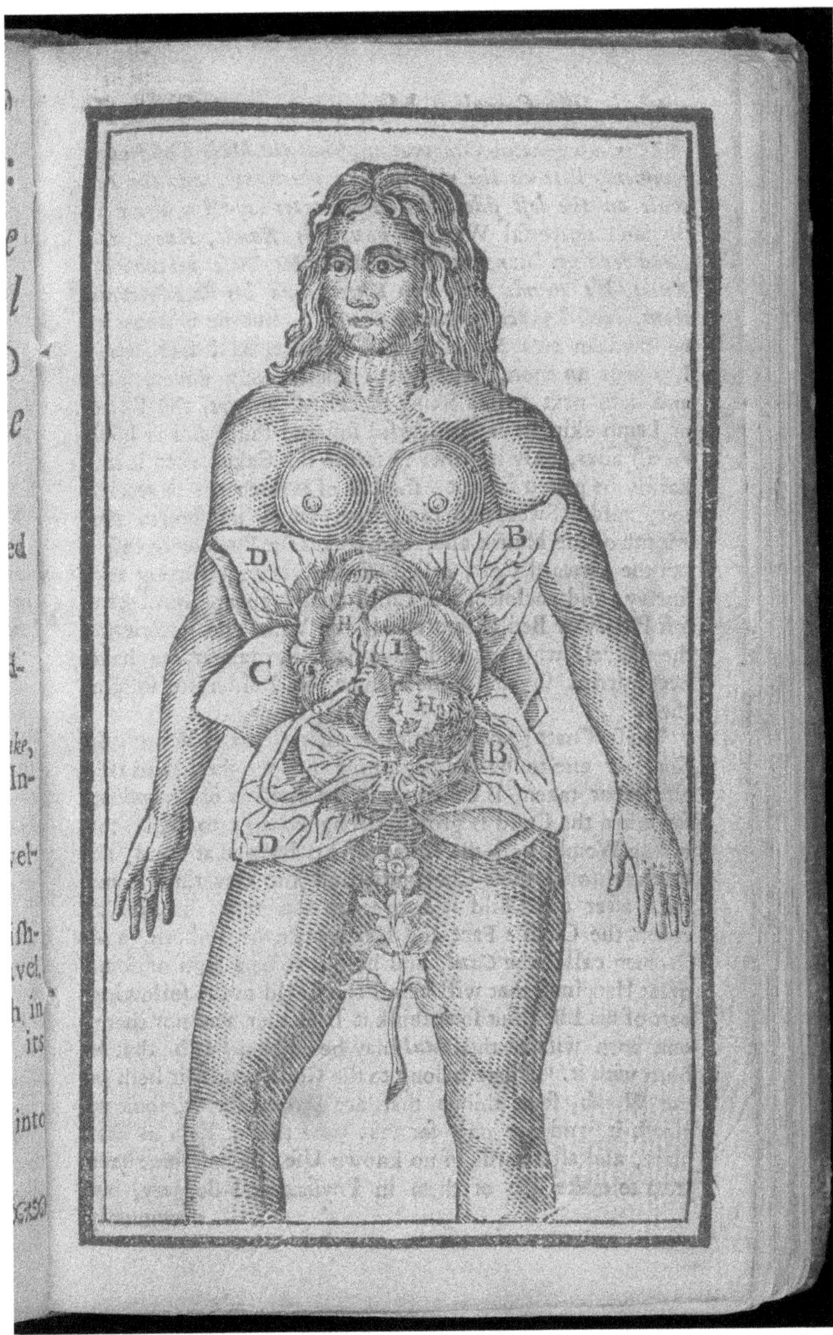

Figure 17.4 Anon. "[Pregnant Anatomy]," woodcut, 9 × 15.5 cm [page]. In Jane Sharp, *The Compleat Midwife's Companion* (London: J. Marshall, 1724). Wellcome Collection.

The plates did not last as long, but the resulting images could be finer and more detailed. The hatching, cross-hatching, and layering of many lines allowed engravings to create contour and tone.[14] Sharp's anatomical figure is not nearly as detailed and fine as some other anatomical illustrations of the period, but it does indicate that the author valued the images and was willing to pay more than the minimum to make them more detailed and prestigious. In the later editions, the illustrations are woodcuts, in which the printmaker cuts away from the surface of a block of wood everywhere they *don't* want ink to print. The block is then rolled with ink and can be printed onto paper using the same kind of press as was used to print text. This is called a "relief" printing technique. Woodblocks are hardy and could be more easily combined with letterpress. However, it is harder to get fine detail and tone with a woodcut, and they were generally associated with cheaper and less prestigious productions.

This use of woodcuts suggests that the 1720s editions of Sharp's book, which were edited and published by John Marshall, were done on a budget, and perhaps aimed at a lower status audience and sold at a cheaper price than the original. By the 1720s, the recycled mixture of ancient classical authors and common medical wisdom would have seemed old-fashioned compared to the newest innovations in midwifery coming from the continent.[15] While such texts were still circulating and popular among lay readers and midwives, a more elite readership of physicians, surgeons, and medically trained midwives were turning to new forms of anatomical and medical knowledge, and new techniques of practice.

But can we see the intended audience, and the spheres of knowledge, in the images themselves? Apart from their media, what do they tell us? The 1724 woodcut copy is a reasonably faithful recreation of the 1671 engraving, but there are differences. The earlier image (Figure 17.1) is finer in detail and tone, the woman has a more distinct hairstyle, and the image has been signed "J.D. *f*." This is short for "J.D. *fecit*," which is Latin for "J.D. *made it*." The phrasing was commonly used by engravers signing their work. Sometimes the original draftsperson would also be credited with the Latin word "invenit" but here they are not mentioned because this is actually a copy of an existing image. The original image is a large, expensive anatomical plate from a much more prestigious book called *De Formato Foetu* by Adriaan van den Spieghel (Figure 17.5). Published in Latin, it was aimed at a readership of learned physicians. The image was part of a series showing different layers of pregnant anatomy, but this one was the most widely copied, reproduced, and adapted. In some cases, the copies were relatively close, in others the image was reduced to just a torso, or even just the fetus (Figure 17.6).[16]

The core of this image is the anatomy of pregnancy – the torso opened, the layers of the uterus and amniotic sac peeled back, the fetus and placenta displayed. This is the element usually privileged in copies, when the background, and even the pregnant woman's body, has been excised (Figures 17.1, 17.4, 17.6). Such images formed part of a new kind of visual anatomy, most famously associated with the anatomical atlas *De Humani Corporis Fabrica* by Andreas Vesalius.[17] It might be termed "observational" anatomy, in contrast to earlier anatomical images which tended to be more abstract and diagrammatic. The new observational

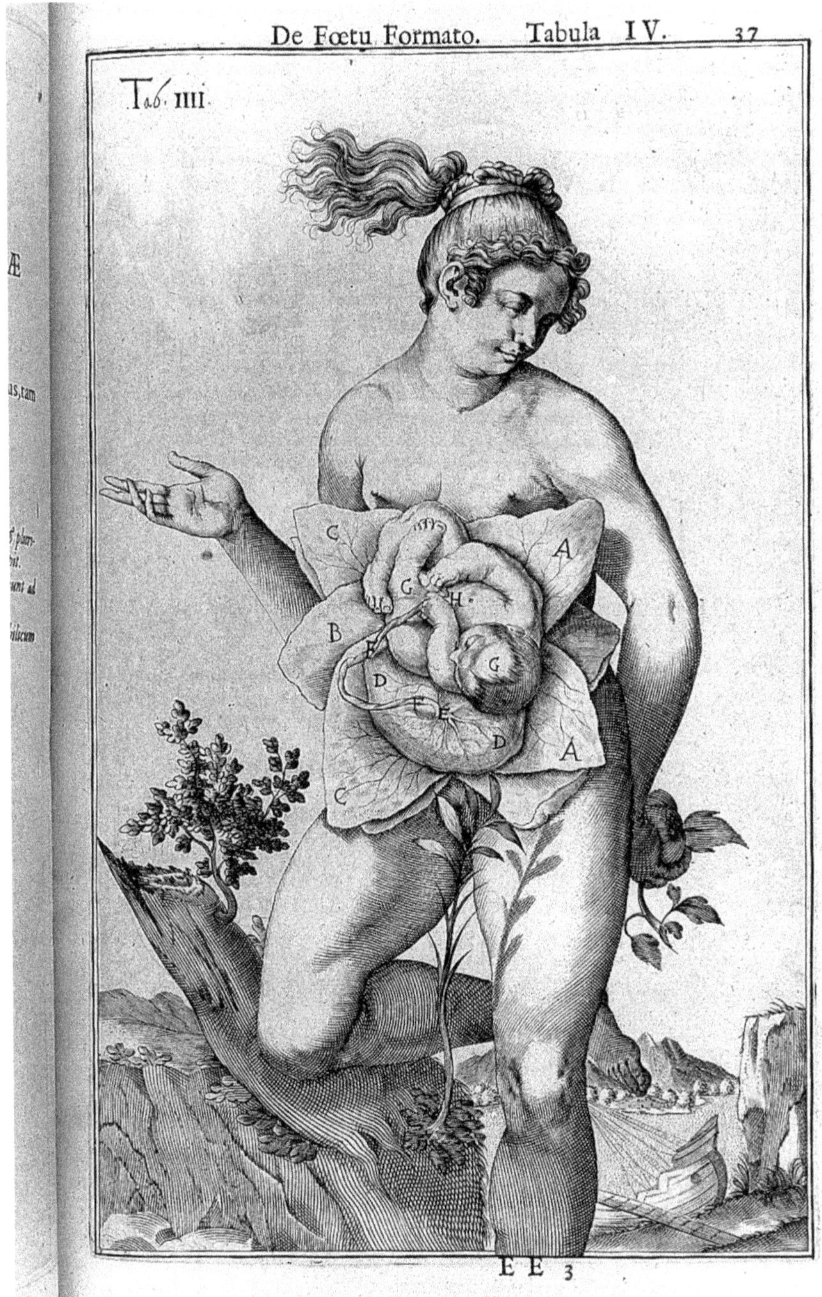

Figure 17.5 Odoardo Fialetti, *Table 4*, engraving, 27 × 43 cm [page]. In Adriaan van de Spieghel, *Opera quae extant omnia* (Amsterdam: Johannes Blaeu, 1645). Wellcome Collection.

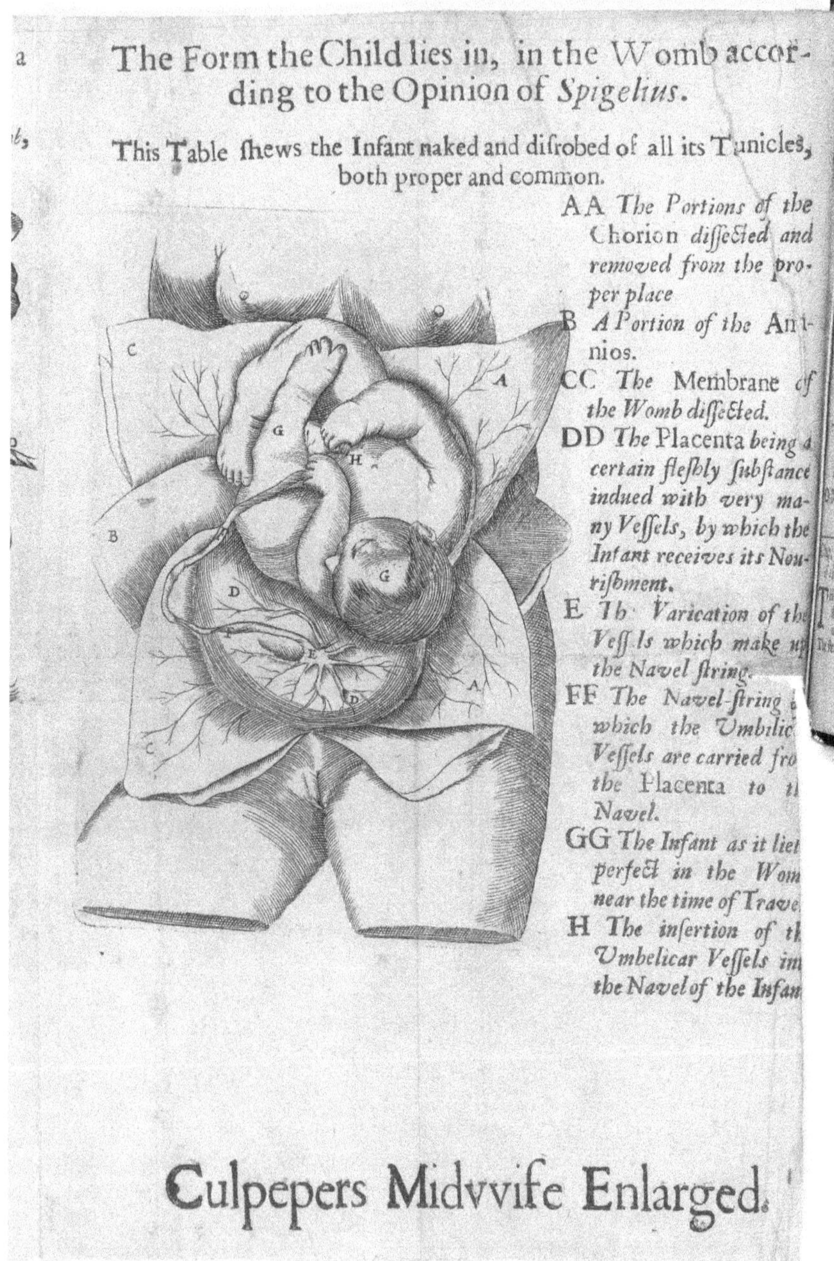

The Form the Child lies in, in the Womb according to the Opinion of *Spigelius*.

This Table ſhews the Infant naked and diſrobed of all its Tunicles, both proper and common.

AA *The Portions of the* Chorion *diſſected and removed from the proper place*

B *A Portion of the* Amnios.

CC *The* Membrane *of the Womb diſſected.*

DD *The* Placenta *being a certain fleſhly ſubſtance indued with very many Veſſels, by which the Infant receives its Nouriſhment.*

E *Th Varication of th Veſſ ls which make u the Navel ſtring.*

FF *The Navel-ſtring i which the Umbilic Veſſels are carried fro the* Placenta *to t Navel.*

GG *The Infant as it lies perfect in the Wom near the time of Trave*

H *The inſertion of th Umbelicar Veſſels in the Navel of the Infan*

Culpepers Midvvife Enlarged.

Figure 17.6 Anon., "[Pregnant Anatomy]," engraving, 32 × 25 cm [page]. In Nicholas Culpeper, *A Directory for Midwives* (London: John Streater, 1671). Wellcome Collection.

anatomical image used perspective, tone, and detail to make an argument for recording what was actually seen in anatomical dissection.[18] Indeed, these images developed alongside the increased practice of dissection in European universities in the sixteenth century, and a shift in which dissectors began to privilege their own discoveries over the established wisdom of ancient authors.[19] Spieghel's pregnant anatomy (Figure 17.5) is part of this visual and intellectual movement but, like all anatomical images in this period, it was not actually drawn from a single dissection, and it was not meant to look like it either. Such images are anatomical knowledge interpreted: they were intended to present an ideal view of anatomy, both because it was felt to be more helpful knowledge for students, and because it demonstrated the author's and artist's skills in synthesizing the knowledge they gained in the dissection room.

Looking for how and why medical images in this period idealize the body is crucial – it indicates not only what the image would have told contemporary viewers but also the broader epistemic values of the period. In both the Spieghel image (Figure 17.5) and the Sharp copies (Figures 17.1 and 17.4), the figure is alive, seemingly facilitating the exposure of her interior. This visual trope was common in the period and served many purposes. For instance, it made the image more visually appealing and aligned anatomical imagery with more high-status forms of art, from classical sculpture to contemporary history painting.[20] It also worked against the troubling associations of anatomical knowledge with death, criminality, dirtiness, and manual labor.[21] These figures are opened but not dead, they do not seep or bleed or rot, and the knowledge of anatomy comes to the viewer without the tough and messy work of dissection.

In Sharp's image, the anatomy is very similar to the original, and the figure's pose is simplified but still alert and self-displaying. Anatomical knowledge is, however, not the only kind displayed. By looking at other elements of the image, we can gain new perspectives on the ways it made meaning. One big change between the original and Sharp's copy is the hairstyle. In both images, the hair works to idealize, but in different times and contexts, it idealizes differently. In the Spieghel original (Figure 17.5), the hairstyle looks rather classical. In Sharp's copy, the hairstyle is one fashionable in England in the 1660s (Figure 17.1).[22] While Spieghel's original links the anatomical image to contemporary fine art styles, Sharp's image links to its viewers, including practicing midwives and lay women. For them, the fact that the woman looks like someone they might know was important, because the image was describing a physical state that they themselves would likely experience, but which they could not see. The image layers the hidden anatomical knowledge of pregnancy with the outward, social aspect of the seventeenth-century body. In the woodcut copy made for the 1720s editions (Figure 17.4), the figure is simplified again and the hair is less obviously styled. Perhaps Marshall, the editor, was less keen to make direct social connections with contemporary women readers, opting for a more abstract anatomical body than a specific social body. Or perhaps the decision was financial and the woodcut was created so it could continue to be used as fashions changed.

Another non-anatomical element worth paying attention to is the use of landscape and plants in the images. The verdant landscape in Spieghel's original, reduced in the copies to the flower that covers the figure's genitals, expresses the widespread theory of the microcosmic body.[23] This theory proposed that the human body worked as a kind of miniature universe, so knowledge of the way things worked in the world was reflected in the body. Pregnancy was often understood as a microcosmic version of the growing of plants, crops, and fruits in the world, indeed the fetus was often referred to as "the fruit."[24] In the original engraving from Spieghel's book (Figure 17.5), the woman holds a fruit in one hand and gestures didactically with the other, indicating the way the fruitful landscape mirrors her fruitful body. This period was one in which modes of knowing and treating the body were layered and pluralistic, where even seemingly contradictory theories could coexist.[25] As Lorraine Daston and Peter Galison put it, "Epistemic virtues do not replace one another like a succession of kings. Rather, they accumulate into a repertoire of possible forms of knowing."[26] Indeed, even the observationally styled anatomy is inflected by microcosmic analogy: the way the membranes and uterus have been cut and fanned out, the way the fetus seems to sit atop the uterus, rather than being nestled within it, draws a visual association between fetus and fruit, gestating body and verdant tree. While the allusion is less strong in the Sharp copies, the floral opening of the body and the flower covering the genitals would have been more than enough to remind early modern viewers of the microcosmic body, primed as they were to think in these terms as much as in mechanical anatomical ones.

Birth Figures

The other set of images produced in every edition of Sharp's book are birth figures – images of the fetus in the uterus that describe the different positions in which a fetus can present for birth (Figures 17.2 and 17.7).[27] These images need to be looked at in a different way. They are not primarily anatomical, like the images discussed above, rather they are "practitional" – images that primarily describe the body as experienced in medical practice, rather than in anatomical dissection.[28] Historians of medicine have, in times past, tended to be rather scathing about these images, pointing out how much space they leave in the uterus, how the fetuses seem to tumble about, and how they often look more like children or even miniature adults than fetuses.[29] However, birth figures were extremely popular and widely produced in the seventeenth century. Sharp's were one of many sets based on the images originally made by Jos Murer for Jakob Rüff (Figure 17.8).[30] So we need to ask: if they were so inaccurate compared to other anatomical images, why were they so widely reproduced? We can assume that images that were produced widely were felt to have some value, or why do it?

I argue that these images are not intended to show how the fetus is curled up tight in the uterus by the end of pregnancy (something that is shown in the anatomical image discussed above). Rather, they are meant to help midwives to understand the different positions of the fetus and how they might correct malpresentations (those not presenting headfirst) by turning the fetus. By looking at the context of medical practice, and particularly the points of change and debate, we can often

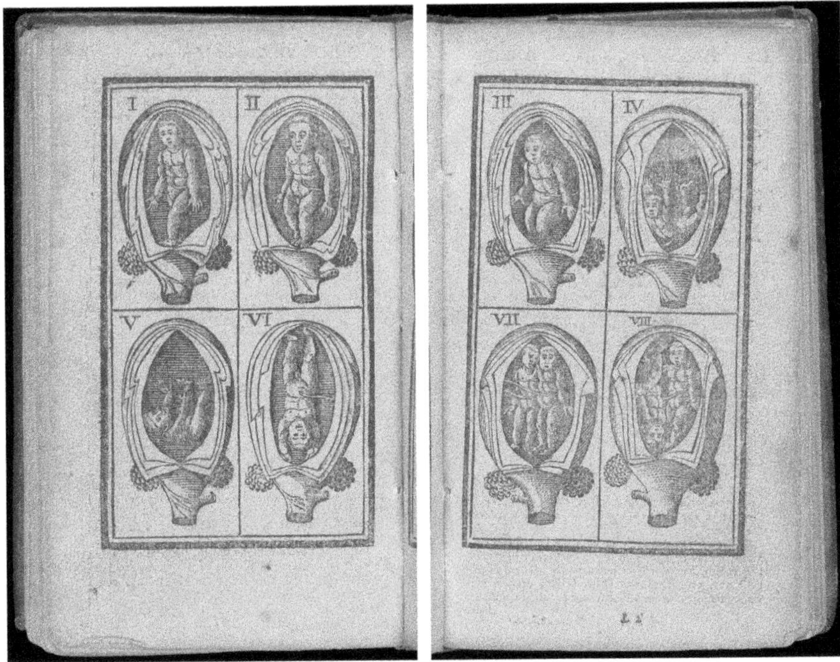

Figure 17.7 Anon. "[Birth Figures]," woodcut, 9 × 15.5 cm [page]. In Jane Sharp, *The Compleat Midwife's Companion* (London: J. Marshall, 1724). Wellcome Collection.

gain a new understanding of the agency of an image. In seventeenth-century midwifery, for example, a new technique called "podalic version" – which involved inserting a hand into the uterus, finding the feet of a malpresenting fetus, and then turning and delivering them by exerting traction on the feet – began to spread in practice and in texts.[31] Birth figures certainly predate this innovation (they are present in many medieval gynecological manuscripts), but they seem to have exploded in number along with the rise of this new intervention, and the vernacular midwifery manuals that described it.[32] An image that was more diagrammatic and less observationally accurate, that privileged being clear about the position of the fetus and their limbs, was likely of great use to midwives trying to learn and use podalic version. By thinking about contemporary changes in medical practices, we can gain an insight into how images at the time were read and used. Conversely, the images give us insights into practice: that they were so widespread suggests that podalic version was an important shift, but also possibly a tricky one for people to get their heads around.

But images can always be read in different ways, by different people, with different preoccupations and needs. If these birth figures were "practitional" images for midwives, for some pregnant women, they were images that had the power to shape and protect their unborn children. Look closely at the fetuses in Sharp's images, and those made for Rüff (Figures 17.2, 17.7 and 17.8). They are not scrawny

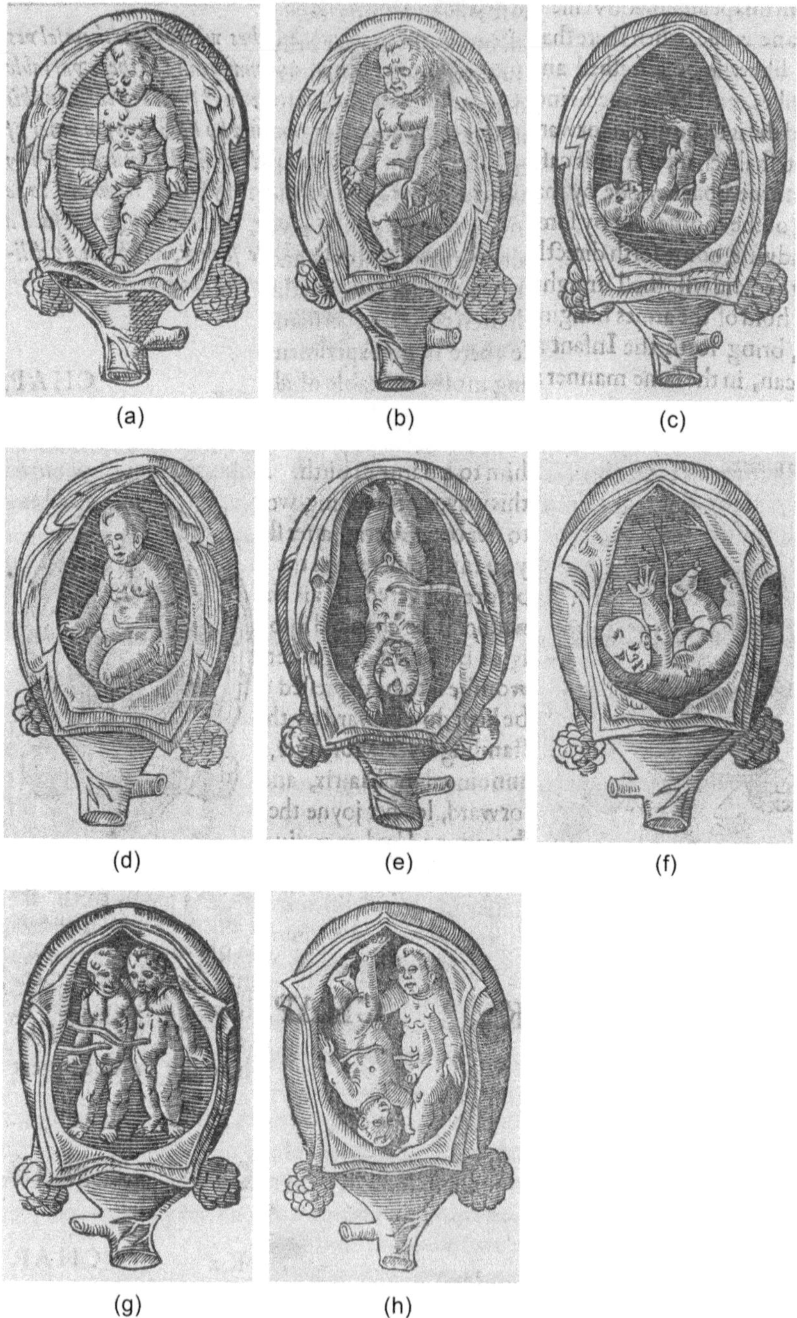

Figure 17.8 Jos Murer, "[Birth Figures]," woodcut, 4.5 × 7 cm [figures]. In Jakob Rüff, *The Expert Midwife* (London: E.G., 1637). Copyright of the University of Manchester.

and vulnerable neonates, but chubby, active toddlers. They are also largely identifiably male and look very similar to the cherubs or *putti* that decorated paintings, furniture, and prints in many genres.[33] Indeed, this is no accident: adopting the visual language of *putti*, birth figures present a positive outlook on what could be a time of danger, sickness, and death for both the pregnant woman and fetus.[34]

In many aspects of our lives today, including in medicine, images shape our perceptions of our bodies. We often imagine our interiors using the forms of medical and anatomical imagery we access in school or on the internet. In the early modern period, images did this and more: they had the power not only to shape perceptions of the body but also to shape the body itself. Maternal imagination was a well-known phenomenon in this period, through which pregnant women imprinted or shaped their unborn children after seeing or experiencing things that caused strong emotional reactions. Most recorded cases were of negative outcomes – women startled by hares who gave birth to babies with "hare lips," or who craved a particular food and gave birth to babies with birthmarks shaped like that food.[35] But some art historians have argued that maternal imagination could also be used positively, indeed that pretty much any image of a beautiful infant – from a cherub or putto to the Christ child – could be meditated upon by pregnant women in order to ensure their own child would be healthy, beautiful, and safe.[36] Birth figures are no exception. While for some the variety of positions spoke of danger in labor, for others they might have been read as the playful acrobatics of energetic children, reflecting both the sensations women felt as their fetuses kicked inside and their desires that their children survive long enough to learn to run and tumble on the outside.

Remember, when you are looking at illustrations in medical books, to keep an open mind about the visual associations they are making, and the uses to which they might have been put. Medicine and medical knowledge did not exist in a bubble, and images printed under the cover of a medical book were not always used in ways that the author would have sanctioned.[37] Medicine in the period incorporated many different practices, only some of which would be recognizably "medical" to us today. But that does not mean they were not important, serious, or powerful to early modern viewers.

Childbirth Scenes

The history of medicine is not just about medical knowledge. It also covers the social and cultural manifestations of medicine. Midwifery, for instance, involved bringing new life into the world and was important for maintaining family structures, inheritance, and lineage. In this period, midwives were expected not only to safely deliver infants but also to ensure that they were not switched or swapped; that no magic was done over them or using the umbilical cord, placenta, or amniotic sac; and that women pregnant out of wedlock disclosed the name of the father.[38] Within their communities, they were women of authority who not only kept laboring women and infants healthy and safe but also ensured legitimacy, upheld the practices of the Church, and, where possible, ensured that the infants were supported by their fathers rather than the parish. Historically, midwives had even been authorized to baptize infants when they seemed likely to die before a priest could be called. While this practice was discouraged and eventually forbidden by the Church of England in the seventeenth century, it probably continued as an illicit emergency practice in England, and as a legitimate one in other parts of Europe.[39] Midwives were also called on to testify in court cases that involved issues of sex and reproduction. Midwives were, therefore, respected members of their community, invested with jobs of great importance, and, within specific settings, holding authority over their social superiors.

This social aspect of the midwife's role is expressed in the three woodcut scenes reproduced in the 1720s editions of Sharp's book (Figure 17.3). The three woodblocks were combined and printed as a frontispiece illustration and used individually as headpieces (illustrations printed in the blank space above a new chapter). The first shows the social space of the lying-in chamber after the birth, with the gossips gathered around the infant in their cradle, the mother tucked up in bed, and the midwife offering her some caudle. The second shows a procession of well-dressed men and women off to church for the infant's baptism. At the front, walks the midwife holding the infant. The third shows a celebratory feast at the home of the parents, probably held after the baptism, though social gathering and sharing food was also a more general part of the mother's lying-in month.[40] In this image we see the clergyman in the center, with his black robes and white preaching bands, and the midwife on the right. In each image, the midwife can be identified as the older, slightly beaky woman wearing a sober headdress and gown. She embodies the convention, oft repeated in midwifery guides, that midwives should be women of middle years, of excellent social standing, and with lots of experience of childbirth, sober, clean, and religious.[41]

No image, however, should be treated as simple documentary evidence of the past. They are always interpretations of and comments on the cultures that made them. In this case, the image is, I argue, both idealizing and nostalgic. It certainly depicts social rituals that did occur, but they did not always look like this. For instance, only reasonably wealthy people would have been able to conduct ceremonies on this scale, with smart clothing, dedicated domestic spaces, and all the necessary furnishings for childbirth, from bed, linens, and cradle to food, drink, and tableware.[42] Poorer people adapted these expectations to their means, borrowing from neighbors, using shared spaces, and gathering what food, drink, fuel, and linens they could afford.[43] For those not in the Anglican church, ceremonies were shaped differently.[44] And, indeed, not all midwives were the picture of respectability and sobriety shown here, in fact differing greatly in age, status, and wealth, and not always on such good terms with the families they attended.[45] And, perhaps most significantly for this image and its cultural context, by the 1720s, surgeons and man-midwives were beginning to attend some women in their labors, particularly if they were difficult. Moreover, discourse around their suitability and credentials for attending laboring women was gaining traction both within and beyond medical communities.[46] That this figure of the "man-midwife" is *not* present in these images is significant.

As well as presenting an ideally affluent, respectable, conforming view of English social childbirth rituals, these little scenes also present a nostalgic view of social practices that were already changing and fragmenting. Baptism, particularly, was often pushed back by the early eighteenth century so the parents could attend, following the mother's month of recovery or "lying-in."[47] And, by this time, it was less common for the midwife to hold such a prominent role.[48] The rather traditionalist view presented in this illustration might have been intended specifically to appeal to viewers uneasy with the recent changes in childbirth rituals.

The images were also nostalgic in their very presence in the midwifery manual. Many of the earliest printed midwifery manuals produced such scenes, most commonly of the lying-in chamber. These images depicted the female space of the lying-in chamber, focusing on the nursing care and community that was part of the recovery process for women after childbirth. In a woodcut from the first edition of Jakob Rüff's manual (Figure 17.9), published in Latin in 1554, we see all the familiar elements: a roaring fire, gossips socializing, the new mother receiving caudle, the infant being washed and swaddled. Such early texts were produced by men who had no access to these spaces, so visual revelations of the spaces of childbirth were arguably just as intriguing as visual revelations of the body's hidden interior. But by the early eighteenth century, these social scenes had largely been excised from new midwifery manuals. Authors, both male and female, were more likely to have experience of the space and wanted to frame their practice in more exclusively medical terms.

So, what are these three woodcut scenes doing in the 1720s editions of Sharp's manual? They do not appear in the 1671 edition, so they are an innovation of the publisher John Marshall. And, judging by the fashions, they look to have been made around the time of publication. I think they indicate a definite shift in audience: Sharp's first edition was scholarly, aimed at educating midwives in the newest medical knowledge and midwifery techniques. By the 1720s, Sharp was certainly dead, and her reissued book was old-fashioned. Midwifery manuals had become more technical, more focused on the processes of birth, and took an approach that was less humoral or holistic, and more completely mechanistic. Indeed, as Elaine Hobby has shown, some of the most out-of-date sections of Sharp's text were removed in the later editions, though it still would have seemed more traditional compared to the cutting-edge new texts by authors such as Hendrik van Deventer.[49]

While the new "man-midwives," and those women midwives who sought a more "professionalized" status through medical training, were turning to new kinds of midwifery books, many more midwives and their clients preferred the older and more accessible books, their mixture of social, medical, and surgical content, their humoral and pluralistic outlook.[50] If Sharp's original book was aimed at the higher status and more ambitious midwife, the 1720s editions had become "popular" in a new way, distinctly different to the newest cutting-edge medical texts in content, in price, and in their illustrations. Well into the nineteenth century, traditional practices in midwifery, midwifery books that had their origins in the first vernacular works of the seventeenth century, and illustrations from that same period, remained popular outside of elite, educated, and urban circles.

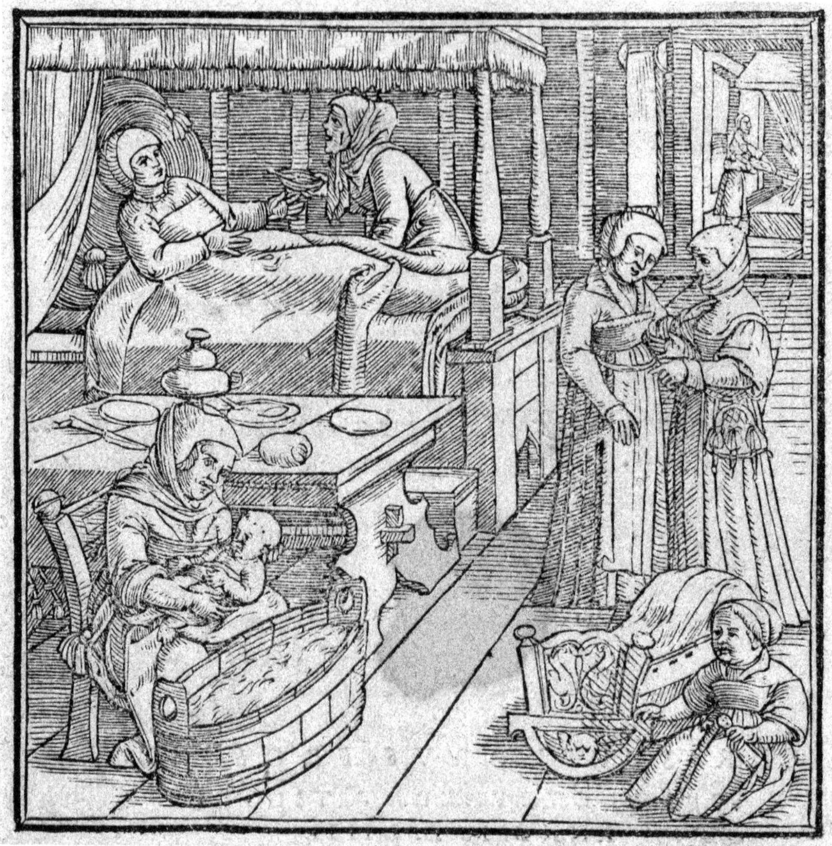

Figure 17.9 Anon., "[Lying-in scene]," woodcut, 10 × 9.9 cm [block]. In Jakob Rüff, *De Conceptu et generatione hominis* (Zurich: Christophorus Froschhoverus, 1554). Wellcome Collection.

The reissued copies of Sharp's manual, with their new childbirth scenes, consciously played to readers who wanted the old systems, the old forms of knowing the body, and the old social rituals. Particularly, I think, the images were meant to appeal to midwives who rejected the newly masculine and medical perspectives on their profession. The three scenes seem carefully chosen to highlight the importance of the traditional midwife. The first scene, showing the lying-in chamber, is conventional for such books. The second less so, but it highlights one of the aspects of the midwife's job – carrying the child to their baptism and handing them to the priest – which had traditionally been central but was increasingly eroded by the diversification of denominations and religious practices, and the increased involvement of the parents in baptism. In the final scene, again we see a picture appealing to a midwife – not only has she attended a family wealthy enough to hold a baptismal feast but she is also treated with deference and respect. It is she and the clergyman whom the other guests face and listen to. It was in the eighteenth century that the social status of the midwife began to be eroded, both by the rise of the "man-midwife" and as the gentry class withdrew socially from their less exulted neighbors, including their local midwives.[51]

Contemporary viewers would have read nuances in how nostalgic such scenes were that we simply cannot see today. But by digging into the history of this kind of image and looking at past and contemporary cultures of books and of midwifery, we can see that this image worked in response both to an existing visual corpus and new changes in the culture of midwifery.

Conclusion

This chapter has shown just a few ways in which medical book illustrations can be analyzed to understand different parts of medical culture. By following the footnotes in this chapter, readers will find more examples of how early modern images created meaning and knowledge and more approaches for studying them. Studying book illustrations can enrich research and lead to new discoveries and conclusions. Indeed, if you are going to work with medical books, you need to look at the images if you want to fully address the sources. And, because relatively few scholars have done this, there is a lot to discover! Images are always rich, complex representations, never simple documentary evidence of what things were like in the past. Treat them with caution, ask how they represent and why, who they were for, what cultural contexts they were working within, and how they might have looked *different* to various kinds of viewers. Doing so will allow you to write thoughtful, rigorous, and original visual histories of medicine.

Sources

Below are some digital resources which include medical book illustrations. They are great for finding material, surveying lots of material, and accessing material that is far away. But there are downsides: digital archives do not give a sense of the materiality of the object; not all digitized editions include the illustrations; and illustrations differ between copies as well as editions. It is always wise to consult physical copies where possible, as you never know what unique placement, printing, or annotation you might discover!

Wellcome Collection: https://wellcomecollection.org/collections

Historical Anatomies on the Web: https://www.nlm.nih.gov/exhibition/historicalanatomies/home.html

Science Museum Collections: https://collection.sciencemuseumgroup.org.uk/

National Library of Medicine: https://www.ncbi.nlm.nih.gov/nlmcatalog/

Early English Books Online (paid resource, most universities will have subscriptions, check your library catalog)

Eighteenth Century Collections Online (paid resource, most universities will have subscriptions, check your library catalog)

Internet Archive: https://archive.org/

Hathi Trust Digital Library: https://www.hathitrust.org/

Google Books: https://books.google.com/

Notes

1 Susan Dackerman, ed., *Prints and the Pursuit of Knowledge in Early Modern Europe* (New Haven, CT: Yale University Press, 2011); Antony Griffiths and Robert A. Gerard, *The Print in Stuart Britain, 1603–1689* (London: British Museum Press, 1998); Michael Hunter, ed., *Printed Images in Early Modern Britain: Essays in Interpretation* (Farnham: Ashgate, 2010); Suzanne Karr Schmidt, *Altered and Adorned: Using Renaissance Prints in Daily Life* (New Haven, CT: Yale University Press, 2011); Sachiko Kusukawa, *Picturing the Book of Nature: Image, Text, and Argument in Sixteenth-Century Human Anatomy and Medical Botany* (Chicago, IL: University of Chicago Press, 2012).

2 Lorraine Daston, "Epistemic Images," in *Vision and Its Instruments: Art, Science and Technology in Early Modern Europe*, ed. Alina Payne (University Park: Pennsylvania State University Press, 2015), 13–35; James Elkins, "Art History and Images That Are Not Art," *The Art Bulletin* 77, no. 4 (1995): 553–71; Alexander Marr, "Knowing Images," *Renaissance Quarterly*, no. 69 (2016): 1000–13.

3 Horst Bredekamp, Vera Dünkel, and Birgit Schneider, eds., *The Technical Image: A History of Styles in Scientific Imagery* (Chicago, IL: University of Chicago Press, 2015); Dackerman, *Prints and the Pursuit of Knowledge*; Lorraine Daston and Peter Galison, *Objectivity* (New York: Zone Books, 2010); Matthew C. Hunter, *Wicked Intelligence: Visual Art and the Science of Experiment in Restoration London* (Chicago, IL: University of Chicago Press, 2013); Kusukawa, *Picturing the Book of Nature*; Wolfgang Lefèvre, Jürgen Renn, and Urs Schoepflin, eds., *The Power of Images in Early Modern Science* (Basel: Birkhäuser, 2003); Brian W. Ogilvie, *The Science of Describing: Natural History in Renaissance Europe* (Chicago, IL: University of Chicago Press, 2006).

4 See Elaine Hobby, "Note on the Text," in *The Midwives Book: Or the Whole Art of Midwifry Disocvered*, ed. Elaine Hobby (Oxford: Oxford University Press, 1999), xxxviii–xxxiv.

5 Lori Anne Ferrell, "Page Techne: Interpreting Diagrams in Early Modern English 'How-To' Books," in *Printed Images in Early Modern Britain: Essays in Interpretation*, ed. Michael Hunter (Farnham: Ashgate, 2010), 113–26; Mary E. Fissell, "Readers, Texts, and Contexts: Vernacular Medical Works in Early Modern England," in *The Popularization of Medicine, 1650–1850*, ed. Roy Porter (London & New York: Routledge, 1992), 72–98; Melissa Lo, "The Picture Multiple: Figuring, Thinking, and Knowing in Descartes's Essais (1637)," *Journal of the History of Ideas* 78, no. 3 (2017): 369–99; Renée Raphael, "Teaching through Diagrams: Galileo's Dialogo and Discorsi and His Pisan Readers," in *Observing the World Through Images: Diagrams and Figures in the Early-Modern Arts and Sciences*, ed. Isla Fay and Nicholas Jardine (Leiden: Brill, 2014), 201–30.

6 Monica Green, *Making Women's Medicine Masculine: The Rise of Male Authority in Pre-Modern Gynaecology* (Oxford: Oxford University Press, 2008).

7 Mary E. Fissell, *Vernacular Bodies: The Politics of Reproduction in Early Modern England* (Oxford: Oxford University Press, 2004); Adrian Wilson, *The Making of Man-Midwifery: Childbirth in England 1660–1770* (London: UCL Press, 1995).

8 Jennifer Wynne Hellwarth, "'I Wyl Wright of Women Prevy Sekenes:' Imagining Female Literacy and Textual Communities in Medieval and Early Modern Midwifery Manuals," *Critical Survey* 14, no. 1 (2002): 44–63; Jennifer Richards, "Reading and Hearing *The Womans Booke* in Early Modern England," *Bulletin of the History of Medicine* 89 (2015): 434–62.

9 Fissell, *Vernacular Bodies*, 51–52; Elaine Hobby, "Introduction," in *The Midwives Book: Or the Whole Art of Midwifry Discovered*, ed. Elaine Hobby (Oxford: Oxford University Press, 1999), xi–xxxi.

10 Caroline Bicks, "Stones Like Women's Paps: Revising Gender in Jane Sharp's Midwives Book," *Journal for Early Modern Cultural Studies* 7, no. 2 (2007): 1–27; Elaine Hobby, "'Secrets of the Female Sex:' Jane Sharp, the Reproductive Female Body, and Early

Modern Midwifery Manuals," *Women's Writing* 8, no. 2 (2001): 201–12; Eve Keller, "Mrs Jane Sharp: Midwifery and the Critique of Medical Knowledge in Seventeenth-Century England," *Women's Writing* 2, no. 2 (1995): 101–11.

11 Katharine Phelps Walsh, "Marketing Midwives in Seventeenth-Century London: A Re-Examination of Jane Sharp's *The Midwives Book*," *Gender & History* 26, no. 2 (2014): 223–41.

12 Nick Hopwood, *Haeckel's Embryos: Images, Evolution and Fraud* (Chicago, IL: University of Chicago Press, 2015), 2–4; Fabian Krämer, "The Persistent Image of an Unusual Centaur: A Biography of Aldrovandi's Two-Legged Centaur Woodcut," *Nuncius* 2 (2009): 313–40; Kusukawa, *Picturing the Book of Nature*, 64–69; Melissa Lo, "Cut, Copy, and English Anatomy: Thomas Geminus and the Reordering of Vesalius's Canonical Body," in *Andreas Vesalius and the Fabrica in the Age of Printing: Art, Anatomy, and Printing in the Italian Renaissance*, ed. Rinaldo Fernando Canalis and Massimo Ciavolella (Turnhout: Brepols, 2018), 225–56; Kärin Nickelsen, *Draughtsmen, Botanists and Nature: The Construction of Eighteenth-Century Botanical Illustrations* (Dordrecht: Springer, 2006), 185–228.

13 Roger Gaskell, "Printing House and Engraving Shop: A Mysterious Collaboration," *The Book Collector* 53 (2004): 213–51.

14 See Bamber Gascoigne, *How to Identify Prints: A Complete Guide to Manual and Mechanical Processes from Woodcut to Inkjet* (London: Thames and Hudson, 2004).

15 Rebecca Whiteley, *Birth Figures: Early Modern Prints and the Pregnant Body* (Chicago, IL: University of Chicago Press, 2023), 87-136.

16 See also Nicholas Culpeper, *A Directory for Midwives: Or, a Guide for Women, in Their Conception, Bearing and Suckling Their Children* (London: Peter Cole, 1651), 40.

17 Kusukawa, *Picturing the Book of Nature*, 178–248; Gianna Pomata, "Observation Rising: Birth of an Epistemic Genre, 1500–1650," in *Histories of Scientific Observation*, ed. Lorraine Daston and Elizabeth Lunbeck (Chicago, IL: University of Chicago Press, 2011), 45–80; Jonathan Sawday, *The Body Emblazoned: Dissection and the Human Body in Renaissance Culture* (London: Routledge, 1995), 105.

18 Martin Kemp, "Taking It on Trust: Form and Meaning in Naturalistic Representation," *Archives of Natural History* 17, no. 2 (1990): 127–88; Martin Kemp, "Style and Non-Style in Anatomical Illustration: From Renaissance Humanism to Henry Gray," *Journal of Anatomy* 216 (2010): 192–208; See also Mechthild Fend, "Drawing the Cadaver 'Ad Vivum:' Gérard de Lairesse's Illustrations for Govard Bidloo's Anatomia Humani Corporis," in *Ad Vivum? Visual Materials and the Vocabulary of Life-Likeness in Europe before 1800*, ed. Thomas Balfe, Joanna Woodall, and Claus Zittel (Leiden: Brill, 2019), 294–327.

19 Andrew Cunningham, *The Anatomist Anatomis'd: An Experimental Discipline in Enlightenment* (Farnham: Ashgate, 2010); Sawday, *The Body Emblazoned*, 64–65.

20 Elizabeth Hallam, *Anatomy Museum: Death and the Body Displayed* (London: Reaktion Books, 2016), 97–123; Lyle Massey, "Against the 'Statue Anatomized:' The 'Art' of Eighteenth-Century Anatomy on Trial," *Art History* 40, no. 1 (2017): 68–103; Sawday, *The Body Emblazoned*, 101–02.

21 Cynthia Klestinec, "Renaissance Surgeons: Anatomy, Manual Skill and the Visual Arts," in *Early Modern Medicine and Natural Philosophy*, ed. Peter Distelzweig, Benjamin Goldberg, and Evan R. Ragland (Dordrecht: Springer, 2016), 43–58; Sawday, *The Body Emblazoned*, 54–84.

22 Fashion History Timeline, 1660–1670. https://fashionhistory.fitnyc.edu/1660-1669/ [accessed April 11, 2021].

23 Michel Foucault, *The Order of Things: An Archaeology of the Human Sciences* (London: Routledge, 2005), 19–50.

24 David Cressy, *Birth, Marriage and Death: Ritual, Religion and the Life-Cycle in Tudor and Stuart England* (Oxford: Oxford University Press, 1997), 18; Kathleen

Crowther-Heyck, "'Be Fruitful and Multiply:' Genesis and Generation in Reformation Germany," *Renaissance Quarterly* 55, no. 3 (2002): 908; See also Jane Sharp, *The Midwives Book: Or the Whole Art of Midwifry Discovered* (London: Simon Miller, 1671), 119.

25 Katherine Eggert, *Disknowledge: Literature, Alchemy and the End of Humanism in Renaissance England* (Philadelphia: University of Pennsylvania Press, 2015).

26 Daston and Galison, *Objectivity*, 113.

27 Whiteley, *Birth Figures*.

28 Rebecca Whiteley, "Figuring Pictures and Picturing Figures: Images of the Pregnant Body and the Unborn Child in England, 1540–c.1680," *Social History of Medicine* 32, no. 2 (2019): 241–66.

29 Lawrence D. Longo and Lawrence P. Reynolds, *Wombs with a View: Illustrations of the Gravid Uterus from the Renaissance through the Nineteenth Century* (Cham: Springer, 2016), 2; K. B. Roberts and J. D. W. Tomlinson, *The Fabric of the Body: European Traditions of Anatomical Illustration* (Oxford: Clarendon Press, 1992), 15.

30 Jennifer Spinks, "Jakob Rueff's 1554 Trostbüchle: A Zurich Physician Explains and Interprets Monstrous Births," *Intellectual History Review* 18, no. 1 (2008): 41–59.

31 The technique was first published by Ambroise Paré, see Janet Doe, *A Bibliography, 1545–1940, of the Works of Ambroise Paré, 1510–1590: Premier Chirurgien & Conseiller Du Roi* (Amsterdam: Gérard Th. van Heusden, 1976), xiii–xiv; it was first published in English by Paré's pupil Guillemeau, and was slowly disseminated in other texts throughout the century: Jacques Guillemeau, *Child-Birth, or the Happy Deliverie of Women* (London: Printed by A. Hatfield, 1612), 127, 136, 154, 162–63; see also Sharp, *The Midwives Book*, 201–05.

32 Green, *Making Women's Medicine Masculine*, 118–62; Whiteley, "Figuring Pictures and Picturing Figures," 250–53.

33 Charles Dempsey, *Inventing the Renaissance Putto* (Chapel Hill: The University of North Carolina Press, 2001); John Heilbron, "Domesticating Science in the Eighteenth Century," in *Science and the Visual Image in the Enlightenment*, ed. W.R. Shea (Canton, MA: Science History Publications, 2000), 1–24.

34 Lianne McTavish, *Childbirth and the Display of Authority in Early Modern France* (Aldershot: Ashgate, 2005), 192.

35 Paul-Gabriel Boucé, "Imagination, Pregnant Women, and Monsters in Eighteenth-Century England and France," in *Sexual Underworlds of the Enlightenment*, ed. G.S. Rousseau and Roy Porter (Manchester: Manchester University Press, 1987), 86–100; Lorraine Daston and Katharine Park, *Wonders and the Order of Nature: 1150–1750* (New York: Zone Books, 1998), 173–214; Katharine Park, "Impressed Images: Reproducing Wonders," in *Picturing Science, Producing Art*, ed. Caroline A. Jones and Peter Galison (New York: Routledge, 1998), 254–71; See also Sharp, *The Midwives Book*, 116–19.

36 Frances Gage, *Painting as Medicine in Early Modern Rome: Giulio Mancini and the Efficacy of Art* (University Park: Pennsylvania State University Press, 2016), 115; Morten Steen Hansen, "The Infant Christ with the 'Arma' Christi: François Duquesnoy and the Typology of the Putto," *Zeitschrift Für Kunstgeschichte* 71, no. 1 (2008): 133; Jacqueline Marie Musacchio, *The Art and Ritual of Childbirth in Renaissance Italy* (New Haven, CT: Yale University Press, 1999), 125–30.

37 See Roger Chartier, "Texts, Printing, Readings," in *The New Cultural History: Essays*, ed. Lynn Hunt (Berkeley: University of California Press, 1989), 154–75; William H. Sherman, *Used Books: Marking Readings in Renaissance England* (Philadelphia: University of Pennsylvania Press, 2008).

38 Cressy, *Birth, Marriage and Death*, 60–62; Jean Donnison, *Midwives and Medical Men: A History of Inter-Professional Rivalries and Women's Rights* (London: Heinemann, 1977), 1–20; Laura Gowing, *Common Bodies: Women, Touch and Power in Seventeenth-Century England* (New Haven, CT: Yale University Press, 2003), 149–76; David Harley, "Provincial Midwives in England: Lancashire and Cheshire, 1660–1760," in *The*

Art of Midwifery: Early Modern Midwives in Europe, ed. Hilary Marland (London: Routledge, 1993), 27–48; Adrian Wilson, *Ritual and Conflict: The Social Relations of Childbirth in Early Modern England* (Farnham: Ashgate, 2013), 153–210.

39 Cressy, *Birth, Marriage and Death*, 118–23.

40 Cressy, 480–81; Sarah Fox, *Giving Birth in Eighteenth-Century England* (London: University of London Press, 2022), 110–15; Wilson, *Ritual and Conflict*, 153–58.

41 See, for example, Thomas Dawkes, *The Midwife Rightly Instructed: Or, the Way, Which All Women Desirous to Learn, Should Take, To Acquire the True Knowledge and Be Successful in the Practice of, the Art of Midwifery* (London: Printed for J. Oswald, 1736), ix–xii; Guillemeau, *Child-Birth*, 84–85.

42 Cressy, *Birth, Marriage and Death*, 50–54; Fox, *Giving Birth in Eighteenth-Century England*, 51–77.

43 Fox, *Giving Birth in Eighteenth-Century England*, 51–77; Wilson, *Ritual and Conflict*, 179.

44 Emily Vine, "Birth, Death, and Domestic Religion in London c.1600–1800" (Queen Mary University of London, PhD Diss., 2019), chap. 2.

45 Sarah Fox, "'Contrary to Her Profession as a Midwife:' Skill, Scandal, and the Licensing of Early Modern Midwives," Seminar Paper, *IHR Women's History Seminar Series*, London, Nov. 13, 2021; Karen O'Brien, "Sexual Impropriety, Petitioning and the Dynamics of Ill Will in Daily Urban Life," *Urban History* 43, no. 2 (2016): 177–99; Wilson, *Ritual and Conflict*, 167.

46 Mary E. Fissell, "Man-Midwifery Revisited," in *Reproduction: Antiquity to the Present Day*, ed. Nick Hopwood, Rebecca Flemming, and Lauren Kassell (Cambridge: Cambridge University Press, 2018), 319–32; Wilson, *The Making of Man-Midwifery*.

47 Will Coster, *Baptism and Spiritual Kinship in Early Modern England* (Oxford: Routledge, 2016), 73; Cressy, *Birth, Marriage and Death*, 480–81; Wilson, *Ritual and Conflict*, 190.

48 Coster, *Baptism and Spiritual Kinship in Early Modern England*, 65–68; Cressy, *Birth, Marriage and Death*, 188–94.

49 Hobby, "Note on the Text." Hendrik van Deventer, *The Art of Midwifery Improv'd: Fully and Plainly Laying Down Whatever Instructions Are Requisite to Make a Compleat Midwife and the Many Errors in All the Books Hitherto Written Upon This Subject Clearly Refuted* (London: E. Curll, J. Pemberton and W. Taylor, 1716).

50 See Whiteley, *Birth Figures*, 87-136.

51 Cressy, *Birth, Marriage and Death*, 61; Harley, "Provincial Midwives in England: Lancashire and Cheshire, 1660–1760," 42–43.

Bibliography

Bicks, Caroline. "Stones Like Women's Paps: Revising Gender in Jane Sharp's Midwives Book." *Journal for Early Modern Cultural Studies* 7, no. 2 (2007): 1–27.

Boucé, Paul-Gabriel. "Imagination, Pregnant Women, and Monsters in Eighteenth-Century England and France." In *Sexual Underworlds of the Enlightenment*, edited by G.S. Rousseau and Roy Porter, 86–100. Manchester: Manchester University Press, 1987.

Bredekamp, Horst, Vera Dünkel, and Birgit Schneider, eds. *The Technical Image: A History of Styles in Scientific Imagery*. Chicago, IL: University of Chicago Press, 2015.

Chartier, Roger. "Texts, Printing, Readings." In *The New Cultural History: Essays*, edited by Lynn Hunt, 154–75. Berkeley: University of California Press, 1989.

Coster, Will. *Baptism and Spiritual Kinship in Early Modern England*. Oxford: Routledge, 2016.

Cressy, David. *Birth, Marriage, and Death: Ritual, Religion and the Life-Cycle in Tudor and Stuart England*. Oxford: Oxford University Press, 1997.

Crowther-Heyck, Kathleen. "'Be Fruitful and Multiply:' Genesis and Generation in Reformation Germany." *Renaissance Quarterly* 55, no. 3 (2002): 904–35.
Culpeper, Nicholas. *A Directory for Midwives: Or, a Guide for Women, in Their Conception, Bearing and Suckling Their Children*. London: Peter Cole, 1651.
Cunningham, Andrew. *The Anatomist Anatomis'd: An Experimental Discipline in Enlightenment*. Farnham: Ashgate, 2010.
Dackerman, Susan, ed. *Prints and the Pursuit of Knowledge in Early Modern Europe*. New Haven, CT: Yale University Press, 2011.
Daston, Lorraine. "Epistemic Images." In *Vision and Its Instruments: Art, Science and Technology in Early Modern Europe*, edited by Alina Payne, 13–35. University Park: Pennsylvania State University Press, 2015.
Daston, Lorraine and Peter Galison. *Objectivity*. New York: Zone Books, 2010.
Daston, Lorraine and Katharine Park. *Wonders and the Order of Nature: 1150–1750*. New York: Zone Books, 1998.
Dawkes, Thomas. *The Midwife Rightly Instructed: Or, the Way, Which All Women Desirous to Learn, Should Take, To Acquire the True Knowledge and Be Successful in the Practice of, the Art of Midwifery*. London: Printed for J. Oswald, 1736.
Dempsey, Charles. *Inventing the Renaissance Putto*. Chapel Hill: The University of North Carolina Press, 2001.
Doe, Janet. *A Bibliography, 1545–1940, of the Works of Ambroise Paré, 1510–1590: Premier Chirurgien & Conseiller Du Roi*. Amsterdam: Gérard Th. van Heusden, 1976.
Donnison, Jean. *Midwives and Medical Men: A History of Inter-Professional Rivalries and Women's Rights*. London: Heinemann, 1977.
Eggert, Katherine. *Disknowledge: Literature, Alchemy and the End of Humanism in Renaissance England*. Philadelphia: University of Pennsylvania Press, 2015.
Elkins, James. "Art History and Images That Are Not Art." *The Art Bulletin* 77, no. 4 (1995): 553–71.
Fend, Mechthild. "Drawing the Cadaver 'Ad Vivum:' Gérard de Lairesse's Illustrations for Govard Bidloo's Anatomia Humani Corporis." In *Ad Vivum? Visual Materials and the Vocabulary of Life-Likeness in Europe before 1800*, edited by Thomas Balfe, Joanna Woodall, and Claus Zittel, 294–327. Leiden: Brill, 2019.
Ferrell, Lori Anne. "Page Techne: Interpreting Diagrams in Early Modern English 'How-To' Books." In *Printed Images in Early Modern Britain: Essays in Interpretation*, edited by Michael Hunter, 113–26. Farnham: Ashgate, 2010.
Fissell, Mary E. "Man-Midwifery Revisited." In *Reproduction: Antiquity to the Present Day*, edited by Nick Hopwood, Rebecca Flemming, and Lauren Kassell, 319–32. Cambridge: Cambridge University Press, 2018.
———. "Readers, Texts, and Contexts: Vernacular Medical Works in Early Modern England." In *The Popularization of Medicine, 1650–1850*, edited by Roy Porter, 72–98. London & New York: Routledge, 1992.
———. *Vernacular Bodies: The Politics of Reproduction in Early Modern England*. Oxford: Oxford University Press, 2004.
Foucault, Michel. *The Order of Things: An Archaeology of the Human Sciences*. London: Routledge, 2005.
Fox, Sarah. "'Contrary to Her Profession as a Midwife:' Skill, Scandal, and the Licensing of Early Modern Midwives," Paper presented at the *IHR Women's History Seminar Series*, London, Nov. 13, 2021.
———. *Giving Birth in Eighteenth-Century England*. London: University of London Press, 2022.

Gage, Frances. *Painting as Medicine in Early Modern Rome: Giulio Mancini and the Efficacy of Art*. University Park: Pennsylvania State University Press, 2016.

Gascoigne, Bamber. *How to Identify Prints: A Complete Guide to Manual and Mechanical Processes from Woodcut to Inkjet*. London: Thames and Hudson, 2004.

Gaskell, Roger. "Printing House and Engraving Shop: A Mysterious Collaboration." *The Book Collector* 53 (2004): 213–51.

Gowing, Laura. *Common Bodies: Women, Touch and Power in Seventeenth-Century England*. New Haven, CT: Yale University Press, 2003.

Green, Monica. *Making Women's Medicine Masculine: The Rise of Male Authority in Pre-Modern Gynaecology*. Oxford: Oxford University Press, 2008.

Griffiths, Antony and Robert A. Gerard. *The Print in Stuart Britain, 1603–1689*. London: British Museum Press, 1998.

Guillemeau, Jacques. *Child-Birth, or the Happy Deliverie of Women*. London: Printed by A. Hatfield, 1612.

Hallam, Elizabeth. *Anatomy Museum: Death and the Body Displayed*. London: Reaktion Books, 2016.

Hansen, Morten Steen. "The Infant Christ with the 'Arma' Christi: François Duquesnoy and the Typology of the Putto." *Zeitschrift Für Kunstgeschichte* 71, no. 1 (2008): 121–33.

Harley, David. "Provincial Midwives in England: Lancashire and Cheshire, 1660–1760." In *The Art of Midwifery: Early Modern Midwives in Europe*, edited by Hilary Marland, 27–48. London: Routledge, 1993.

Heilbron, John. "Domesticating Science in the Eighteenth Century." In *Science and the Visual Image in the Enlightenment*, edited by W.R. Shea, 1–24. Canton, MA: Science History Publications, 2000.

Hellwarth, Jennifer Wynne. "'I Wyl Wright of Women Prevy Sekenes:' Imagining Female Literacy and Textual Communities in Medieval and Early Modern Midwifery Manuals." *Critical Survey* 14, no. 1 (2002): 44–63.

Hobby, Elaine. "Introduction." In *The Midwives Book: Or the Whole Art of Midwifry Discovered*, edited by Elaine Hobby, xi–xxxi. Oxford: Oxford University Press, 1999.

———. "Note on the Text." In *The Midwives Book: Or the Whole Art of Midwifry Disocvered*, edited by Elaine Hobby, xxxvii–xliii. Oxford: Oxford University Press, 1999.

———. "'Secrets of the Female Sex:' Jane Sharp, the Reproductive Female Body, and Early Modern Midwifery Manuals." *Women's Writing* 8, no. 2 (2001): 201–12.

Hopwood, Nick. *Haeckel's Embryos: Images, Evolution and Fraud*. Chicago, IL: University of Chicago Press, 2015.

Hunter, Matthew C. *Wicked Intelligence: Visual Art and the Science of Experiment in Restoration London*. Chicago, IL: University of Chicago Press, 2013.

Hunter, Michael, ed. *Printed Images in Early Modern Britain: Essays in Interpretation*. Farnham: Ashgate, 2010.

Karr Schmidt, Suzanne. *Altered and Adorned: Using Renaissance Prints in Daily Life*. New Haven, CT: Yale University Press, 2011.

Keller, Eve. "Mrs Jane Sharp: Midwifery and the Critique of Medical Knowledge in Seventeenth-Century England." *Women's Writing* 2, no. 2 (1995): 101–11.

Kemp, Martin. "Style and Non-Style in Anatomical Illustration: From Renaissance Humanism to Henry Gray." *Journal of Anatomy* 216 (2010): 192–208.

———. "Taking It on Trust: Form and Meaning in Naturalistic Representation." *Archives of Natural History* 17, no. 2 (1990): 127–88.

Klestinec, Cynthia. "Renaissance Surgeons: Anatomy, Manual Skill and the Visual Arts." In *Early Modern Medicine and Natural Philosophy*, edited by Peter Distelzweig, Benjamin Goldberg, and Evan R. Ragland, 43–58. Dordrecht: Springer, 2016.

Krämer, Fabian. "The Persistent Image of an Unusual Centaur: A Biography of Aldrovandi's Two-Legged Centaur Woodcut." *Nuncius* 2 (2009): 313–40.

Kusukawa, Sachiko. *Picturing the Book of Nature: Image, Text, and Argument in Sixteenth-Century Human Anatomy and Medical Botany*. Chicago, IL: University of Chicago Press, 2012.

Lefèvre, Wolfgang, Jürgen Renn, and Urs Schoepflin, eds. *The Power of Images in Early Modern Science*. Basel: Birkhäuser, 2003.

Lo, Melissa. "Cut, Copy, and English Anatomy: Thomas Geminus and the Reordering of Vesalius's Canonical Body." In *Andreas Vesalius and the Fabrica in the Age of Printing: Art, Anatomy, and Printing in the Italian Renaissance*, edited by Rinaldo Fernando Canalis and Massimo Ciavolella, 225–56. Turnhout: Brepols, 2018.

———. "The Picture Multiple: Figuring, Thinking, and Knowing in Descartes's Essais (1637)." *Journal of the History of Ideas* 78, no. 3 (2017): 369–99.

Longo, Lawrence D. and Lawrence P. Reynolds. *Wombs with a View: Illustrations of the Gravid Uterus from the Renaissance through the Nineteenth Century*. Cham: Springer, 2016.

Marr, Alexander. "Knowing Images." *Renaissance Quarterly* 69 (2016): 1000–13.

Massey, Lyle. "'Against the "Statue Anatomized:' The 'Art' of Eighteenth-Century Anatomy on Trial." *Art History* 40, no. 1 (2017): 68–103.

McTavish, Lianne. *Childbirth and the Display of Authority in Early Modern France*. Aldershot: Ashgate, 2005.

Musacchio, Jacqueline Marie. *The Art and Ritual of Childbirth in Renaissance Italy*. New Haven, CT: Yale University Press, 1999.

Nickelsen, Kärin. *Draughtsmen, Botanists and Nature: The Construction of Eighteenth-Century Botanical Illustrations*. Dordrecht: Springer, 2006.

O'Brien, Karen. "Sexual Impropriety, Petitioning and the Dynamics of Ill Will in Daily Urban Life." *Urban History* 43, no. 2 (2016): 177–99.

Ogilvie, Brian W. *The Science of Describing: Natural History in Renaissance Europe*. Chicago, IL: University of Chicago Press, 2006.

Park, Katharine. "Impressed Images: Reproducing Wonders." In *Picturing Science, Producing Art*, edited by Caroline A. Jones and Peter Galison, 254–71. New York: Routledge, 1998.

Pomata, Gianna. "Observation Rising: Birth of an Epistemic Genre, 1500–1650." In *Histories of Scientific Observation*, edited by Lorraine Daston and Elizabeth Lunbeck, 45–80. Chicago, IL: University of Chicago Press, 2011.

Raphael, Renée. "Teaching through Diagrams: Galileo's Dialogo and Discorsi and His Pisan Readers." In *Observing the World through Images: Diagrams and Figures in the Early-Modern Arts and Sciences*, edited by Isla Fay and Nicholas Jardine, 201–30. Leiden: Brill, 2014.

Richards, Jennifer. "Reading and Hearing *The Womans Booke* in Early Modern England." *Bulletin of the History of Medicine* 89 (2015): 434–62.

Roberts, K. B., and J. D. W. Tomlinson. *The Fabric of the Body: European Traditions of Anatomical Illustration*. Oxford: Clarendon Press, 1992.

Sawday, Jonathan. *The Body Emblazoned: Dissection and the Human Body in Renaissance Culture*. London: Routledge, 1995.

Sharp, Jane. *The Midwives Book: Or the Whole Art of Midwifry Discovered.* London: Simon Miller, 1671.

Sherman, William H. *Used Books: Marking Readings in Renaissance England.* Philadelphia: University of Pennsylvania Press, 2008.

Spinks, Jennifer. "Jakob Rueff's 1554 Trostbüchle: A Zurich Physician Explains and Interprets Monstrous Births." *Intellectual History Review* 18, no. 1 (2008): 41–59.

van Deventer, Hendrik. *The Art of Midwifery Improv'd: Fully and Plainly Laying Down Whatever Instructions Are Requisite to Make a Compleat Midwife and the Many Errors in All the Books Hitherto Written Upon This Subject Clearly Refuted.* London: E. Curll, J. Pemberton and W. Taylor, 1716.

Vine, Emily. "Birth, Death, and Domestic Religion in London c.1600–1800." PhD Dissertation. Queen Mary University of London, 2019.

Walsh, Katharine Phelps. "Marketing Midwives in Seventeenth-Century London: A Re-Examination of Jane Sharp's The Midwives Book." *Gender & History* 26, no. 2 (2014): 223–41.

Whiteley, Rebecca. *Birth Figures: Early Modern Prints and the Pregnant Body.* Chicago, IL: University of Chicago Press, 2023.

———. "Figuring Pictures and Picturing Figures: Images of the Pregnant Body and the Unborn Child in England, 1540–c.1680." *Social History of Medicine* 32, no. 2 (2019): 241–66.

Wilson, Adrian. *The Making of Man-Midwifery: Childbirth in England 1660–1770.* London: UCL Press, 1995.

———. *Ritual and Conflict: The Social Relations of Childbirth in Early Modern England.* Farnham: Ashgate, 2013.

18 Medicine Containers and Healing Vessels

Anna Winterbottom[1]

Introduction

Open your bathroom closet and take out a bottle of pills or a box of tablets. The packaging will be a neutral color or, for a bottle, semi-transparent, bearing the logo of the manufacturer and a list of ingredients. These conventions seem obvious to us: they tell us about the contents (although, to most of us, that list of ingredients means very little) and the semi-transparent bottle helps us to see when our pills need replenishing. In the early modern period, however, boxes, bottles, and packaging for pills, lotions, and other substances used for healing looked quite different. These containers could be highly decorative and ornate objects, sometimes made from valuable materials. They might resemble jewelry or ritual objects and indeed, they often overlapped in their functions with these items. This trend was not confined to one part of the world but was a feature of several very different societies. This is perhaps not surprising. Medicine containers and healing objects relate to three key aspects of global early modernity. First, there was an increase in the production and ownership of "things," including luxury objects.[2] Medicines that were packaged and sold or gifted, rather than made at home or by a local healer, count among these luxuries. Second, there was a heightened interest in the mental, bodily, and social implications of "drugs," a category that was not as clearly divided between the medicinal and the recreational as it is today.[3] Packaging could reflect excitement about new and "exotic" drugs or assuage worries about the effects of consuming foreign substances. Third, there was increased connectivity as more people and goods traveled long distances.[4] Medicine containers also implied mobility and were sometimes made specifically for long-distance travel, as in the case of ships' medicine chests.

Medicine containers and healing vessels exist from long before the early modern period: for example, some ancient Egyptian containers have survived that were associated with healing. These include examples shaped like the pomegranate (Figure 18.1) and the water lily, both of which have medicinal virtues, and jars perhaps imported from Asia Minor and thought to have held opium.[5] Containers for medicines from other pre-modern societies also indicate cross-cultural exchanges. For example, Persian medicine jars and Chinese ceramics were found among the ruins of the hospital of Mihintale in Sri Lanka, built in the ninth or tenth century.[6]

DOI: 10.4324/9781003094876-23

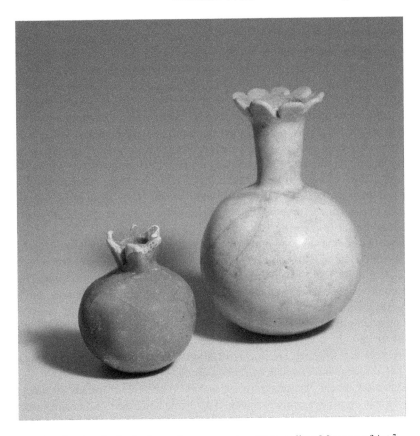

Figure 18.1 Two bottles in the form of pomegranates, Metropolitan Museum of Art.[7]

Although these and other early examples point to wide-ranging premodern exchanges in healing vessels, many more medicine containers survive from after the sixteenth century than from before. After the early nineteenth century, the industrial production of medicine containers led to greater uniformity in the way medicines were packaged and labeled.[8] These new standards soon applied not only to biomedicine but also to the reimagined versions of "traditional" healing practices including Ayurveda, traditional Chinese medicine, and traditional African medicine.[9] The early modern period therefore stands out as one in which a large number of high-quality, individually crafted medicine containers and healing vessels were produced and exchanged.

As a starting point, let us briefly examine some medicine containers from different parts of the early modern world: East Asia, North America, West Africa, Europe, and South Asia. *Inrō* were small Japanese containers with multiple compartments designed to be hung from the sash of the kimono. They were first made during the Momoyama period (1573–1615) when they were used to carry seals but were most popular during the Edo period (1615–1868), when they were used as medicine boxes.[10] "Octopus bags" and "panel bags" were produced in northern parts of Turtle Island (North America) from at least the late fifteenth century, by speakers of Algonquian and Iroquois languages.[11] They were originally used to carry medicines and later tobacco and paraphernalia (this gave rise to another name, "fire bags"). Healing vessels fashioned from brass in Benin City (in modern Nigeria) were marks of status for *ebo* (doctors) and were used for divination and as charms as well as for administrating herbal medicines.[12] Cups for medicines made from exotic materials such as coconut, ostrich egg, and "unicorn's horn" (usually narwhal tusk) were used in several parts of early modern Europe, where these materials were considered to be effective against poison.[13] The collection of healing vessels that I studied most closely is from Kandyan period (c. 1595–1815) Sri Lanka. They are made from materials including ivory, horn, coconut, brass, and other metals, some carved or decorated with lacquer. They were used to contain medicines or in connection with healing ceremonies aimed at casting out demons considered to cause sickness.[14]

These objects are diverse, but they have a few things in common, aside from their use as containers for medicinal or healing substances. First, they were all considered to play an active role in healing that went beyond merely preserving drugs. Their power could derive from the materials from which they were made or from the symbols with which they were decorated. Second, all demonstrate borrowing from other cultures combined with culturally specific symbolism. Finally, in the case of the inrō, the octopus bags, and the Benin brass containers, by the nineteenth century, they had lost their specific association with medicine and become objects designed for local and global markets in craft objects.

Despite the recent "material turn" of history in general, historians of medicine and pharmacy have generally overlooked medicine containers and healing vessels as sources. In this chapter, I will discuss how to access objects like these; how to find out more about them; some potential problems and challenges involved in using them as sources; and what these objects might tell us about medicine, early modernity, and early modern medicine. I will draw mainly on my own experience studying Sri Lankan medicine containers but will also refer to several examples from other parts of the early modern world for comparison and to suggest avenues for future research.

Locating Medicine Containers and Healing Vessels

Like other material objects, medicine containers and healing vessels can mainly be accessed through museum collections, although private collections and the archives of pharmaceutical companies may also contain relevant objects.[15] Museum collections vary in their extent and scope, but in most cases, the items that are displayed make up only a small proportion of the total collection. Usually, some proportion of the items in the collection have been cataloged, and, in some cases, these catalogs are available online, some accompanied by images and details about the object. Even so, most museum objects remain invisible and uncataloged. For example, the British Museum holds at least 8 million objects. Roughly 80,000 objects, or 1 percent of the collection, are on display at any one time and 2 million objects can be accessed through the online catalog.[16] While not exhaustive, online catalogs are a good starting point, and it is useful to try several different related search terms to locate objects that might be described differently. Smaller museums are less likely to host their catalogs online, but they may be available within the library in print or digital form. Most museums welcome researchers and the curator will usually be a first point of contact and a valuable source of information.

Where catalogs exist, they will usually contain a title and description of the object, information about its provenance (where it came from, its previous owners, and its acquisition by the museum), and sometimes references for further details. When objects are featured in museum exhibitions, they may be described in more detail in museum catalogs, which are often available in digital form on museum websites. Some museums also publish their own journals or newsletters, which are good sources of information. When objects are not cataloged, information about them can often be found in accession registers. Accession registers will typically contain a brief description of the object, information about the previous owner of an object, the date of its acquisition and sometime the amount for which it was purchased. Often the information that the museum holds about its objects will be derived from the original collector.[17] Where they are available, the archives of the collector can reveal additional information about the objects as well as about the collector's priorities (which objects they were particularly interested in, and why, and other types of objects they may have overlooked or excluded) and collecting strategies (how and where objects and information about them were acquired).

When using museum collections, it is important to consider the layers of meaning that were added to the objects at different stages through the processes of assembling the collection, labeling, and cataloging the objects, and displaying them. The short text on a museum label or within a catalog entry can be used to frame an object in different ways. In the case of a medicine container or healing vessel, the collector or curator might choose to treat it as a functional object, a work of art, as representative of a particular culture or period, or as part of a larger story about medicine or pharmacy. These brief texts themselves are representative of a particular time and place, which are usually different from the context in which the object itself was made. For example, the Sri Lanka objects I studied were collected in the early twentieth century by Casey Wood, a medical doctor, who saw them as part of the prehistory of modern medicine. Similar objects were collected in and around the same period by the art historian Ananda Coomaraswamy, who framed them instead as representing an Indigenous tradition of South Asian arts and crafts that was lost with the coming of modernity. How an object is interpretated in a museum context depends on the nature and aims of the museum and on the other objects with which it is juxtaposed to form a collection or display.

Specialized collections that include medicine containers and healing vessels include pharmacy and medical museums. One of the largest such collections was the museum established by Henry Wellcome (1853–1936), which opened in 1913 and by the 1930s contained an estimated 1 million objects.[18] Wellcome classified a large number of these objects as "anthropological" and they were at one time displayed in a gallery of "primitive medicine."[19] Wellcome, like other nineteenth-century collectors, saw such objects as representing both the prehistory of "modern medicine" and the present mindset of colonialized peoples in Sudan (where he personally collected the largest number of objects) and elsewhere. The Wellcome museum was later dispersed between the British Museum, the Science Museum, and the Wellcome Trust. Another large collection of medicine containers and healing vessels, in this case relating mainly to Europe, is in the Pharmacy Museum of the University of Basel, originating from the private collections of the pharmacist Josef Anton Häfliger (1873–1954).[20] In Japan, the Naito Museum of Pharmaceutical Science and Industry was similarly begun by the founder of a pharmaceutical company, Toyoji Naito, in 1971.[21] Private collections of prominent doctors and pharmacists formed the nucleus of museum collections, large and small, in many other parts of the world as well.[22]

Pharmaceutical collections are useful sources of medicine containers and related objects, and they sometime also house libraries. However, they sometimes focus on telling a teleological story about how pharmacy arrived where it is today, and the arrangement of the objects within the collection can reflect this. Displays often represent a linear development over the science over time, albeit with certain setbacks (like the forgotten technology of glass for containers).[23] In the past, "universal" collections like Wellcome's tended to present "western" medicine as a process of historical development that was separate from a series of "traditional" or "folk" forms of medicine that have remained largely unchanging. Returning to the objects in these collections from a different perspective or considering other objects can sometimes help to challenge these ideas. For example, the persistence of the "witch bottle" (discussed below) in England up to the beginning of the twentieth century calls into question the idea that supernatural or "superstitious" elements of medicine were confined to non-Western societies in the post-medieval period.

Medicine containers and healing objects also feature among the collections of national museums. National museums are institutions created to embody and engender a sense of national identity.[24] While many were created during the nineteenth century, others are more recent. For example, the Edo Museum of West African Art is currently being created specifically as a destination for repatriated Edo bronzes and aims at "an undoing of the objectification that has happened in the West" by reconstructing scenes from precolonial Benin.[25] The National Museum of the American Indian – which has one of the best collections of medicine bags from the region – aims to act as a resource for Native cultures within North America as well as a holding place for material culture.[26] In the context of a national museum, medical containers and healing vessels appear as part of assemblages meant to construct a national story. Looking at medicine containers in the context of other contemporary objects can be useful because it reveals how they were embedded in the material culture of a particular period. For instance, many of the small ivory pill containers from Sri Lanka that I studied were decorated with a red-lacquered design based on the leaf of the bo-tree, a symbol that is important in Buddhism (Figure 18.2). Looking at the larger collections in the Kandyan National Museum, I noticed that the same design often appeared on relic containers. This emphasized for me that medicine containers could also be considered sacred objects. Seeing

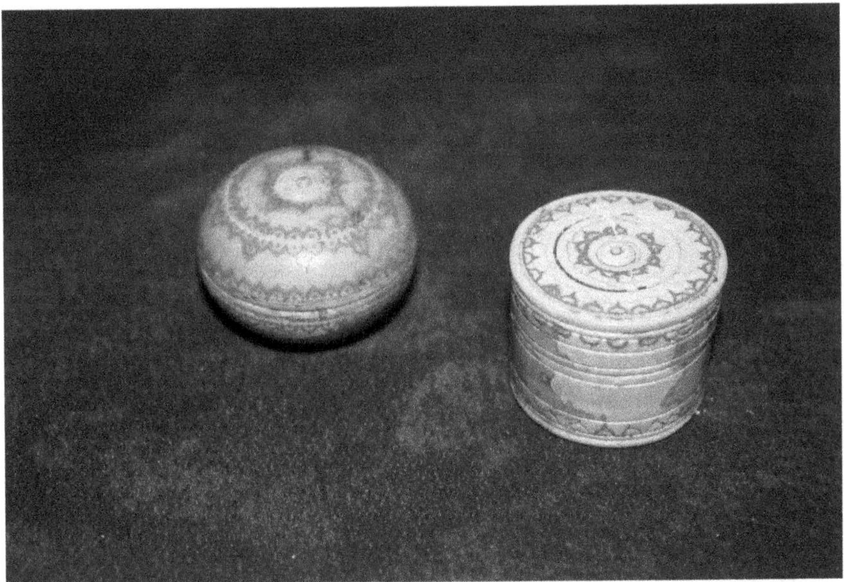

Figure 18.2 Small ivory boxes for medicines, Redpath Museum, McGill.

medicine containers in the context of other contemporary objects rather than within a dedicated collection can also raise problems. For example, in the Sri Lankan context, cattle horns were used to contain medicines, but they also held gunpowder. Small pillboxes could also have held small items of jewelry. So, what is distinctive about a medicine container or healing vessel? Sometimes, the answer can be nothing except for its designated use.

National museums' collections can also pose problems to do with selection. In telling stories about national identity, these museums tend to prioritize majority narratives and often exclude objects connected with minorities, less wealthy groups, and women.[27] In the case of objects associated with medicine and healing, more ornate items belonging to elites are often privileged for collection and display over more quotidian objects or those used in household medicine. In the Colombo National Museum, ornate medical objects from the Kandyan period (1595–1815) were on display, while less ornate but similarly formed objects from the more recent past were kept in the ethnography department of the same museum and not displayed. Often, such objects are omitted from museum collections altogether. Museum collections that originated in colonial settings (like the Colombo Museum) also tended to be informed by Western interpretations of the boundaries between medicine and magic or "superstition" and these prejudices were often reflected in the choice of which objects were displayed and how they were contextualized. While national museums tend to focus on elites, folk museums lean in the opposite direction, focusing on everyday life and sometimes presenting an idealized vision of past simplicity and social harmony.[28] For example, Martin Wickramasinghe Folk Museum in Sri Lanka contains some healing objects and contextual information that I had not seen found elsewhere, including mancala boards (also used for a popular game) that Sri Lankan women used for divination connected with preventing smallpox.

Several recent studies have highlighted a general problem with museum collections: in the traditional museum, the multi-sensory aspects of the object are reduced to a solely visual encounter from behind glass.[29] If we could shake pill boxes, peek inside medicine containers to see the remains of wrappers, and smell or even taste the residues of the powders they contained, our encounters with the objects would be different. In the early modern period, healing often took place in ritual contexts, which would have involved music, dance, strong smells, and ritual actions. For example, Benin medicine containers often held burnt materials – herbal medicines were thought to be activated by burning – and would have smelt strongly. The medicine vessel in Figure 18.3 still contains some burnt medicine which leaked out of a small casting flaw. Physical interactions with the containers were also important: healers (ebo) in Benin, often took part in divination ceremonies, which would involve shaking items from healing vessels and spitting chewed up kola nut (a psychoactive substance which also has medical properties) onto them.[30]

Some containers associated with healing worked through touch. They were intended to be worn on the body as charms, sometimes accompanied by the recitation of spells or prayers. These are generally known as "amulets." Amulets were used in many parts of the world from an early period.[31] They range from natural and man-made objects to texts associated with healing. An example from early modern Italy is the "brevi," short texts sealed inside pouches sometimes containing other charms, which were worn by women as protection, including during pregnancy and childbirth. The legend of St Margaret of Antioch, the patron saint of childbirth, was also read or placed on the body of Italian women giving birth, intended to protect them in the event of a difficult birth.[32] Annie Thwaite has recently pointed out in a study of several objects held in London's Science Museum, how healing or safeguarding the wearer from harm (including disease and injury) was one of the most common uses of an amulet. As she also points out, modern museum collections tend to class these objects as merely "lucky," dissociating them from healing.[33]

The emphasis on the visual in museums themselves dates only from the mid-nineteenth century – early museums, cabinets of curiosity, and private collections allowed visitors to interact with their collections in more varied ways.[34] The attributes of objects that were thought to aid in the healing process were often the same as those that made them desirable collectables: novelty, exotic origins, and rarity. For example, Chinese porcelain, which was displayed as a symbol of wealth and good taste across the medieval and early modern world, was also ingested as a medicine.[35] A ceramic of Mexican origin, used to make vessels called *búcaros de Indias*, was similarly ingested by Spanish and Italian elites for its medicinal virtues.[36] In Europe, early modern apothecaries' shops often resembled and overlapped with "cabinets of curiosity," with their displays of exotica meant to attract customers.[37]

Many museums have attempted to rebalance and reinterpret their collections in light of recent critiques. In the global north, recent debates have centered on

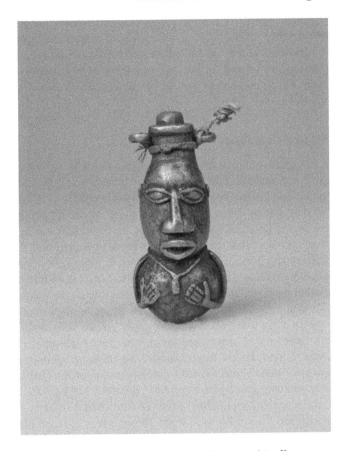

Figure 18.3 Medicine Vessel: Figure, Metropolitan Museum of Art.[38]

"decolonizing" collections.[39] As well repatriation (physical and digital), responses have included relabeling and rearranging collections, conducting detailed provenance research, working with communities in source locations and in diasporas to reinterpret collections, and commissioning new works of art that respond to the original collections. Given the historical entanglement of medicine and ideas about race, these debates are particularly important for institutions that focus on the history of medicine. The Wellcome Collection's recent exhibitions have invited viewers to challenge and question, as well as to view and enjoy their collections.[40] Nonetheless, questions remain about what decolonization means, whether it is appropriate terminology, and how far it is possible. Many western institutions also remain wary of repatriation claims. Despite much discussion, few of the looted Benin "bronzes" have yet been returned.[41] As well as the decolonization movement, museums have sought other ways to reinterpret and refocus their collections, including by rebalancing their traditional focus on elites, men, and able-bodied people and refocusing on sensory aspects of their collections.

Researching medical containers can add to these current debates, for example, by producing more detailed accounts of the provenance of objects and how they were acquired, or by finding new ways to historicize and contextualize them. Researchers also need to look and listen for the gaps and silences in museum collections and to ask which objects and voices were never represented and how far it is possible to recover them.

"Reading" Medical Containers and Healing Vessels

There is now a large literature that focuses on the question of what material culture can reveal about societies, how historians and other scholars should approach objects as sources, and the extent to which objects have effects on history that are independent of their human creators.[42] Although these arguments are important, I will focus here on the practical question of what we could look for in a medical container or healing object that might inform us about its history and significance within the societies which created or preserved it.[43]

Some medicine containers contain quite clear indications of how they were made by, for what purpose, and when. For example, some inrō were signed by their makers or stamped with their personal seals (as mentioned above, another use for inrō was to carry these seals) (Figure 18.4). Artists belonged to schools, often based on families and some were famous for their high-quality work and for specific artistic innovations. For example, the Shunshō school of inrō artists were known for their contributions to the technique of togidashi, in which the design appears flush with its background.[44] Because inrō became collectors' items, there are resources (including some in European languages) designed to identify artists and their schools.[45] When these details are available, textual sources can be used to find out more about the artists' influences, materials, and patrons. However, these resources usually have less to say about inrō as medicine containers.

A rare indication of the medicinal substances that an inrō contained occurs in a four-case inrō made by Shunshō Kagemasa, an early eighteenth-century member of the Shunshō school. This case still contains labels attached to the internal compartments which specify their contents, in this case: kumo-no-i-gan, tablets of bear's gallbladder for curing stomachache, emmei-gan tablets for prolonging life, and so-kō-san, a powder for curing coughs.[46] This combination of general tonics and cures for minor complaints appears appropriate for the contents of a case carried by an elite man concerned with the preservation of his good health and perhaps required to travel as part of his duties. While medicines like bear's gallbladder were widely used across East Asia, the packaging of them in the inrō was unique to Japan.

Most medicine containers provide far less information, bearing no signature or date or indication of the medicines they contained. How might we "read" an object like this? Things to consider include the material it is made from, its shape and size, and its decoration. The features of the object can be "read" alongside

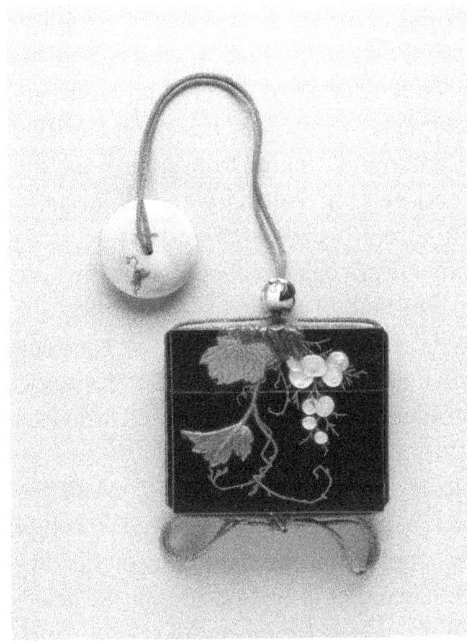

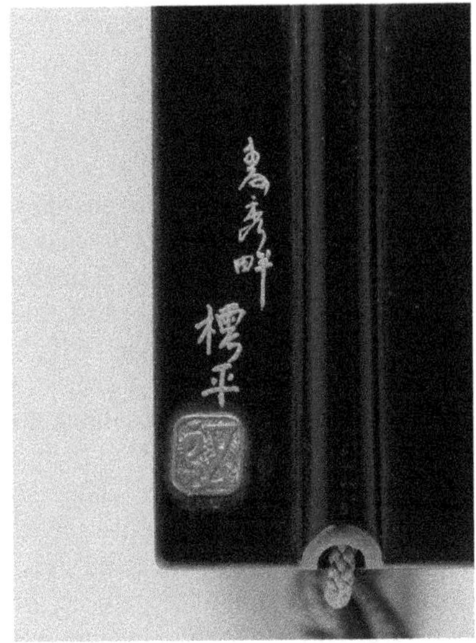

Figure 18.4 Inrō with Grapevine, bearing the sign and seal of the artist Nomura Choheisai, Metropolitan Museum of Art.[47]

textual evidence. For example, in Sri Lanka, manuals for craftsmen provide an important source of evidence about how medicine containers (and other objects) were produced.

The materials that were chosen to craft medicine containers often matched the type of materia medica that was being stored. Dioscorides – whose work was influential in many parts of the early modern world – recommended using thick vessels of glass, horn, or silver for most medicines, wooden boxes for botanicals and aromatics, storing liquids in brass vessels, gums in goatskins, and fats and resins in tin boxes.[48] Horn was mentioned in early Sri Lankan chronicles as a container for medicines as well as gunpowder. Chinese porcelain and imitations of it made elsewhere were used to store medicines from Persia to Holland.[49] Paper wrappers and labels were also a Chinese innovation that traveled to Japan (as seen in the inrō container discussed above) and to Europe.[50]

Materials can have symbolic meanings too. High-status materials tend to indicate that the object was made for a wealthy patron, although which materials were considered valuable can vary between different cultures. Several of the Sri Lankan containers I looked at were made from ivory. In Sri Lanka, where most elephants lack tusks, ivory was a rare commodity and as such was reserved for the royal court. This tells us that the pill boxes were produced by artisans associated with the court. Similarly, in Benin, brass and bronze objects were produced almost exclusively for the court. These objects conveyed the centrality and power of the king and his divine nature.[51] In Benin, many rituals connected with kingship involved the consumption of medicine. Among them is "Igue," which aimed to strengthen the King's mystical powers by applying medicinal substances to his body.[52] In another ritual honoring the King's ancestor, Ugie Erha Oba, members of the herbalist guild, Ewaise, would bring a specially designed brass vessel filled with medicine to the king.[53] In both Sri Lanka and Benin, thinking about the material from which medicine containers and healing vessels were made demonstrates how material culture as well as ritual reinforced perceived connections between kingship and healing. Similar connections can be observed elsewhere in the early modern world. For example, in England, after being touched by the monarch to cure scrofula or the "King's Evil," sufferers would receive a golden coin known as an "angel," strung on a ribbon and tied around the sufferer's neck. The "angel" was thought to continue the protection against sickness afforded by the monarch's touch.[54]

In cases like the ivory or coconut cups used in Europe to repel poison or the beads strung on North American medicine bags, materials acquired through long-distance trade were used in fabricating containers for medicine or healing substances. The appeal of the "exotic" was widespread in this period, in the sense that objects acquired from elsewhere were often valued for more than their use or monetary worth. As the anthropologist Mary Helms points out, in many early modern societies, objects acquired through long-distance trade could be invested with status and ritual or cosmological power like that of objects crafted for use in courtly settings.[55] The meaning and value attached to objects often shifted in the process of exchange. For example, beads of European manufacture used on medicine bags made by First Nation and Métis people had a spiritual significance and an association with long life and well-being that they did not possess in Europe.[56] Similarly, in Europe, coconut was invested with special powers, such as the ability to repeal poison, which were not associated with it in societies like Sri Lanka where it was a more familiar material. Often, foreign objects were combined with more familiar decorative themes, as shown in the example in Figure 18.5, in which the coconut has been carved with figures from the Old Testament. This process, which can also be observed in medicine containers from other parts of the early modern world, was perhaps a means of assimilating novel sources of healing power (including foreign *materia medica*) through crafting.

Like its material, the shape of a medicine container or healing vessel also tends to be determined partly by practical needs, while also having symbolic elements. Sometimes, the medicine containers used by merchants and medical professionals differed from those intended for patients, most obviously by being larger. For example, whereas inrō were small containers designed for patients, doctors during the Edo period in Japan carried larger cases featuring several compartments and containing up to 30 medicinal drugs, each wrapped in paper.[57] The large "martaban" jars – thick stoneware jars glazed inside and out (made in China and Southeast Asia and named after a port in modern Myanmar/Burma) – were used over several centuries to transport medicine – from mercury to opium – as well as oil, wine, and other provisions on long voyages, are an example. Martaban jars also acquired spiritual significant in parts of Indonesia, and, in Borneo, parts of old pots were ground into powder and used as medicine.[58] In England and America, the

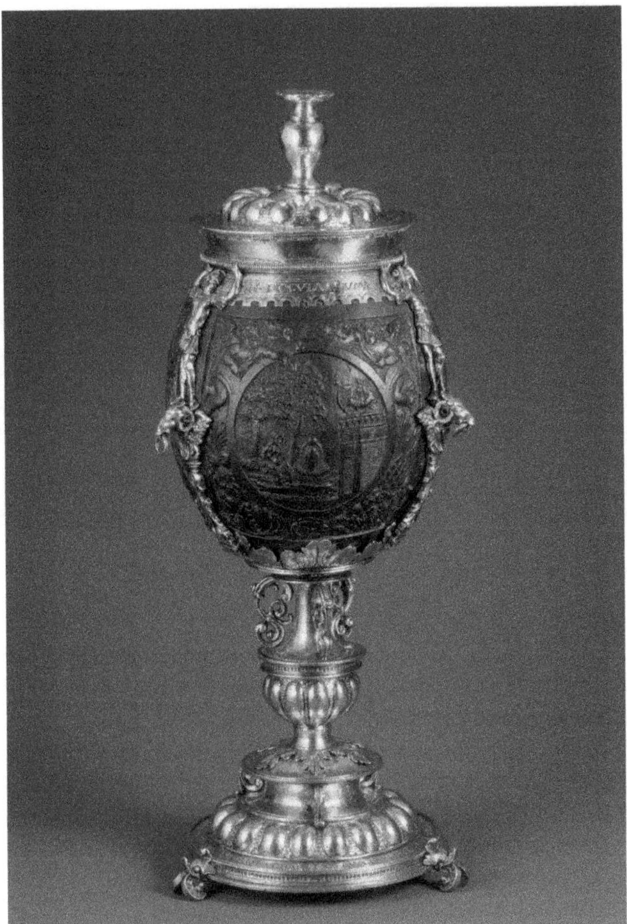

Figure 18.5 "Cup with cover," made by Hans van Amsterdam in c. 1533/1534, Metropolitan Museum of Art.[59]

"apothecary's show globe," a large glass vessel often hung outside the shop that acted as a symbol of pharmacy, developed out of large containers used to display medicines.[60]

Several types of early modern medicine containers feature separate compartments for different medicines. Inrō have between two and five compartments. The distinctive form of the "octopus bag," with its four distinctive tabs or "fingers," hanging below the main body of the bag, also results from the desire to transport several medicinal substances separately.[61] Several horn staffs belonging to Sri Lankan *vaidyavarayā* (physicians) are made up from several detachable compartments, each designed to carry a different medicine. Similar forms can be seen in pill boxes made for individuals in nineteenth-century Britain and France.[62] Such similarities across different cultures could reflect the same response to a common problem (like how to transport several medicines simultaneously). But similarities

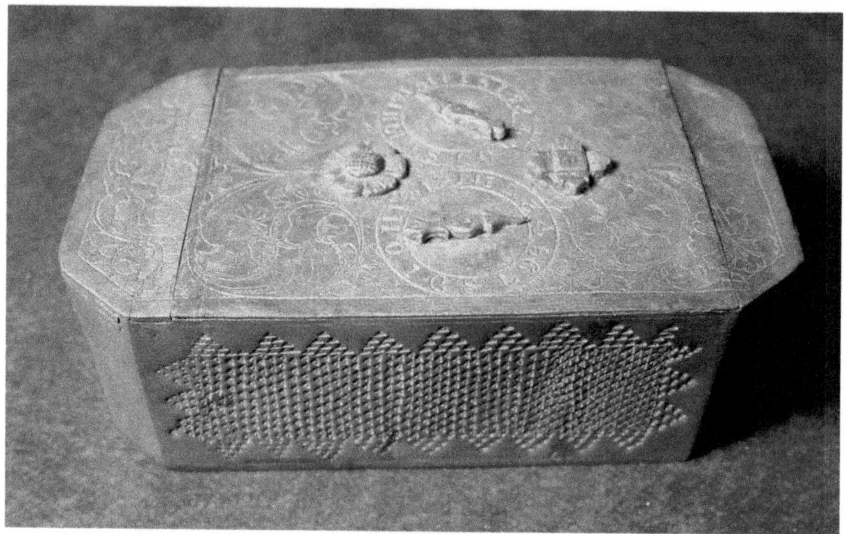

Figure 18.6 Clock-faced locking box, Redpath Museum, McGill.

often developed from cross-cultural contact. For example, Kandyan copper boxes meant for storing dried medicines strongly resemble Dutch tobacco boxes. This resemblance results from the presence of the Dutch East India Company (VOC) in Sri Lanka in the early modern period, where Sri Lankan craftsmen produced tobacco boxes, as well as several other objects, for the Dutch settlers. Sri Lankan craftsmen also creatively reworked European objects, as in the example of a box for medicines (perhaps dangerous or expensive preparations) in which a clock-face functions as a lock (Figure 18.6). Clocks were popular items of European manufacture in Asia, but its reuse in this way is thoroughly unique.

Some of the most distinctively shaped objects among the Sri Lankan collections that I have studied are containers associated with the consumption of areca nut, betel leaves, and slaked lime (made from crushed shells). In Sri Lanka, these containers resemble (and predate) European pocket watches and are similarly designed to be hung on the clothing. Looking at these objects demonstrated to me how borrowing between early modern medical cultures was multi-directional, including in colonial settings. The form of the Sri Lankan betel containers themselves drew on earlier precedents from Southeast Asia, where the practice of consuming betel is very old. Containers for the different ingredients of the betel chew, as well as items like lime spatulas, cutters for the areca nut, and mortar and pestles for pounding it have survived from the region dating from as early as 500 BCE.[63] The betel chew is one of many substances that straddle the boundaries between drugs taken for pleasure and those taken for medicinal purposes. In combination, betel, areca, and lime are thought to have medicinal benefits, including improving dental health and digestion. Betel leaves are a traditional gift to a physician or astrologer in Sri Lanka and other parts of Asia. At the same time, the use of betel and areca were central to social interactions, including marriages and the reception of guests. New drugs like tobacco also generated new containers for storing it in its different forms. One example is the highly decorative Chinese snuff bottle, which developed during the Qing period.[64]

Occasionally, the shape of a medicine container matches the medicine it is intended to contain, like the pomegranate-shaped vessels discussed above (Figure 18.1). The Sri Lanka medicine containers I studied included one shaped like a medicinal fruit. Anthropomorphic or animal shapes for medicine containers and healing vessels are also common across cultures. The example from Benin shown in Figure 18.3 is in the form of a figure wearing its own small medicine container around its neck.[65] There are also many Southeast Asian examples of anthropomorphic jars for medicines and other substances.[66] Anthropomorphic jars can lend themselves to forms of healing that involve sympathetic magic. An example of this is the "bellarmine" or "greybeard" stoneware vessels that were imported to England in large quantities from the lower Rhineland from the late sixteenth century. These jars had a malicious looking bearded face on the neck and a round "belly." The form of the jars (originally used for storing food, drink, or medicine) apparently suggested their reuse in England as "witch bottles," intended to ward off harm from, or return injury to, a witch. Witch bottles were filled with the urine of the supposed victim of sorcery and other objects, often nails, pins or other sharp objects, and concealed beneath the hearth or elsewhere within a building. Later witch bottles were also constructed using different containers, the tradition enduring up until the twentieth century.[67] While there are only a few surviving references to witch bottles in the literature of the period, numerous discoveries of witch bottles indicate that they retained their popularity through the seventeenth, eighteenth, and nineteenth centuries. This is an example of how a focus on material sources can reveal healing practices that are often unrecorded, but which were apparently practiced by people of different genders and social ranks.

As Ananda Coomaraswamy has pointed out, terms like "decoration" or "ornament" are now often seen as referring to something that adds aesthetic value to an object but is not essential. However, to "decorate" an object or person also means to endow them with the power or status necessary to perform a particular role. Both Coomaraswamy and more recent scholars have pointed out that in Asian contexts, ornamentation (*alaṁkāra*) functions to enhance the efficacy of the thing or person that is adorned and even that to be without ornament is inauspicious or courts danger.[68] In some cultures, therefore, the ornamentation of medicine containers might be considered to actively enhance the power or efficacy of the object in healing. A note of caution is needed here, however, because ornamentation was not always regarded positively. For example, certain schools of Sri Lankan Buddhism associate beautiful objects with attachment to worldly things (which is considered to perpetuate the circle of death and rebirth).

In many cultures, the decoration of medicine containers features themes that are considered auspicious, connected with good health, or longevity. For example, the inrō discussed above made by Shunshō Kagemasa is decorated with an image of a sage under a plum tree, accompanied by a crane. The symbolism of the inrō, deploying well-known East Asian symbols of longevity (the old man, crane, and plum tree), matched well with its contents (tonics aimed at preserving good health). Grapevines were another symbol of longevity that appear on inrō (Figure 18.4). Some medical objects bear symbols that are less easy to interpret or that can be counter-intuitive in their meaning.

The same images can also have different implications in different cultures. For example, Martaban jars made in China were often decorated with dragons, which in China were a symbol of the Chinese Emperor but in Borneo were considered to come from the underworld and represent a source of fertility (similarly to the Indian *makara*).[69] Flowers are among the most common decorative themes across both time and space, but flowers often have specific culture meanings or messages. For example, embroidered "octopus bags" made by Métis women in Turtle Island during the nineteenth century drew on floral motifs acquired from missionary schools and copied from Indian chintz (Figure 18.7).[70] At the same time, the ways in which they depict the parts of the plant (representing the "four states of vegetation") are in line with Ojibwa/Chippewa thought about the four-fold nature of the universe.[71] In this case, the symbolism was deliberately obscured because of the

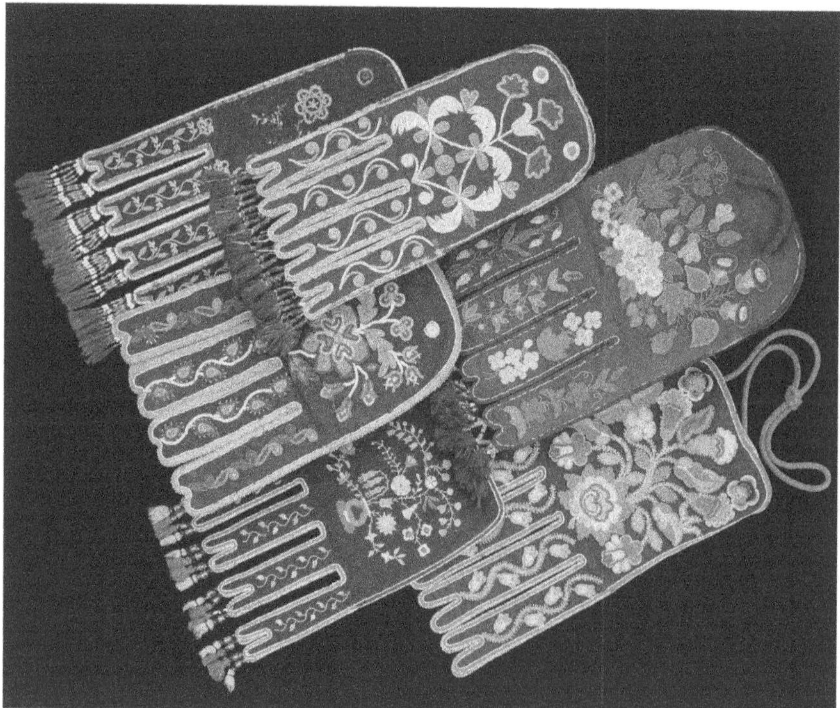

Figure 18.7 Métis "octopus" bags in the Canadian Museum of History.

prohibition under colonial and church rule in Canada of all forms of indigenous spirituality. Writing material culture back into accounts of medicine and healing can sometime help recover perspectives that were lost or, as in this case, had to be concealed. These can include the practices and beliefs of women, whose voices are often missing from other records of early modern medicine.

Examining a medicine container or healing vessel closely can provide insights about its use, value, and about the connections between medicine and other social practices. It can also highlight interactions between different early modern societies. It is also important to be aware of how the meanings of the whole object, the materials from which it was made, and the ways in which it was decorated, could shift as it moved across space and time.

Concluding Thoughts

To conclude, I would like to return to the question of why early modern vessels for medicines and other healing substances look so different from the containers we might find in our medicine cabinets. What changed between now and then? Two key shifts during the nineteenth century were the dissociation of "orthodox" medicine from ritual and religion and the distinction that emerged between "orthodox" medicine, "alternative" medicine, and illicit drugs (despite the movement of substances between these categories).[72] Both these shifts were reflected in – and sometimes aided by – the ways these substances were packaged.

In this chapter, I discussed both medicine containers and healing vessels. Indeed, it was difficult to separate the two. In most parts of the early modern world, medicines were accompanied by healing rituals, from prayer to exorcism. Rituals associated with kingship could also involve healing, performed on or by the ruler. The inextricability of medicine from some form of spiritual healing was a feature of most early modern societies. This is one of the key ways in which early modern medicine differs from global biomedicine. Although, as anthropologists of medicine have shown, biomedicine is replete with its own forms of ritual, these rituals tend to reinforce the power of biomedicine, rather than invoking external forces like gods or demons.[73] Medicine containers still convey messages, often having to do with the transparency and openness of scientific medicine (the clear plastic pill bottle, the long list of ingredients). However, these elements symbolize the power of biomedicine rather than being sources of power themselves. The nineteenth-century dissociation of "orthodox" medicine from overt religious or spiritual associations was one of the ways in which elite merchants and practitioners of medicine sought to distinguish themselves both from what came before and from other forms of healing.

Another difference between past and present is the gap that emerged between drugs that were considered legitimate and those deemed taboo, a distinction that was enacted in law but also in social attitudes and material culture. For example, while opium remained a widely used ingredient in nineteenth-century medicine, smoking it became taboo. The "opium den" was marked out as a place to consume the drug for pleasure by its decorative pipes, trays, lamps, and oriental drapery.

Similarly, from the 1960s onward, a specific material culture developed around the consumption of cannabis as a recreational drug with "headshops" selling pipes, brightly colored boxes for storing the drug, and objects like candles and incense. More recently, as cannabis has been legalized in several areas of the world and retailers advertise it to a broader audience in the form of teas or gummies, new conventions of packaging it have emerged, which are less likely to use counter-cultural symbols and are closer to the ways that "alternative" medicines and foods are packaged.[74] This is an example of how the changing status of a drug is not just reflected but affected by its packaging, making it more palatable for a different group of consumers.

Examining the material culture of early modern medicine demonstrates that drugs we would now consider medicinal, as well as those we now class as recreational or illicit, were regarded as sources of prestige, power, and luxury. Like jewelry, they were often worn on the body and were meant to be decorative items and markers of status. Their decoration, as well as their shape and the materials they were made from were often thought to enhance the curative powers of the medicines they contained. "Reading" these sources closely can provide insights into aspects of early modern medical cultures that are rarely reflected in written sources, including the connections between medicine and ritual and the agency of craftspeople and women in shaping medical cultures. Taking the material culture of medicine seriously can help to challenge common assumptions – such as the uniqueness of "Western" medicine – and can reveal similarities as well as differences across the early modern world.

Notes

1 anna.winterbottom@mcgill.ca. I am grateful to Olivia Weisser for inviting me to contribute and to Sebestian Kroupa for his helpful feedback.

2 Frank Trentmann, *Empire of Things: How We became a World of Consumers, from the Fifteenth Century to the Twenty-First* (New York: Harper Perennial, 2016).

3 Benjamin Breen, *The Age of Intoxication: Origins of the Global Drug Trade* (Philadelphia: University of Pennsylvania Press, 2019); Benjamin Breen, "Drugs and Early Modernity," *History Compass* 15, no. 4 (2017).

4 Felipe Fernández-Armesto, *Pathfinders: A Global History of Exploration* (New York: Norton, 2007).

5 James P. Allen, *The Art of Medicine in Ancient Egypt* (New York: Metropolitan Museum of Art, 2005).

6 C. G. Uragoda, *History of Medicine in Sri Lanka from the Earliest Times to 1948* (Colombo: Sri Lanka Medical Association, 1987), 28.

7 Metropolitan Museum, Acc. nos. left, 44.4.52, right 26.7.1180, https://www.metmuseum.org/art/collection/search/590955 (accessed October 2, 2021). The large yellow jar represents the ripe pomegranate, consumed as a drink while the small green jar represents the unripe fruit, the juice of which had medicinal uses.

8 George B. Griffenhagen and Mary Bogard, *History of Drug Containers and Their Labels* (Madison, WI: American Institute of the History of Pharmacy, 1999).

9 See, for example, Madhulika Banerjee, "Power, Culture and Medicine: Ayurvedic Pharmaceuticals in the Modern Market," *Contributions to Indian Sociology* 36, no. 3 (2002): 435–67.

10 Raymond Bushell, *The Inrō Handbook: Studies of Netsuke, Inrō, and Lacquer* (New York: Weatherhill, 1979).
11 Kate C. Duncan, "So Many Bags, So Little Known: Reconstructing the Patterns of Evolution and Distribution of Two Algonquian Bag Forms," *Arctic Anthropology* 28, no. 1 (1991): 56–66.
12 Kate Ezra, *Royal Art of Benin: The Perls Collection in the Metropolitan Museum of Art* (New York: Metropolitan Museum of Art, 1992).
13 Lydia Mez-Mangold, *A History of Drugs* (Basel: F. Hoffmann-La Roche, 1971), 118.
14 For a detail account of these objects and references, see Anna Winterbottom, "Material Culture and Healing Practice: Museum Objects from Kandyan-Period Sri Lanka (c. 1595–1815)," *Asian Medicine* 15, no. 2 (2020): 251–290.
15 For a general guide to using museum collections, Leonie Hannan and Sarah Longair, *History Through Material Culture* (Manchester: Manchester University Press, 2017), 95–120.
16 The British Museum, *British Museum Collection,* fact sheet, 2019, https://www.britishmuseum.org/sites/default/files/2019-10/fact_sheet_bm_collection.pdf accessed August 23, 2021.
17 Clare Wintle, "Consultancy, Networking, and Brokerage: The Legacy of the Donor in Museum Practice," *Journal of Museum Ethnography* 23, no. 23 (2010): 72–83.
18 Ken Arnold and Danielle Olsen, eds., *Medicine Man: The Forgotten Museum of Henry Wellcome* (London: BMP, 2003).
19 John Mack, "Medicine and Anthropology in Wellcome's Collection," in Arnold and Olson eds., *Medicine Man,* 213–33.
20 Mez-Mangold, *A History of Drugs.*
21 Sami Khalaf Hamarneh, *Temples of the Muses and a History of Pharmacy Museums* (Naito Foundation, 1972).
22 See, for example, the case studies of the historical practice of pharmacy and pharmaceutical museums in Bulgaria, Lithuania, Latvia, and Estonia in Regine Pötzsch and Alain Touwaide, *The Pharmacy: Windows on History* (Basel: Editiones Roche, 1996), 91–101.
23 For example, Griffenhagen and Bogard, *History of Drug Containers and Their Labels.*
24 Fiona McLean, "Museums and the Construction of National Identity: A Review," *International Journal of Heritage Studies* 3, no. 4 (1998): 244–52.
25 Edo Museum of West African Art (EMOWAA), press release, https://www.adjaye.com/work/edo-museum-of-west-african-art/ (accessed September 21, 2021).
26 Many digital images are available from https://americanindian.si.edu/explore/collections/search.
27 McLean, "Museums and the Construction of National Identity."
28 McLean, "Museums and the Construction of National Identity."
29 Nina Sobol Levent and Alvaro Pascual-Leone, *The Multisensory Museum: Cross-Disciplinary Perspectives on Touch, Sound, Smell, Memory, and Space* (Lanham, MD: Rowman and Littlefield, 2014).
30 Ezra, *Royal Art of Benin,* 215–25. On kola nut, Edmund Abaka, "Kola Nut," in Kenneth F. Kiple and Kriemhild Coneè Ornelas ed., *The Cambridge World History of Food* (Cambridge: Cambridge University Press, 2000), 684–92.
31 For a detailed study of amulets from between the fourth and seventh centuries, see Joseph Naveh and Shaul Shaked. *Amulets and Magic Bowls: Aramaic Incantations of Late Antiquity,* 3rd ed. (Jerusalem: Magnes Press, 1998).
32 Katherine M. Tycz, "Material Prayers and Maternity in Early Modern Italy: Signed, Sealed, Delivered," Maya Corry et al. eds., *Domestic Devotions in Early Modern Italy,* vol. 59 (Leiden: Brill, 2018), 244–71.
33 Annie Thwaite, "A History of Amulets in Ten o\Objects," *Science Museum Group Journal* 11 (2019). http://dx.doi.org/10.15180/191103.

34 C. Classen, "Museum Manners: The Sensory Life of the Early Museum," *Journal of Social History* 40, no. 4 (2007): 895–914.
35 Oliver Kahl, *The Dispensary of Ibn al-Tilmid* (Leiden: Brill, 2007), 260–64.
36 See Metropolitan Museum of Art, "Covered Jar," Acc. no. 2015.45.2a, b.
37 Classen, "Museum Manners." Patrick Wallis, "Consumption, Retailing, and Medicine in Early-Modern London," *The Economic History Review* 61, no. 1 (2008): 26–53; Breen, *Age of Intoxication*, 46–54.
38 Metropolitan Museum of Art, "Medicine Vessel: Figure," Acc. no. 1991.17.37, https://www.metmuseum.org/art/collection/search/316508 (accessed October 2, 2021).
39 For a collection of resources on this topic, see the Museum Association website, https://www.museumsassociation.org/campaigns/decolonising-museums/resources/# (accessed January 18, 2022).
40 See for example, the website for the exhibition 'Ayurvedic Man', Encounters with Indian Medicine, November 16, 2017–April 8, 2018, https://wellcomecollection.org/exhibitions/WduTricAAN7Mt8yY (last accessed January 18, 2022). See also Wellcome Trust, "The colonial roots of our collections, and our response," June 4, 2021, https://wellcomecollection.org/pages/YLnsihAAACEAfsuu (last accessed January 18, 2022).
41 Dan Hicks, *The Brutish Museums: The Benin Bronzes, Colonial Violence and Cultural Restitution* (London: Pluto Press, 2020).
42 For a summary of the philosophical arguments, see Christopher Y. Tilley, *Reading Material Culture: Structuralism, Hermeneutics, and Post-Structuralism* (Oxford: Blackwell, 1990); for a review of recent approaches, Dan Hicks and Mary Carolyn Beaudry, *The Oxford Handbook of Material Culture Studies* (Oxford: Oxford University Press, 2010).
43 For a useful diagram showing many of the possible questions to ask about an object, Hannan and Longair, *History Through Material Culture,* 47.
44 Bushall, *Inrō Handbook*, 31.
45 Laurance P. Roberts, *A Dictionary of Japanese Artists: Painting, Sculpture, Ceramics, Prints, Lacquer* (Toyko: Weatherhill, 1976); Philip Schneider, *The Japanese Signature Handbook* (Hollywood, FL: Schneider, 1978).
46 Bushall, *Inrō Handbook*, 36.
47 Metropolitan Museum of Art Acc. no. 29.100.883, https://www.metmuseum.org/art/collection/search/58803 (accessed October 2, 2021).
48 Griffenhagen and Bogard, *History of Drug Containers and Their Labels.*
49 On Dutch Delftware, see Griffenhagen and Bogard, *History of Drug Containers and Their Labels.*
50 Some of the earliest printed pharmacy labels are in the Vincenzo Giustiniani medicine chest, c. 1562–1566, in the Wellcome collection in the Science Museum. This chest holds 126 glass vials with individual handwritten paper labels. It can be seen at https://wellcomecollection.org/works/t548n8xc (accessed October 2, 2021).
51 Barbara Plankensteiner, "Benin: Kings and Rituals: Court Arts from Nigeria," *African Arts* 40, no. 4 (2007): 74–87.
52 Ezra, *Royal Art of Benin.*
53 See for example, British Museum object no. Af1954, 23.296.a–b, https://www.britishmuseum.org/collection/object/E_Af1954-23-296-a-b (accessed September 24, 2021).
54 Thwaite, "A History of Amulets in Ten Objects."
55 Mary W. Helms, "Long-Distance Contacts, Elite Aspirations, and the Age of Discovery in Cosmological Context," in E.M. Schortman and P.A. Urban eds., *Resources, Power, and Interregional Interaction: Interdisciplinary Contributions to Archaeology* (Boston, MA: Springer, 1992), 157-174; Mary W. Helms, *Craft and the Kingly Ideal: Art, Trade, and Power* (Austin: University of Texas Press, 1993), 6.
56 George R. Hamell, *Trading in Metaphors: The Magic of Beads: Another Perspective Upon Indian-European Contact in Northeastern North America* (Albany: New York State Museum, 1983).

57 Akira Hattori, "Medicine Box in the Edo Era," *The Japanese Journal for the History of Pharmacy* 52 (2017): 16–20. (Text in Japanese with an English summary.)
58 Eva Ströber, "The Collection of Chinese and Southeast Asian Jars (martaban, martvanem) at the Princessehof Museum, Leeuwarden, the Netherlands" (2016), unpublished research downloadable from https://princessehof.nl/en/collection/research (accessed September 29, 2021), 27–33.
59 Metropolitan Museum of Art, "Cup with cover," made by Hans van Amsterdam in c. 1533/4, Acc. no. 17.190.622a, b, https://www.metmuseum.org/art/collection/search/193595 (last accessed October 4, 2021).
60 Griffenhagen and Bogard, *History of Drug Containers and Their Labels.*
61 Duncan, "So Many Bags, So Little Known."
62 See for example, Science Museum, "Pill box in three sections, hallmarked silver, English, 19th century" (Image accessible via the Wellcome Trust: https://wellcomecollection.org/works/sqtt4esg and https://wellcomecollection.org/works/parud9n9 (accessed September 29, 2021). This object bears the motto *Prius quam factum considera* ("think before you act"), the motto of the English Reeve family. The Science Museum also has similar objects from nineteenth-century France.
63 For example, Metropolitan Museum of Art: Box for Betel Leaves, Acc. no. 2000.284.47a, b, https://www.metmuseum.org/art/collection/search/37747 (accessed September 27, 2021); Anthropomorphic lime container, Acc. no. 2000.284.44, https://www.metmuseum.org/art/collection/search/37750 (accessed September 27, 2021).
64 C. F. K., "Chinese Snuff Bottles and Miniature Porcelains," *Bulletin of the Art Institute of Chicago* 18, no. 6 (1924): 77–79; Lucie Olivova, "Tobacco Smoking in Qing China," *Asia Major* 18, no. 1 (2005): 225–60.
65 Ezra, *Royal Art of Benin,* 215–225.
66 Ströber, "The Collection of Chinese and Southeast Asian Jars (martaban, martvanem) at the Princessehof Museum, Leeuwarden, the Netherlands."
67 Ralph Merrifield, "Witch Bottles and Magical Jugs," *Folklore* 66.1 (1955): 195–207; Brian Hoggard, "The Archaeology of Counter-Witchcraft and Popular Magic," in Owen Davies and Willem de Blécourt eds., *Beyond the Witch Trials: Witchcraft and Magic in Enlightenment Europe* (Manchester: Manchester University Press, 2004), 167–87.
68 Ananda Coomaraswamy, "Ornament," *Art Bulletin* 21, no. 4 (1939): 375–82, 377; Vidya Dehejia, *The Body Adorned: Dissolving Boundaries between Sacred and Profane in Indian Art* (New York: Columbia University Press, 2009), 24.
69 Ströber, "The Collection of Chinese and Southeast Asian Jars (martaban, martvanem) at the Princessehof Museum, Leeuwarden, the Netherlands," 34.
70 David W. Penney, "Floral Decoration and Culture Change: An Historical Interpretation of Motivation," *American Indian Culture and Research Journal* 15, no. 1 (1991): 53–78. https://doi.org/10.17953/aicr.15.1.m4j88474t4m28736.
71 Barkwell, "Metis Octopus Bags."
72 Roberta Bivins, *Alternative Medicine? A History* (Oxford: Oxford University Press, 2010), Breen, *Age of Intoxication.*
73 John S. Welch, "Ritual in Western Medicine and Its Role in Placebo Healing," *Journal of Religion and Health* 42, no. 1 (2003): 21–33.
74 On this subject, see Ann Miles, "Science, Nature, and Tradition: The Mass-Marketing of Natural Medicine in Urban Ecuador," *Medical Anthropology Quarterly* 12, no. 2 (1998): 206–25.

Bibliography

Abaka, Edmund. "Kola Nut." In *The Cambridge World History of Food,* edited by Kenneth F. Kiple and Kriemhild Coneè Ornelas, 684–92. Cambridge: Cambridge University Press, 2000.

Allen, James P. *The Art of Medicine in Ancient Egypt.* New York: Metropolitan Museum of Art, 2005.

Arnold, Ken and Danielle Olsen, eds. *Medicine Man: The Forgotten Museum of Henry Wellcome.* London: BMP, 2003.

Banerjee, Madhulika. "Power, Culture and Medicine: Ayurvedic Pharmaceuticals in the Modern Market." *Contributions to Indian Sociology* 36, no. 3 (2002): 435–67.

Bivins, Roberta. *Alternative Medicine? A History.* Oxford: Oxford University Press, 2010.

Breen, Benjamin. *The Age of Intoxication: Origins of the Global Drug Trade.* Philadelphia: University of Pennsylvania Press, 2019.

———. "Drugs and Early Modernity." *History Compass* 15, no. 4 (2017).

Bushell, Raymond. *The Inrō Handbook: Studies of Netsuke, Inrō, and Lacquer.* New York: Weatherhill, 1979.

C. F. K. "Chinese Snuff Bottles and Miniature Porcelains." *Bulletin of the Art Institute of Chicago* 18, no. 6 (1924): 77–79.

Classen, C. "Museum Manners: The Sensory Life of the Early Museum." *Journal of Social History* 40, no. 4 (2007): 895–914.

Coomaraswamy, Ananda. "Ornament." *Art Bulletin* 21, no. 4 (1939): 375–82.

Corry, Maya, ed. *Domestic Devotions in Early Modern Italy.* Leiden: Brill, 2018.

Davies, Owen and Willem de Blécourt. *Beyond the Witch Trials: Witchcraft and Magic in Enlightenment Europe.* Manchester: Manchester University Press, 2004.

Dehejia, Vidya. *The Body Adorned: Dissolving Boundaries between Sacred and Profane in Indian Art.* New York: Columbia University Press, 2009.

Duncan, Kate C. "So Many Bags, So Little Known: Reconstructing the Patterns of Evolution and Distribution of Two Algonquian Bag Forms." *Arctic Anthropology* 28, no. 1 (1991): 56–66.

Ezra, Kate. *Royal Art of Benin: The Perls Collection in the Metropolitan Museum of Art.* New York: Metropolitan Museum of Art, 1992.

Fernández-Armesto, Felipe. *Pathfinders: A Global History of Exploration.* New York: Norton, 2007.

Griffenhagen, George B. and Mary Bogard. *History of Drug Containers and Their Labels.* Madison, WI: American Institute of the History of Pharmacy, 1999

Hamarneh, Sami Khalaf. *Temples of the Muses and a History of Pharmacy Museums.* Naito Foundation, 1972.

Hamell, George R. *Trading in Metaphors: The Magic of Beads: Another Perspective Upon Indian-European Contact in Northeastern North America.* Albany: New York State Museum, 1983.

Hannan, Leonie and Sarah Longair. *History Through Material Culture.* Manchester: Manchester University Press, 2017.

Hattori, Akira. "Medicine Box in the Edo Era." *The Japanese Journal for the History of Pharmacy* 52, no. 1 (2017): 16–20.

Helms, Mary W. "Long-Distance Contacts, Elite Aspirations, and the Age of Discovery in Cosmological Context." In *Resources, Power, and Interregional Interaction: Interdisciplinary Contributions to Archaeology*, edited by E.M. Schortman and P.A. Urban, 157–74. Boston, MA: Springer, 1992.

———. *Craft and the Kingly Ideal: Art, Trade, and Power.* Austin: University of Texas Press, 1993.

Hicks, Dan. *The Brutish Museums: The Benin Bronzes, Colonial Violence and Cultural Restitution.* London: Pluto Press, 2020.

Hicks, Dan and Mary Carolyn Beaudry. *The Oxford Handbook of Material Culture Studies.* Oxford: Oxford University Press, 2010.

Hoggard, Brian. "The Archaeology of Counter-Witchcraft and Popular Magic." In *Beyond the Witch Trials: Witchcraft and Magic in Enlightenment Europe*, edited by Owen Davies and Willem de Blécourt, 167–87. Manchester: Manchester University Press, 2004

Kahl, Oliver. *The Dispensary of Ibn al-Tilmid.* Leiden: Brill, 2007.

Kapferer, Bruce. *A Celebration of Demons*, revised edition. London: Routledge, 2021.

Kiple, Kenneth F. and Kriemhild Coneè Ornelas, ed. *The Cambridge World History of Food.* Cambridge: Cambridge University Press, 2000.

Levent, Nina Sobol and Alvaro Pascual-Leone. *The Multisensory Museum: Cross-Disciplinary Perspectives on Touch, Sound, Smell, Memory, and Space.* Lanham, MD: Rowman and Littlefield, 2014.

Mack, John. "Medicine and Anthropology in Wellcome's Collection." In *Medicine Man: The Forgotten Museum of Henry Wellcome,* edited by Ken Arnold and Danielle Olsen, 213–33. London: BMP, 2003.

McLean, Fiona. "Museums and the Construction of National Identity: A Review." *International Journal of Heritage Studies* 3, no. 4 (1998): 244–52.

Merrifield, Ralph. "Witch Bottles and Magical Jugs." *Folklore* 66, no. 1 (1955): 195–207.

Mez-Mangold, Lydia. *A History of Drugs.* Basel: F. Hoffmann-La Roche, 1971.

Miles, Ann. "Science, Nature, and Tradition: The Mass-Marketing of Natural Medicine in Urban Ecuador." *Medical Anthropology Quarterly* 12, no. 2 (1998): 206–25.

Naveh, Joseph, and Shaul Shaked. *Amulets and Magic Bowls: Aramaic Incantations of Late Antiquity*. Jerusalem: Magnes Press, Hebrew University, 1998.

Olivova, Lucie. "Tobacco Smoking in Qing China." *Asia Major* 18, no. 1 (2005): 225–60.

Penney, David W. "Floral Decoration and Culture Change: An Historical Interpretation of Motivation." *American Indian Culture and Research Journal* 15, no. 1 (1991): 53–78

Plankensteiner, Barbara. "Benin: Kings and Rituals: Court Arts from Nigeria." *African Arts* 40, no. 4 (2007): 74–87

Pötzsch, Regine and Alain Touwaide. *The Pharmacy: Windows on History.* Basel: Editiones Roche, 1996.

Roberts, Laurance P. *A Dictionary of Japanese Artists: Painting, Sculpture, Ceramics, Prints, Lacquer.* Toyko: Weatherhill, 1976.

Schneider, Philip. *The Japanese Signature Handbook.* Hollywood, FL: Schneider, 1978.

Schortman, E.M. and P.A. Urban, eds. *Resources, Power, and Interregional Interaction. Interdisciplinary Contributions to Archaeology.* Boston, MA: Springer, 1992.

Seneviratne, H. L. *Rituals of the Kandyan State*. Cambridge: Cambridge University Press, 1978.

Thwaite, Annie, "A History of Amulets in Ten Objects." *Science Museum Group Journal* 11 (2019). https://journal.sciencemuseum.ac.uk/article/history-of-amulets/

Tilley, Christopher Y. *Reading Material Culture: Structuralism, Hermeneutics, and Post-Structuralism.* Oxford: Blackwell, 1990.

Trentmann, Frank. *Empire of Things: How We became a World of Consumers, from the Fifteenth Century to the Twenty-First.* New York: Harper Perennial, 2016.

Tycz, Katherine M. "Material Prayers and Maternity in Early Modern Italy: Signed, Sealed, Delivered," In *Domestic Devotions in Early Modern Italy*, edited by Maya Corry et al, 244–71. Vol. 59. Leiden: Brill, 2018.

Uragoda, C. G. *History of Medicine in Sri Lanka from the Earliest Times to 1948.* Colombo: Sri Lanka Medical Association, 1987.

Wallis, Patrick. "Consumption, Retailing, and Medicine in Early-Modern London." *The Economic History Review* 61, no. 1 (2008): 26–53.

Welch, John S. "Ritual in Western Medicine and Its Role in Placebo Healing." *Journal of Religion and Health* 42, no. 1 (2003): 21–33.

Winterbottom, Anna. "Material Culture and Healing Practice: Museum Objects from Kandyan-Period Sri Lanka (c. 1595–1815)." *Asian Medicine* 15, no. 2 (2020): 251–90.

Wintle, Clare. "Consultancy, Networking, and Brokerage: The Legacy of the Donor in Museum Practice." *Journal of Museum Ethnography* 23, no. 23 (2010): 72–83.

Index

Note: **Bold** page numbers refer to tables; *Italic* page numbers refer to figures and page numbers followed by "n" denote endnotes.

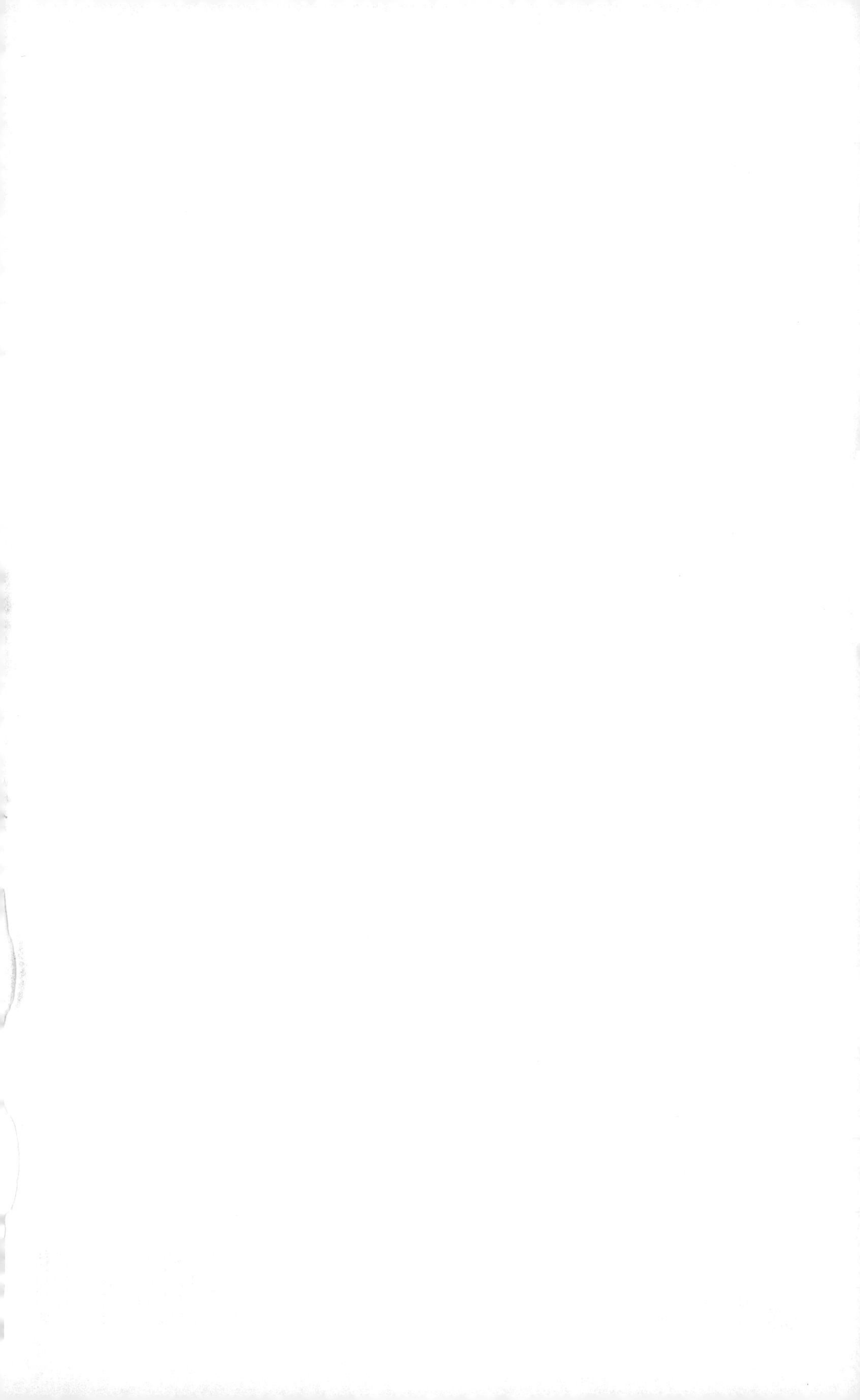

Milton Keynes UK
Ingram Content Group UK Ltd.
UKHW031536071024
449327UK00024B/1876